Benign Postreproductive Gynecologic Surgery

NOTICE

Medicine is an ever-changing science. As new research and clinical experience broaden our knowledge, changes in treatment and drug therapy are required. The authors, editor, and publisher of this work have checked with sources believed to be reliable in their efforts to provide information that is complete and generally in accord with the standards accepted at the time of publication. However, in view of the possibility of human error or changes in medical sciences, neither the editor nor the publisher nor any other party who has been involved in the preparation or publication of this work warrants that the information contained herein is in every respect accurate or complete, and they are not responsible for any errors or omissions or for the results obtained from use of such information. Readers are encouraged to confirm the information contained herein with other sources. For example and in particular, readers are advised to check the product information sheet included in the package of each drug they plan to administer to be certain that the information contained in this book is accurate and that changes have not been made in the recommended dose or in the contraindications for administration. This recommendation is of particular importance in connection with new or infrequently used drugs.

Benign Postreproductive Gynecologic Surgery

Editor

Marvin H. Terry Grody, M.D.

Professor, Department of Obstetrics,
Gynecology, and Reproductive Sciences
Temple University School of Medicine
Philadelphia, Pennsylvania

McGRAW-HILL, INC.
Health Professions Division

New York   St. Louis   San Francisco   Auckland   Bogotá   Caracas
Lisbon   London   Madrid   Mexico City   Milan   Montreal
New Delhi   San Juan   Singapore   Sydney   Tokyo   Toronto

BENIGN POSTREPRODUCTIVE GYNECOLOGIC SURGERY

1 2 3 4 5 6 7 8 9 0   DOCDOC 9 9 8 7 6 5 4

ISBN 0-07-105460-X

The editors were Gail Gavert and Susan Finn.
The production supervisor was Gyl A. Favours.
This book was set in Times Roman by J.M. Post Graphics,
    a division of Cardinal Communications Group, Inc.
R. R. Donnelley & Sons Company was printer and binder.

The book is printed on acid-free paper

Library of Congress Cataloging-in-Publication Data

Benign postreproductive gynecologic surgery/edited by Marvin H. Terry Grody.
p. cm.
Includes bibliographical references and index.
ISBN 0-07-105460-X
1. Generative organs, Female—Surgery.   2. Geriatric gynecology.
3. Urogynecologic surgery.   4. Middle aged women—Surgery.   5. Aged
women—Surgery.   I. Grody, Marvin H. Terry.
[DNLM: 1. Genital Diseases, Female—surgery.   2. Genital Diseases.
Female—in middle age.   3. Genital Diseases, Female—in old age.
WP 660 B467 1994]
RG104.B37 1994
618.'059—dc20
DNLM/DLC
for Library of Congress   93-40645

Susan B. Grody

*A loving companion of
infinite tolerance,
boundless encouragement,
undying devotion, and
remarkable inspiration.*

CONTENTS

CONTRIBUTORS

James L. Breen, M.D.

Chairman, Department of Obstetrics
and Gynecology
St. Barnabas Medical Center
Clinical Professor of Obstetrics and
Gynecology
UMDNJ-New Jersey Medical
School
Clinical Professor of Obstetrics and
Gynecology
Thomas Jefferson University School
of Medicine
Livingston, NJ   [17]

J. Michael Breen, M.D.

Assistant Professor of Obstetrics and
Gynecology
Director of Gynecology
Chief, Section of Urogynecology
Department of Obstetrics and
Gynecology
University of Tennessee School of
Medicine (Chattanooga Unit)
Chattanooga, Tennessee   [17]

Ashwin J. Chatwani, M.D.

Associate Professor of Obstetrics
and Gynecology
Temple University School of
Medicine
Director of Residency Training
Temple University Hospital
Philadelphia, Pennsylvania   [15]

Elizabeth B. Connell, M.D.

Professor of Gynecology and
Obstetrics
Emory University School of
Medicine
Atlanta, Georgia   [1]

Marvin H. Terry Grody, M.D.

Professor of Obstetrics and
Gynecology
Director of Education in Obstetrics
and Gynecology
Temple University School of
Medicine
Director of Gynecology
Temple University Hospital
Philadelphia, Pennsylvania
      [1,3,4,7,9,10,11,16,18,19]

Parviz Hanjani, M.D.

Professor of Obstetrics and
Gynccology
Temple University School of
Medicine
Director of Gynecologic Oncology
Abington Memorial Hospital
Abington, Pennsylvania   [13]

C. William Helm, M.D.

Consultant in Gynecological
Oncology
Christie Cancer Hospital
Manchester, England   [12]

John H. Isaacs

Emeritus Chairman and Professor
Department of Obstetrics and
Gynecology
Loyola University School of
Medicine
Maywood, Illinois   [14]

Carolyn V. Kirschner, M.D.

Assistant Professor of Obstetrics and
Gynecology
Rush-Presbyterian-St. Luke's
Medical Center
Chicago, Illinois   [14]

Robert E. Rogers, M.D.

Professor of Obstetrics and
  Gynecology
Indiana University School of
  Medicine
Director of Gynecology
Indiana University Hospital
Indianapolis, Indiana   [4]

Stanley F. Rogers, M.D.

Clinical Professor of Obstetrics and
  Gynecology
Baylor University College of
  Medicine
Director of Education in Gynecology
Women's Hospital of Texas
Houston, Texas   [8]

Richard J. Scotti, M.D.

Director, Department of Obstetrics
  and Gynecology
Mount Sinai Hospital
Hartford, Connecticut
Associate Professor of Obstetrics
  and Gynecology
Director of Urogynecology
University of Connecticut School of
  Medicine
Farmington, Connecticut   [5,6]

Bob L. Shull, M.D.

Professor of Obstetrics and
  Gynecology
Texas A. and M. School of Medicine
Director of Gynecology
Scott and White Clinic and Hospital
Temple, Texas   [2]

PREFACE

As we approach the twenty-first century, hardly any publication could be more timely than one concerning the health care of women in their later years. When Robert Browning wrote, "Grow old along with me, the best is yet to be!" 150 years ago, to be 40 years old and still in good health was a great feat. Our projections are far beyond any of Browning's dreams.

The average life expectancy of women in the United States now approaches 80, 7.5 years longer than that for men. The fastest growing segment of our population is women over 50, burgeoning from 21 million in 1960 to well over 40 million in the 1990s. Congress gives top priority to social security, and the administration in Washington has placed health care, with emphasis on the elderly and Medicare, at the top of the list. Today, in an established gynecologist's office, 80% of patient visits are by postreproductive women. A growing, more significant number of these women present with benign symptomatic pelvic lesions requiring surgical correction for relief. More pointedly and specifically related to the critical need for texts on this subject is the startling fact that today's gynecologic surgical schedules list more than 20% of the procedures as corrections of prolapsed pelvic structures, most of them in postmenopausal women. Since this trend is steadily increasing, obviously knowledgeable, skillful gynecologic surgeons must be available to serve this older female population well.

Creating such a competent surgical force for the future has become a major dilemma. Because of remarkable scientific and technical advances across the full spectrum of obstetrics and gynecology, spawning such subdivisions as perinatology, reproductive biology, and oncology, residency programs are spread far too thin for concentration on reconstructive and urogynecologic, much less vaginal, surgery. At best there is just enough time to teach the basics of simple extirpative surgery, such as abdominal hysterectomy. Compounding the problem is an astonishing paucity of experienced surgeons who can teach the art of reconstructive surgery and generate interest in this special area.

The major diversionary stumbling block is the virtual stampede to use the laparoscope. Young people in training seem enamored of this remarkable instrument, a technical advance that unquestionably has added to our gynecologic capabilities. However, both respected gynecologic leaders and organizations are objectively questioning the results and impact of this intoxication with endoscopic surgery. The major issues are surgical overuse (overkill might be more to the point) and manpower distraction, in that order.

There is widespread general agreement that laparoscopic surgery has been extended far beyond practical and logical limits in terms of cost, time, efficacy, and safety compared to more traditional surgical approaches. This applies even when—and perhaps especially when—using the advanced techniques presented in this book. And this leads to the second problem, i.e., the limited capacity of the relatively few "traditional" experts, to train the new generation of gynecologists in this mainstream, vaginal route operative technique. The number of surgical cases available for teaching is far too constricted as it is. Because the learning curve for laparoscopic surgery is so long and so wide, situations that should be treated by traditional methods are often diverted, leaving even fewer educational opportunities to learn the types of surgery encompassed by this volume. This is indeed a terrible plight!

It has been recognized that benign gynecologic surgery beyond abdominal excisional procedures is being done relatively inferiorly because of lack of training. What will become of the steadily enlarging army of incontinent, prolapsing, elderly women who are subjected to endoscopic reparative procedures only because their doctors were not trained adequately in alternative, more appropriate surgical techniques?

Which brings me to the goals behind the creation of this book: Major medical organizations and resident training centers seem finally to have recognized how ill-equipped health care professionals are today in the management of older people, especially women. *Benign Postreproductive Gynecologic Surgery* will provide residents and practitioners with the information they need when they must operate on the older woman vaginally or in more traditional ways.

The text begins by making a strong case for the use of estrogen preoperatively. It is firmly advocated that, with few exceptions, most women will live happier, healthier lives if given hormones postmenopausally—and that their ability to tolerate surgery is greatly improved. Much information can be found concerning the anatomy of the pelvis and how best to approach incontinence. Vaginal hysterectomy, paravaginal defects, and massive vaginal vault eversion are covered, as are enterocele and rectocele repairs. Management of premalignant lesions in the older patient is discussed fully. Endoscopy, which is after all one of the many weapons we can use to improve health, is shown as a means for postmenopausal diagnosis and treatment. Comprehensive chapters cover wound healing and suture selection, surgical complications, and postoperative management, because aging tissue and organs require different techniques and observations.

Those who view the septuagenarian patient as an object of pity, inevitably dying of cancer, must be trained—or retrained—to recognize her as someone seeking a better quality of life, able to participate positively and as fully as she is able in her community. Gynecologists can contribute so much, perhaps more than any group of physicians, to the welfare of the elderly. Good surgery with good outcomes, using the best means possible, can often facilitate such a goal.

M.H.T.G.

ACKNOWLEDGMENTS

To those who have taught me so much and are, in one way or another, directly and indirectly, responsible for the creation of this volume.

Willard M. Allen, M.D.

William H. Masters, M.D.

Harry Fields, M.D.

Jonathan Rhoads, M.D.

Eugene Bricker, M.D.

George W. Morley, M.D.

David H. Nichols, M.D.

Henry Falk, M.D.

Abraham Lash, M.D.

M. Herbert Marbach, M.D.

M. Leon Tancer, M.D.

John D. Thompson, M.D.

Raymond A. Lee, M.D.

James L. Breen, M.D.

John H. Isaacs, M.D.

Byron J. Masterson, M.D.

Wayne Baden, M.D.

A. Cullen Richardson, M.D.

Bob L. Shull, M.D.

E. Albert Reece, M.D.

Benign
Postreproductive
Gynecologic
Surgery

Estrogen: Major Factor in Pelvic Reconstructive and Urogynecologic Surgery

Elizabeth B. Connell
Marvin H. Terry Grody

ESTROGEN MAINTENANCE: HALLMARK OF HEALTH IN THE POSTREPRODUCTIVE WOMAN

There is no more appropriate way to open a book covering any aspect of postreproductive welfare in women than by a discussion of the powerful impact of estrogen replacement therapy (ERT). The major general issues unquestionably concern maintenance or restoration of total body health and quality of life. Under this broad umbrella, pelvic reconstructive and urogynecologic surgery in the geriatric woman occupy a prominent position because its success depends on an effective estrogen presence.

In a volume dedicated to major surgical procedures in older women, the importance of bringing such patients to the operating room in the best physical and physiologic condition cannot be overemphasized. Although the initial objective must never be less than optimal survival from the operation, achieving the best lasting results in restoration of anatomy and function are the particular targets of almost all benign gynecologic procedures performed on the postmenopausal woman. None of this can be accomplished without estrogen. There is no substitute. Nothing else can do it.

This chapter reviews estrogen first as to its general sphere of positive influence on the body as a whole. Then estrogen is explored in respect to its profound effect on the vitality of the tissues of the pelvis in the environment of which all the operations described in this book take place. Not anywhere will there be any letup on the importance of estrogen in its crucial role in helping all good surgical things happen in the geriatric patient.

Background

Tremendous changes have occurred in the lives of American women in just the last few generations.[1-3] Not too many years ago, our ancestors lived primarily in hunting and gathering societies. Their menarche occurred between the ages of 15 and 17 as compared to 12 to 13 today and they had only a total of 4 or 5 years of menstrual periods, whereas young women today can expect to menstruate for about 35 years. They were pregnant for about 5 to 10 years whereas, with our current desire for smaller families, today's women have on average only one to 2 years of pregnancy. Whereas the age of first pregnancy used to be in the late teens and early 20s, we are now seeing more in their younger teens and, because of the delay of pregnancy, more women in their late 20s, 30s, and even 40s.

Lactation consumed up to 15 years of our ancestors' lives. Breast-feeding also provided a major form of contraception, which is now being lost, even in developing countries. Today, despite an increased interest in breast-feeding, most women in developed countries lactate either not at all or very briefly, only a year or so. Clearly, as has been vividly reinforced by recent regulatory events, breasts in this country are more regarded as a means of ornamentation than lactation.

The life expectancy of our ancestors was approximately 35 years. Today's American women, now better nourished and healthier, can anticipate living into their 70s, 80s, 90s, or even over the age of 100. Contemplation of the lives of our female predecessors can lead to only one conclusion: they were pregnant, lactating, or dead! This is clearly not the case for women today.

Whereas only a few generations ago she could anticipate spending at best about a third of her life after her last menstrual period, this has changed dramatically; the average young woman today can assume that the likelihood of experiencing almost half of her life after menopause is increasingly great. This fact has innumerable and extremely important personal, social, and medical implications, the latter a major factor in the creation of this book.

Age of Menopause

Although there has been considerable debate in recent years, it would appear that, despite the gradually decreasing age of menarche, the average age of menopause is slightly over 50, and that no major changes have occurred in several centuries.[4,5] Many cultural, economic, and medical factors have been investigated to see whether or not they play a role in the precise age of the menopause. Conversely, the interrelationship of the age at menarche and menopause and certain diseases has been studied. For example, it has been noted that women who develop carcinoma of the breast and endometrium tend to be obese, are of low parity, and have, on average, a somewhat earlier menarche and later menopause[5] than those who do not develop these problems. Ovarian cancer is associated with low parity, late menopause, and uninterrupted ovulation. It was thought for a while that long-term use of oral contraceptives might block the normal reduction in ovarian follicles that occurred with ovulation, making pregnancy possible in women 50 to 70 years old. However, this has not been the case, the usual follicular attrition continuing to take place along with a lowered risk of cancer of the ovary.[5] The environmental factor that has been established in a key role in determining the precise age of a woman's menopause is her injudicious use of cigarettes. The earlier she began smoking and the more she has smoked, the earlier her menopause is apt to be[5] along with more profound physical defects both in her appearance and in her inner structures.

Implications of Longer Life

The gradual increase in the life expectancy of women in the United States has many implications. The recognition that a considerable proportion of a woman's life probably lies ahead of her after her last menstrual period usually colors her attitudes and behavior. Objectively speaking, a long-term view with appropriate multifaceted planning becomes essential, stressing life-style and health. For financial and psychological reasons, younger women have increasingly active roles outside their homes. Once established, this pattern tends to continue into the older age group as women acknowledge their need and desire to remain both productive and socially involved long past the age when their ancestors would have dared think this way.

Thus, long-term health and preventive medicine have become major concerns of today's postreproductive woman. Over the past three decades, through individual and community education and general public awareness, simultaneous with a steady and substantial increase in life expectancy, a new approach to medical care for older women has emerged. Previous emphasis, not that long ago, on care and treatment limited to acute medical conditions, has shifted drastically to a broad spectrum of prophylactic, investigative, and maintenance practices as the female presence has asserted itself.

From a public health perspective, we now recognize that multiple factors are of key importance if an individual is to enjoy a long, healthy, and satisfying older age.[6] For example, the medical profession for quite some time has been aware of the important need for proper dietary intake, particularly calcium, during pregnancy. However, grossly inadequate attention has been given to the fact that after the age of 35 to 40 no significant amounts of new bone will be laid down. In fact, it has been well documented that American women are grossly calcium deficient. However, because they are concerned about their weight, lipid levels, and cholesterol intake, they tend to stop using dairy products and fail to substitute for this loss. Therefore, it becomes imperative that women, long before the menopause, be taught about practical dietary alterations that keep their food intake in balance without sacrificing one essential for another, in this case, adequate calcium to keep the cholesterol level down. It is a reasonable assumption that inadequate diet, particularly food suppliers of collagen building blocks, takes its toll on the supportive and suspensory connective tissues of the pelvis well before the actual menopause occurs, only to be magnified further during the climacteric.

It is now firmly established that much of the morbidity and mortality associated with fractures due to osteoporosis could well have been avoided if proper emphasis had been placed on good nutrition in the younger age groups. In the same category, dissolution of other body tissues such as those of the cardiovascular system and of the pelvis might have been prevented through healthier habits and nutrition at a younger age level. Fortunately attitudes are now emerging through public health promotions that stress exercise and diet as vital factors toward a sustained sound mind and body.[7] Sadly the general response to campaigns advancing good health, particularly with emphasis on the detrimental effects of smoking, are far less effective than authorities would like. As compared to their hunter-gatherer forebears, today's women with not enough exceptions, exercise less, consume more fat and less fiber, and have higher risks for developing malignancies in their reproductive tracts.[5]

Although many environmental factors have been recognized as important in the long-term health of women, one of the most destructive of these, now extensively documented, is cigarette smoking,[8] which unfortunately is apparently increasing. This practice is associated with innumerable pathologic situations, including cancer of the lung, bladder, colon, and cervix. It also induces numerous degenerative changes in the pulmonary, cardiovascular, and digestive systems as well as in the connective tissue of the body as a whole, and this includes bone. The specific relevance of cigarette smoking to the major theme of this book will be developed later in this chapter, as will also be done with estrogen deficiency. It is germane to conjecture that, despite the burgeoning size of the older female population segment and the progressively longer life expectancy in this group, how much larger and longer would they be if smoking were entirely eliminated?

TABLE 1-1 Early to Intermediate Endocrine Deficiency Signs and Symptoms

Target Organ	Results
Genital tract	Vulvar pruritus
	Vaginal atrophy
	Vaginal discharge
	Dyspareunia
Urinary tract	Urinary frequency
	Urge incontinence
	Stress incontinence
Central nervous system	Insomnia
	Depression
	Irritability
	Mood changes
	Hot flashes
	Flushes, night sweats

Postmenopausal Events

Early Changes

Whereas it was once considered to be "normal" for women to stop having menstrual periods for variable lengths of time before they died, the view that the postmenopausal woman is basically in a continuous state of hormonal deficiency is of much more recent origin. With the discovery of the importance of estrogen in the biologic and physiologic maintenance of women's tissues, ERT has been increasingly used. For many years it has been accepted that the early and intermediate signs and symptoms of the climacteric are common (Table 1-1).[9] Treatment of these conditions on a short-term basis has long been accepted by the medical profession, but its attitude toward long-term benefits of continued ERT has been considerably less enthusiastic.

Late Changes

With the advancement of life expectancy, the development of both bone and cardiovascular disease states has become steadily more important among the conditions now recognized to be related to endocrine deficiency (Table 1-2).

The major causes of morbidity and mortality for older women are osteoporosis and cardiovascular disease. For a number of years the evidence has been strong that it is possible to maintain and perhaps even slightly improve the strength of bone in these individuals by the use of ERT, thus reducing the high incidence of fractures.[10–21]

TABLE 1-2 Late Endocrine Deficiency Signs and Symptoms

Target Organ	Results
Skeleton	Osteoporosis
	Fractures
	Wrist, spine, hip
Cardiovascular system	Atherosclerosis
	Angina
	Coronary heart disease
Pelvic floor	Uterovaginal prolapse
Breast	Reduced size
	Drooping
Skin	Dryness
	Wrinkling
	Easily traumatized
	Hair loss
	Less pliable

More recent evidence suggests that, of equal or probably even greater importance, is the prevention of cardiovascular disease, particularly myocardial infarction.[21–48] Although women themselves and their health care providers have been preoccupied with fear about the risk of possible estrogen-promoted malignancy of the uterus and breast,[49–102] major benefits to female cardiovascular systems that far outweigh such risks have not been emphasized enough. This trepidation persists despite the addition of progesterone[103–109] as effective opposition to adverse estrogen effects on the endometrium and mega-analyses revealing no increase in breast cancer at the standard low-dose levels of estrogen required for adequate therapeutic replacement. Unfortunately, the increased risk of endometrial carcinoma associated with the use of unopposed estrogen, often at higher than necessary doses, in the 1970s still colors the attitudes of women and their health care providers and still tends to limit markedly the number of women being given or willing to take hormone replacement therapy (HRT; combined estrogen-progesterone). The use of progestins in association with estrogen has been thoroughly documented in the reduction of endometrial hyperplasia and malignancy and is no longer a source of major concern.[103–109] The correct balanced dosage yields no greater incidence of endometrial lesions than in the general population.[100]

The frightening specter of breast cancer, even though not augmented by HRT, and even though it statistically presents a significantly lesser threat than death from coronary artery disease, which can be halved by HRT, is too powerful a psychological barrier to overcome with too many patients and too many doctors, particularly general surgeons. As a result, it is speculated that only 10% of women in the United States take HRT beyond the short-term phase of relief from hot flashes.

Epilogue

This brings us to the two obvious concluding sequential questions, both pertinent to rendering the vital tissue support so necessary to optimal outcomes in the surgery described in this volume. First, is the menopause, as an unquestioned hormone-deficiency state, a true disease? Many experts think so. Certainly simply because it is an inevitable consequence of aging, we cannot allow it to be classified as "normal" any more than diabetes, an insulin-deficient problem, or hypothyroidism, a thyroid-deficient syndrome, or Addison's disease, an adrenal-deficient dilemma, can be called normal. In the menopause, estrogen disappears and progressive, often profound, deterioration occurs throughout the body, just as changes occur in the deficiency diseases named above. And as with these diseases, when replacement is administered, the disease process is stopped and reversed. Considering not only prevention of life-threatening cardiovascular disease and osteoporosis, but the goals to be achieved in all the pages to follow herein, we who do pelvic reconstructive and urogynecologic surgery at Temple University Hospital (TUH) consider the menopause to be a disease and further, one that is treatable.

The second question, then, particularly within the context of this book, asks whether or not all women who enter the menopause should be offered and encouraged to take HRT? If we grant that estrogen plays a major role in the sustenance and integrity of pelvic tissues, as will be discussed in the ensuing pages of this chapter, consider the following observations on menopausal women. It is estimated that at least 50% of women have some degree of pelvic relaxation. Of these, 20% of the cases involve symptoms significant enough to cause a quest for help.[111] An assumption may be made that many more cases could be symptomatic enough to cause some degree of disability but for one reason or another never reach the doctor's office. Also, further statistics show that pelvic prolapse accounts for about 20% of patients scheduled for gynecologic operations and that 60% of major gynecologic surgery at the geriatric level is performed for prolapse of pelvic organs.[112,113] Although one accepts that other factors contribute to loss of pelvic support, who knows how much surgery could be prevented, or at least made easier, if HRT would be routinely instituted at the outset of the menopause? So, our answer to this question at TUH is a resounding affirmative, especially because we will not operate on anyone not already established on HRT together with a lifetime commitment to it.

ESTROGEN: SURGICAL CATALYST, LIFETIME CONSTANT

Background

Anatomic problems and abnormalities of the female pelvis that reach fruition or develop to levels sufficient to interfere with normal function and quality of life in the menopausal state are almost invariably associated with estrogen deficiency. Recognition and acceptance of this relationship has only come in recent years on the heels of, first, definite scientific documentation that estrogen deprivation is the major factor in osteoporosis and, second, perhaps much more importantly, that it is a principal player in cardiovascular disease in aging women. The influence of estrogen, or the lack of it, we learn more and more, is reflected on all the body tissues, particularly on connective tissue, the "glue" that holds the body together and comprises 30% to 35% of the total body substance. But nowhere is its effect so acutely dominant as it is in the connective tissue and organs in the female pelvis. When its influence wanes as the menopause deepens, atrophy sets in and the pelvis degenerates into disability and forced distasteful changes in life-style. Crucial supports lose their blood supply, become denervated, and thin out and weaken. Muscle tone disappears, epithelial surfaces dry up, and paradoxical contractures and attenuations develop simultaneously. Organs hang out, coitus becomes impractical or impossible, urine involuntarily escapes, anal gas punctuates and embarrasses, and aches and pains and irritations make life miserable.

To be sure, the hypoestrogenism of the menopause is not solely responsible for this kind of deterioration, which has just been described in its extreme and occurs most often, fortunately, in lesser degrees of severity over a broad spectrum of the older population. Other major causative factors of varying importance from one woman to another include the direct trauma of previous childbirth, the progressive wear and tear of aging with associated denervation, and congenital factors in collagen synthesis deficiency. Yet, in all cases, the presence or absence of estrogen plays a key role in the determination of whether or not defects can be compensated for, partially or almost completely. For example, despite symptomatic urethral hypermotility with rotational descent of the urethrovesical junction, surgery can be avoided by tissue rejuvenation and subsequent cessation of incontinence in a small but significant number of cases simply through the introduction of estrogen. Similarly, one can believe that many women who require surgical repair in the seventh through ninth decades of life could have avoided such an experience if only ERT had been initiated early in the sixth decade at the outset of menopause and natural ovarian failure. This section explores the roles that various factors, beginning with estrogen, play in determining the quality of the tissue with which one works in pelvic surgery. Stress will be placed most of all on the need for lifetime ERT combined with good diet and nonsmoking commitment to achieve lasting good results. The common complication of breast cancer is confronted with relation to ERT, necessitating patient participation in all decision-making in choosing the appropriate clinical approach that seems to offer the least risk and fear in individual cases.

Estrogen Receptors in Pelvic Tissues

Mounting evidence has established the presence of estrogen receptors (ER) throughout a variety of tissues in the female pelvis. As expected, the earliest studies have revealed a strong concentration of ER in the uterus, particularly the endometrium.

Strong suspicions that ER have existed in other organs and in the pelvic connective tissues have been present through most of this century simply as a result of clinical observation. Foremost in this regard has been the dryness of the vagina that develops so often within a few years of menopausal onset and then disappears so quickly when ERT is instituted, especially if mediated topically. Microscopically this waxing and waning in the vagina has been established conclusively through the progressively decreasing level of squamous cell cornification as the menopause deepens over time. Similarly the return of mature cornified cells is a guaranteed picture through the lens once regular estrogen reenters the scene through exogenous portals. As already implied, urinary problems such as urethral syndrome and urge incontinence often develop as menopausal hypoestrogenism sets in. Then, when ERT is instituted, in so many cases the annoying urinary symptoms disappear. Additional accountings are not uncommonly related to sluggish rectal evacuating activity that began after menses vanished for good and then picked up to normal bowel movement rhythm simultaneous with ERT.

Over the past 20 years, specific investigative accounts identifying ERs in the pelvic tissues have sporadically appeared in the medical literature. Among the earliest, Schreiter and colleagues in 1976 reported strong evidence that ERT in the menopause could improve the sensitivity of α-adrenergic receptors in the lower urinary tract.[114] In 1981, Iosif and coworkers firmly documented high-affinity estradiol receptors located in the urethra. Although lower in concentration than in the urethra, these researchers clearly showed ER in the bladder also.[115] Smith and colleagues positively quantitated ER in the female pelvic floor muscles, urogenital ligaments, and ureters.[116] They were unable to demonstrate ER in the rectus abdominis muscles, strengthening the concept of special affinity of estrogen to pelvic structures. In a study to help determine the cause of anal incompetence in menopausal women where none of the usual causes could be implicated, Haadem and coworkers in Sweden in 1991 worked on the hypothesis that the general reduction of anal competence after age 50 in women might be due to absence of estrogen.[117] These investigators discovered substantial ER concentrations in the external anal sphincters of women. The male controls, in contrast, showed either no or few such receptors. In animal laboratory experiments in 1992, Batra and Iosef were able to demonstrate ERs in the vagina as well as in the uterus and urogenital tissue.[118] At the time of the publication of this book, with improved methods of detection of ERs, studies are being conducted in multiple centers to advance further the concept of ERs throughout the pelvic tissue of women.

At TU Hospital, a referral center for pelvic reconstructive and urogynecologic surgery, we see substantial numbers of cases of one or more previous failed surgeries. A high percentage of these have never been under the influence of ERT. Before reoperating, all of these patients are placed on estrogen priming regimens for a minimum of 6 weeks and are concomitantly pledged to a lifetime commitment to ERT postoperatively in concordance with the discoveries. Additionally, urodynamics testing is not done until after at least 5 weeks of estrogen priming.

Collagen Synthesis

Defects in connective tissue have been indicted as the principal cause of prolapse of organs within the pelvis. How much of this is due to the destructive effects of delivery, to innate inherited deficiencies, to the wear and tear of aging, and to chronic conditions (ie, constipation or pulmonary disease) that repetitively increase intra-abdominal pressure cannot be precisely delineated. All of these factors certainly play significant causative roles. In women, estrogen, long suspect and now defined, apart from these other factors, exerts dominant influence on connective tissue in a different and singular manner. In many cases the presence of estrogen can compensate for deficiencies wrought by these destructive elements, and its absence can exaggerate them.

Studies taking place and reported during the 15 years prior to the publication of this book indicate rather conclusively the profound effect of estrogen on connective tissue in general and collagen, its largest component, in particular. The latter fact is most important because collagen is responsible for most of the mechanical strength of connective tissue and represents 50% of the total protein in repair tissue,[119,120] as noted in recovery from vaginal delivery or colpoperineorrhaphy. Because elastin, another important constituent of connective tissue, is difficult to study secondary to its lack of general solubility, assessment of estrogen effect on it cannot be determined. Yet one cannot help but postulate that such an influence must exist because elasticity in skin is relatively stable until its deterioration in the fifth and sixth decades[121] as the postmenopause sets in.

It has long been known that collagen, in the clinical configurations of types I and III, is the principal component of the connective tissue of skin. Also, skin thickness has traditionally been taken to reflect body connective tissue generally.[122] Furthermore, it has been established that both skin thickness and skin collagen diminish steadily as the menopause develops.[122,123] Studies also indicate that the collagen framework of the urethra is relatively analogous to that of the skin.[124] Thus researchers have capitalized on this similarity to measure both the effects of estrogen deficiency and estrogen restoration on the connective tissue of the urethra, and presumably of the pelvis in general. This postulation is based on the work reported by Brincat and coworkers in 1983 that showed a direct correlation between menopausal skin thickness and collagen content and estrogen levels, that is, thicker and greater when ERT is administered than before in menopausal women.[125] This study was confirmed by the results of an investigation published in 1993 by Savvas and colleagues.[126]

How these facts relate to the urethra comes together with recognition that (1) the incidence of incontinence rises with age,[127] (2) continence is upheld if urethral pressure remains normally stable,[128] and (3) connective tissue is intricately involved with urethral function.[129] In 1987, Ulmsten and coinvestigators showed that the skin of women afflicted with stress incontinence contained 40% less collagen than skin of continent women.[130] Using this information, Versi and colleagues in 1988 devised an important investigation to check the association between urethral pressure and urethral collagen.[131] Direct experimentation by urethral biopsy, obviously unethical, was bypassed in favor of skin biopsies to reflect changes in connective tissue in the urethra. The biopsies in turn were correlated with measurements of urethral pressure. Drawing from the already documented proof that both skin collagen and urethral pressure are dependent on estrogen,[132–140] the results of this work seem to indicate that the positive effects on urethral function by estrogen could be mediated via collagen.

Extrapolating from these studies, one can make logical assumptions that the collagen of the urethra, the easiest pelvic tissue on which to conduct investigation practically, reflects the properties of collagen throughout the pelvis. Thus we arrive at the probability that the entire pelvic connective tissue network of suspension and support is, to a reasonable degree, dependent on an estrogen presence for continued integrity. Also, we can conjecture further that, since collagen regenerates in the urethra under estrogen stimulation, the same rejuvenation probably occurs in other tissues in the pelvis. So, in conclusion, no urogynecologic or reconstructive surgery should be performed in geriatric women without prior exogenous estrogen priming and a lifetime commitment to ERT to give insurance to the hoped-for lasting effects of any corrective procedure.

Cigarette Smoking

Estrogen and smoking do not mix well. A progressively growing body of literature has emerged that rather conclusively demonstrates the adverse and negating effects of smoking on estrogen, not to mention the direct and indirect detrimental effects of habitual smoking itself on pelvic connective tissue. Baron and coworkers, in a cumulative report in 1990, illustrating the harmful effects of cigarette smoking beyond limitation to tissues in direct contact to smoke (ie, lungs), declared that cigarette-addicted women behave in many ways as though they are estrogen deficient.[141] This has been thought to be due to some extent to alteration of estradiol metabolism, leading to exaggerated formation of the inactive catechol estrogens.[142,143] Also, aromatase is vital in estrogen metabolism and nicotine has been established as a strong inhibitor to the catalyzing activity of aromatase and other enzymes crucial to estrogen deportment in vivo.[144–150] Lower luteal phase urinary excretion of estrone, estradiol, and estriol in premenopausal smokers compared to nonsmokers has been reported.[151] Recent investigations have shown that postmenopausal smokers taking oral estradiol have lower estradiol and estrone levels than postmenopausal nonsmokers on the same ERT.[152,153] Animal experiments have disclosed that cigarette smoke extracts cause ovarian atresia.[154] This seemed to verify previous concepts about antiovarian effects of smoke.[155] Early menopause in women who smoke had been well recognized by 1980 when Mattison reported the possible toxic impact of smoking on the developing graafian follicle.[156] Evidence has steadily accumulated linking smoking, often pinpointed to nicotine, as a formidable inhibitor, in various areas of the brain, of central mechanisms controlling ovarian function.[157–174] These studies could account for both the menstrual irregularities and the premature termination of menses in premenopausal smokers.

From the epidemiologic viewpoint, considerable testimony points to cigarette smoking as the cause of physiologic behavior simulating relative estrogen deficiency. As already mentioned from a laboratory viewpoint, population data substantiate early menopause in smokers. It occurs one to 1.5 years earlier in current smokers than in never-smokers[175–187] and often we see women smokers entering the climacteric at an age 5 to 7 years younger than their nonsmoking mothers did. A cause and effect relationship between early natural menopause and cigarette smoking is firmly accepted, considering the constancy of the finding, the lack of confounding variables, and the obvious dose-related effects, that is, number of cigarettes smoked,[175,178,183,185] strengthening the antiestrogenic concept of smoking.

To emphasize the importance of recognition of the antiestrogenic properties of smoking, since our wide and lengthening experience as a referral center at TUH indicates general neglect of this deterrent factor, it is germane to cite other epidemiologic documentation to this effect that has surfaced in recent years. The risk for endometrial cancer, accepted as a tumor that can be related to estrogen stimulus,[188–190] seems to be considerably decreased, as much as half in some instances in chronic smokers, according to recent reports.[191–194] Reduction in risk of developing uterine fibroids in cigarette-smoking women has been demonstrated.[195–198] Probable lowered risk for endometriosis in women who smoke has been noted.[199,200] A possibility of infertility being more common in smokers has been considered.[201,202] Various reports note estrogen deficiency-related symptoms such as hirsutism, irregular menses, and perimenopausal laments, to be more prominent in smokers.[203–215] Cigarette smoking has been linked to fractures secondary to osteoporosis in a number of studies with reference primarily to the spine and the hip.[216–225] A recent report states that smoking eliminates the protective effect of oral ERT on the risk for hip fracture in women.[226]

In 1983, Zacharin emphasized the substantial contributing role of smoking in stress incontinence and its recurrence after successful continence surgery when smoking was continued.[227] Baron and coworkers reported on the antiestrogenic impact of cigarette smoking in women, alluding to both direct and indirect effects on the function of the bladder and the urethra,[141] thereby amplifying Zacharin's ideas. The antagonistic hormonal effects of smoking were shown to depress the quality of collagen[131,140] and also to weaken smooth muscle tone through muting of α-adrenergic receptor response.[138] Also, smoking habituation was demonstrated to interfere directly with collagen synthesis.[228] In addition, because smoking promotes and provokes habitual, sometimes violent, coughing spells, remarkable increases in intra-abdominal pressure occur repeatedly. The resultant downward bulging of the pelvic floor not only attenuates pelvic connective tissue but probably induces repeated stretching damage to the pudendal and pelvic nerves that supply pelvic skeletal muscle, thus adding further destruction to the support system.[229] As deduced by Bump and McClish,[230] this would only exaggerate further the ongoing progressive denervation of aging that is highlighted in the pelvis by the pathogenesis of stress incontinence.[231–233] In their study of 606 women assessed urogynecologically, Bump and McClish affirmed a strong statistical association between urinary incontinence and smoking. Their intensive investigation revealed striking differences between the study subjects who had ever smoked and those who had never touched a cigarette, that is, 2.2 to 2.5 times the incidence of genuine stress incontinence in the former. The chance for motor incontinence was even stronger in smokers compared to nonsmokers. Such increased prevalence occurred independent of other established risk factors related to incontinence such as heavier weight, greater parity, older age, or more profound hypoestrogenism. In the face of all this accumulating data, at TUH we have established stringent rules about smoking. It must be stopped at once, never to be restarted, from the moment the decision to operate is made. Close relatives as well as the patient are made clearly cognizant of the damage already caused by smoking and the negative impact that any further smoking will exert not only directly on the corrective surgery but also in blocking the supportive effects of ERT. We also emphasize the need for restriction of smoking by all others within the same household as the patient.

Thrombosis

There is widespread belief among physicians that estrogen, even in the relatively low doses currently advised and used in ERT, causes thrombosis. As a result, many women who are thought to be at an increased risk for this problem are deprived of ERT. A growing body of studies reveals that such fear is unfounded.[234–242] Such deprivation is especially devastating to any form of anatomic restorative surgery in the pelvis of climacteric women.

Additionally many gynecologic surgeons deliberately take patients off ERT, often for as much as a month preoperatively and not infrequently for just as long postoperatively, for fear of increased perioperative thrombotic risk. Not one shred of evidence indicates that such worry is justified, especially when both antithromboembolic stockings and sequential compression (pneumatic) devices are in routine use both during and after pelvic operations (see Chapters 3 and 18).

Cancer of the Breast

Having clearly established the prominent role played by estrogen deprivation in the deterioration of the postmenopausal female pelvis and the corollary need for ERT to protect the surgically repaired pelvis from breakdown, the question of management of the climacteric patient afflicted with breast cancer arises when she coincidentally is involved with pelvic surgical restitution. Because it has been epidemiologically firmly determined that, in the United States, one of every 9 women will develop breast carcinoma, the incidence increasing with age, this dilemma arises frequently. The easy way out for the physicians but the one that makes the least sense is the pathway most commonly adopted, namely, no estrogen for anyone with a history of breast cancer. Because considerable authoritative opinion feels that breast cancer can be influenced by hormones, it is understandable that breast surgeons and oncologists almost unanimously preach this negative doctrine. As a result, the individual practitioner, not wishing to be blamed for helping to cause a recurrence in any individual patient, follows the same line.

The truth of the matter is that no data exist in any appreciable numbers to indicate that women who have been treated for breast cancer will experience an increased incidence of recurrence if placed on ERT. Nonetheless there is a steadily growing sentiment, not supported as yet by concrete data but advocated earnestly by respected gynecologic oncologists and endocrinologists, stating that there is considerable more benefit from estrogen than from the risk of cancer recurrence. Such pronouncements are made solely with reference to the misery some women are forced to suffer from the symptoms of the menopause syndrome itself when deprived of ERT and to the significant increase in mortality from cardiovascular disease and hip fracture attributed to estrogen deprivation. If we add the markedly increased chance of deterioration of good corrective surgery in the absence of continued exogenous estrogen support, the argument in favor of giving ERT despite a history of breast cancer is further strengthened. One must consider the statements made by the climacteric patient afflicted with organ prolapse, with or without urinary or fecal incontinence, on the quality of her life: "I can't go on living like this" or "I'd rather die than continue life this way."

It is not within the province of this publication to review the steadily accumulating evidence, direct and indirect, that may eventually lead to universal acceptance that many, if not most, women with previous breast cancer, based on a significantly positive balance of benefits over risks, should be maintained on ERT. We encourage close scrutiny of the opinions of experts such as Creasman, Mishell, Desaia, and Speroff, and of the conclusions of the various meta-analyses that are beginning to appear in print, as well as the relevant data of the US Centers for Disease Control and Prevention. Conveying this information to patients and their families will go a long way to help make all concerned, including the doctor, comfortable with whatever decision is reached regarding continued supportive therapy.

How is the specific situation of extensive pelvic reconstructive surgery in the postreproductive female confounded by breast cancer managed at TUH? We begin with the precept that the patient must be the key figure of the decision-making process after thorough discussion of all benefits and risks with her and appropriate family members. All discussions are documented and the ultimate decision, especially if it directs ERT maintenance, is clearly stated in the chart and signed by the patient. With all elements considered, our principal argument, as tough as it sounds, comes to this: If metastases do exist, they will eventually surface anyhow and the patient will die of them, but if no metastases are present and the patient, from fear, is deprived of the estrogen required to maintain surgical integrity, she may suffer immeasurably and needlessly. No data suggest that estrogen, in the low doses currently advocated for ERT, accelerates the development and proliferation of metastases.

A major element that we bring into discussion at TUH is the question of whether or not estrogen receptors were found in the tissue analysis of the removed breast cancer. If none were uncovered, then our pitch in favor of estrogen therapy becomes even stronger. If such receptors were present, although our entreaties favoring estrogen might be considered more challengeable, the basic situation has not really changed. However, almost invariably in today's total therapeutic regimen for carcinoma of the breast, in the presence of estrogen receptors, the patient is subjected to a course of antiestrogen treatment, most often tamoxifen, which is continued for several years at the least. Such a turn certainly confounds the issue even more since, at the time of this publication, no one seems to know what negative effect, if any, tamoxifen will have on exogenous estrogen. Tamoxifen itself is a mysterious drug because, although scientifically established as an antiestrogen, peculiarly it has been shown recently to cause endometrial hyperplasia, possibly even uterine cancer. No such applicable estrogenic influence has been demonstrated elsewhere in the pelvis. Relative to this problem of tamoxifen therapy interfering with our desire to maintain effective estrogen support of postoperative pelvic tissue, we have studied the pharmacology of tamoxifen and conversed directly with Richard Love of the University of Wisconsin, a well-recognized oncologist with a special interest in tamoxifen. His opinions have helped us reach certain conclusions.

As a result of our ruminations, never drifting from our solid principles of not causing any harm while trying to do good, we have adopted an approach that we feel is the most acceptable at the present time in conjunction with tamoxifen. We will prime the patient's pelvic tissues via oral conjugated estrogens at 0.625 mg daily for 5 to 6 weeks preoperatively, with the assumption that stimulation will get through despite the tamoxifen. Then, postoperatively we ask the patient to insert 1 g conjugated estrogen cream intravaginally twice a week. It is known that estrogen can be absorbed readily through a nonstimulated, thin, atrophic vaginal mucosa to produce relatively high levels of circulating hormone. These may be considerably higher than levels achieved by oral administration. However, often the heavily calloused, highly cornified vaginal mucosa resulting from friction in cases of pelvic prolapse provides a significant barrier to systemic release. In the absence of long-term vaginal eversion and in other cases of atrophic mucosa, it has been shown that maturation can be achieved rather quickly with small doses of vaginal estrogen without appreciable absorption.[243] So, we feel that once we have reached adequate cornification, by either standard oral ERT or very low-dose vaginal estrogen (0.5 g biweekly), a continuing regimen twice a week of 1 g, not the usual 2 g, hormone cream is an acceptable and effective compromise.

When no estrogen receptors are involved, although this situation is far from an absolute barometer, we exert more concerted effort to convince the patient, not only to preserve the integrity of her operation, but on an across-the-board benefit-risk basis, to go to standard low-dose oral ERT.

In conclusion, we strongly urge practitioners to practice humanely and intelligently when the complicating issue of cancer challenges standard therapy. Absolving oneself from responsibility by refusing to give treatment based on fear and false assumption is indeed, in itself, irresponsible. Common sense, bolstered both by subjective and objective comprehension of risks versus benefits, involving both patient and doctor in the formulation of decisions in management, will lead to the ultimate overall best care for any group of patients.

Pelvic Denervation

Although we must depend on ERT in the postmenopausal woman both preoperatively and postoperatively for rejuvenation and maintained high function, it can only do so much in consideration of other factors. Perhaps the most important of these is the status of the pelvic innervation. Aging in itself, combining the wear and tear of time and general steady metabolic deterioration, constitutes a major factor in denervation.[244–247] However, most investigators seem to agree that the principal cause of pelvic denervation, and the single major reason for the differences between nulliparous and multiparous women in pelvic nerve response, is childbirth.[247–250] Without much conjecture, one can easily understand how damage to the pudendal, pelvic, and spinal pelvic nerves is readily sustained from overstretching during the terminal portion of labor as the pelvic floor is forced to descend as much as 3 to 4 cm. A great deal of recovery occurs after delivery, but this seems to apply primarily to the first pregnancy and not so much to subsequent ones, with the permanent injurious effects increasing measurably with each parturition. Additionally, the alteration of the normal vaginal axis (see Chapter 9) secondary to both childbirth and aging, involving muscle and connective tissue attenuation directly, produces continuing and permanent strain on all the nerves of the pelvis.

Obviously it is difficult to discern which comes first and which exerts the greatest individual negative influence in pelvic symptomatic anatomic disruption: neuropathy, muscle and connective tissue attenuation, aging, or estrogen deprivation. Of these contributing detrimental elements only hypoestrogenism is reversible to any significant degree and only neuropathy can be measured directly and objectively. The latter is accomplished by sophisticated neuromyographic methods. However, at TUH, when we perform them, we generally do not order such tests until sufficient ERT has initially been achieved to afford the maximum level of tissue responsiveness. We feel this approach is crucial to accuracy not only in judgment of the extent of neuropathy but also in evaluating urodynamics scores.

One must question, beyond academic information, the value of any neuromyographic testing. At TUH we do not routinely preoperatively test our patients myographically because we feel it is not cost effective nor will it alter our plans for surgical anatomic correction. Also, patient time and discomfort are discouraging factors. Yet the role of neuropathy is always discussed with patients before surgery because of its possible adverse effects over the long term despite the best surgical efforts. We are most likely to seek diagnostic help from neuromyography in special instances of previous not completely explicable surgical failure or those cases of urinary or fecal incontinence not completely compatible with normal or relatively normal physical findings. We feel such testing is indicated in patients who have undergone multiple surgical restorative procedures and display an objective good anatomic result yet persist with symptoms of incontinence. The need for such an examination is suggested by the early studies of Smith and Belentine[251] and Mundy[252] and the more recent findings of Benson and McClellan.[253] These investigations attribute neuropathies to nerve trauma due primarily to pelvic surgery itself. In the latter report, a distinct differentiation is made between the route of the surgery, vaginal or abdominal, the former being the offending entry. We envision a flaw in this evaluation because of the short-term postoperative assessment, apparently only a matter of weeks. Until more long-term data become available, it is logical to assume, in view of the very high percentage of good long-term results we at TUH and others achieve after extensive vaginal reconstruction, that considerable nerve regeneration occurs over time. Therefore, the cases deserving neuromyographic study are the failures for symptom relief after several months, at the least, exhibiting objective good anatomic restitution in an adequately estrogenically stimulated environment.

Conclusion

This opening chapter has made a strong statement: estrogen priming preoperatively and lifetime estrogen commitment postoperatively are crucial to the success of the operations described throughout the balance of this book. Adjunctively the patient will enjoy systemic benefits of markedly significant positive impact on her quality of life, the enhancement of which is the major goal of well-conceived and adroitly performed pelvic surgery.

REFERENCES

1. Treloar AE. Menstrual cyclicity and the premenopause. *Maturitas.* 1981;3:249–252.
2. Treolar AE, Boynton RE, Behn BG, et al. Variation of the human menstrual cycle through reproductive life. *Int J Fertil.* 1967;12:77–126.
3. Vollman RF. *The Menstrual Cycle.* Philadelphia: Saunders, 1977.
4. Tanner JM. Trends towards earlier menarche in London, Oslo, Copenhagen, the Netherlands and Hungary. *Nature.* 1973;243:95–96.
5. Weg RB. Demography. In: Mishell DR, ed. *Menopause: Physiology and Pharmacology.* Chicago: Year Book Medical Publishers; 1987:23–40.
6. Mishell DR, ed. *Menopause: Physiology and Pharmacology.* Chicago: Year Book Medical Publishers; 1987:41–368.
7. Lawrence C, Tesaro I, Durgerian S, et al. Smoking, body weight, and early stage endometrial cancer. *Cancer.* 1987;59:1665–1669.
8. Wilson PWF, Garrison RJ, Castelli WP. Postmenopausal estrogen use, cigarette smoking, and cardiovascular morbidity in women over 50. *N Engl J Med.* 1985;313:1038–1042.

9. Judd HL. The basis of menopausal vasomotor symptoms. In: Mastroianni L, Paulson CA, eds. *Aging, Reproduction and the Climacteric.* New York: Plenum 1986.

10. Hillner BE, Hollenbert JP, Pauker SG. Postmenopausal estrogens in prevention of osteoporosis: Benefit virtually without risk if cardiovascular effects are considered. *Am J Med.* 1986;80:1115–1127.

11. Weiss NS, Ure CL, Ballard JH, et al. Decreased risk of fractures of hip and lower forearm with postmenopausal use of estrogen. *N Engl J Med.* 1980;303:1195–1198.

12. Lindsay R, Hart DM, MacLean A, et al. Bone response to termination of oestrogen treatment. *Lancet.* 1978;1:1325–1327.

13. Christiansen C, Christensen MS, Transból I. Bone mass in postmenopausal women after withdrawal of oestrogen/gestagen replacement therapy. *Lancet.* 1981;1:459–461.

14. Christiansen C, Riis BJ, Nilas L, et al. Uncoupling of bone formation and resorption by combined oestrogen and progestogen therapy in postmenopausal osteoporosis. *Lancet.* 1985;2:800–801.

15. Lindsay R, Hart DM, Purdie D, et al. Comparative effects of oestrogen and a progestogen on bone loss in postmenopausal women. *Clin Sci Mol Med.* 1978; 54:193–195.

16. Dequeker J, De Muylder E. Long-term progesterone treatment and bone remodelling in peri-menopausal women: A longitudinal study. *Maturitas.* 1982; 4:309–313.

17. Selby PL, Peacock M, Barkworth SA, et al. Early effects of ethinyloestradiol and norethisterone treatment in post-menopausal women on bone resorption and calcium regulating hormones. *Clin Sci.* 1985;69:265–271.

18. Crilly RG, Marshall DH, Nordin BC. The effect of oestradiol valerate and cyclic oestradiol valerate/DL-norgestrel on calcium metabolism. *Postgrad Med J.* 1978;54(suppl 2):47–49.

19. Nachtigall LE, Nachtigall RH, Nachtigall RD, et al. Estrogen replacement therapy I: A 10-year prospective study in the relationship to osteoporosis. *Obstet Gynecol.* 1979;53:277–281.

20. Robin JC, Ambrus JL, Ambrus CM. Studies on osteoporosis. X. Effect of estrogen-progestin combination of heparin-induced osteoporosis. *Steroids.* 1983;42:669–675.

21. Grady D, Rubin SM, Petitti DB, et al. Hormone therapy to prevent disease and prolong life in postmenopausal women. *Ann Intern Med.* 1992;117:1016–1037.

22. Jick H, Dinan B, Rothman KJ. Noncontraceptive estrogens and nonfatal myocardial infarction. *JAMA.* 1978;239:1407–1408.

23. Jick H, Dinan B, Herman R, et al. Myocardial infarction and other vascular diseases in young women. Role of estrogens and other factors. *JAMA.* 1978;240:2548–2552.

24. Gordon T, Kannal WB, Hjortland MC, et al. Menopause and coronary heart disease: The Framingham Study. *Ann Intern Med.* 1978;89:157–161.

25. Wilson PW, Garrison RJ, Castelli WP. Postmenopausal estrogen use, cigarette

smoking, and cardiovascular morbidity in women over 50. The Framingham study. *N Engl J Med.* 1985;313:1038–1043.

26. Bush TL. Noncontraceptive estrogen use and risk of cardiovascular disease: An overview and critique of the literature. In: Korenmen SG, ed. *The Menopause. Biological and Clinical Consequences of Ovarian Failure: Evolution and Management.* Norwell, Mass: Sereno Symposia; 1990:211–233.

27. Stampfer MJ, Colditz GA. Estrogen replacement therapy and coronary heart disease: A quantitative assessment of epidemiologic evidence. *Prev Med.* 1991; 20:47–63.

28. Henderson BE, Paganini-Hill A, Ross RK. Decreased mortality in users of estrogen replacement therapy. *Arch Intern Med.* 1991;151:75–78.

29. Adams S, Williams V, Vessey MP. Cardiovascular disease and hormone replacement treatment: A pilot case-control study. *Br Med J.* 1981;282:1277–1278.

30. Bush TL, Barrett-Connor E, Cowan LD, et al. Cardiovascular mortality and noncontraceptive use of estrogen in women: Results from the Lipid Research Clinics program follow-up study. *Circulation.* 1987;75:1102–1109.

31. Criqui MH, Suarez L, Barrett-Connor E, et al. Postmenopausal estrogen use and mortality. Results from a prospective study in a defined, homogeneous community. *Am J Epidemiol.* 1988;128:606–614.

32. Petitti DB, Perlman JA, Sidney S. Noncontraceptive estrogens and mortality: Long-term follow-up of women in the Walnut Creek study. *Obstet Gynecol.* 1987;70:289–293.

33. Ross RK, Paganini-Hill A, Mack TM, et al. Menopausal oestrogen therapy and protection from death from ischemic heart disease. *Lancet.* 1981;1:858–860.

34. Sullivan JM, Vander Zwaag R, Hughes JP, et al. Estrogen replacement and coronary artery disease. Effect on survival in postmenopausal women. *Arch Intern Med.* 1990;150:2557–2562.

35. Talbot E, Kuller LH, Detre K, et al. Biologic and psychosocial risk factors of sudden death from coronary disease in white women. *Am J Cardiol.* 1977;39:858–864.

36. Wolf PH, Madans JH, Finucane FF, et al. Reduction of cardiovascular disease-related mortality among post-menopausal women who use hormones: Evidence from a national cohort. *Am J Obstet Gynecol.* 1991;164:489–494.

37. Stampfer MJ, Colditz GA,Willett WC, et al. Postmenopausal estrogen therapy and cardiovascular disease. Ten-year follow-up from the nurses' health study. *N Engl J Med.* 1991;325:756–762.

38. Cauley JA, LaPorte RE, Kuller LH, et al. Menopausal estrogen use, high density lipoprotein cholesterol subfractions and liver function. *Atherosclerosis.* 1983;49:31–39.

39. Fahraeus L, Wallentin L. High density lipoprotein subfractions during oral and cutaneous administration of 17 beta-estradiol to menopausal women. *J Clin Endocrinol Metab.* 1983;56:797–801.

40. Jensen J, Nilas L, Christiansen C. Cyclic changes in serum cholesterol and lipoproteins following different doses of combined postmenopausal hormone replacement therapy. *Br J Obstet Gynaecol.* 1986;93:613–618.

41. Krauss RM, Perlman JA, Ray R, et al. Effects of estrogen dose and smoking on lipid and lipoprotein levels in postmenopausal women. *Am J Obstet Gynecol.* 1988;158:1606–1611.

42. Barrett-Connor E, Wingard DL, Criqui MH. Postmenopausal estrogen use and heart disease risk factors in the 1980's. Rancho Bernardo, Calif, revisited. *JAMA.* 1989;261:2095–2100.

43. Colditz GA, Willett WC, Stampfer MJ, et al. Menopause and the risk of coronary artery disease in women. *N Engl J Med.* 1987;316:1105–1110.

44. Grimes DA. Prevention of cardiovascular disease in women: Role of the obstetrician-gynecologist. *Am J Obstet Gynecol.* 1988;158:1662–1668.

45. Henderson BE, Paganini-Hill A, Ross RK. Estrogen replacement therapy and protection from acute myocardial infarction. *Am J Obstet Gynecol.* 1988;159:312–316.

46. Henderson BE, Ross RK, Paganini-Hill A, et al. Estrogen use and cardiovascular disease. *Am J Obstet Gynecol.* 1986;154:1181–1184.

47. Ross RK, Paganini-Hill A, Mack TM, et al. Estrogen use and cardiovascular disease. In Mishell DR, ed. *Menopause: Physiology and Pharmacology.* Chicago: Year Book Medical Publishers, 1986:209–224.

48. Stampfer JM, Wilett WC, Colditz GA, et al. A prospective study of postmenopausal estrogen therapy and coronary heart disease. *N Engl J Med.* 1985;313:1044–1047.

49. Mark TM, Pike MC, Henderson BE, et al. Estrogens and endometrial cancer in a retirement community. *N Engl J Med.* 1976;294:1262–1267.

50. Gray LA Sr, Christopherson WM, Hoover RN. Estrogens and endometrial carcinoma. *Obstet Gynecol.* 1977;49:385–389.

51. McDonald TW, Annegers JF, O'Fallon WM, et al. Exogenous estrogen and endometrial carcinoma: Case-control and incidence study. *Am J Obstet Gynecol.* 1977;127:572–579.

52. Weiss NS, Szekely DR, English DR, et al. Endometrial cancer in relation to patterns of menopausal estrogen use. *JAMA.* 1979;242:261–264.

53. Hulka BS, Fowler WC Jr, Kaufman DG, et al. Estrogen and endometrial cancer: Cases and two control groups from North Carolina. *Am J Obstet Gynecol.* 1980;137:92–101.

54. Buring JE, Bain CJ, Ehrmann RL. Conjugated estrogen use and risk of endometrial cancer. *Am J Epidemiol.* 1986;124:434–441.

55. Paganini-Hill A, Ross R, Henderson B. Endometrial cancer and patterns of use of oestrogen replacement therapy: A cohort study. *Br J Cancer.* 1989;59:445–447.

56. Ziel HK, Finkle WD. Increased risk of endometrial carcinoma among users of conjugated estrogens. *N Engl J Med.* 1975;293:1167–1170.

57. Hoogerland DL, Buchler DA, Crowley JJ, et al. Estrogen use-risk of endometrial carcinoma. *Gynecol Oncol.* 1978;6:451–458.

58. Wigle DT, Grace M, Smith ES. Estrogen use and cancer of the uterine corpus in Alberta. *Can Med Assoc J.* 1978;118:1276–1278.

59. Shapiro S, Kaufman DW, Slone D, et al. Recent and past use of conjugated

estrogens in relation to adenocarcinoma of the endometrium. *N Engl J Med.* 1980;303:485–489.

60. Jelovsek FR, Hammond CB, Woodard BH, et al. Risk of exogenous estrogen therapy and endometrial cancer. *Am J Obstet Gynecol.* 1980;137:85–91.

61. Spengler RF, Clarke EA, Woolever CA, et al. Exogenous estrogens and endometrial cancer: a case-control study and assessment of potential biases. *Am J Epidemiol.* 1981;114:497–506.

62. Shapiro S, Kelly JP, Rosenberg L, et al. Risk of localized and widespread endometrial cancer in relation to recent and discontinued use of conjugated estrogens. *N Engl J Med.* 1985;313:969–972.

63. Stampfer M, Colditz G, Willett W, et al. A prospective study of exogenous hormones and risk of endometrial cancer. *Am J Epidemiol.* 1986;124:520. Abstract.

64. Persson I, Adami HO, Berghvist L, et al. Risk of endometrial cancer after treatment with oestrogens alone or in conjunction with progesteogens: results of a prospective study. *Br Med J.* 1989;298:147–151.

65. Kennedy DL, Baum C, Forbes MB. Noncontraceptive estrogens and progestins: use patterns over time. *Obstet Gynecol.* 1985;65:441–446.

66. Antunes CM, Stolley PD, Rosenshein NB, et al. Endometrial cancer and estrogen use. Report of a large case-control study. *N Engl J Med.* 1979;300:9–13.

67. Hulka BS, Kaufman DG, Fowler WC Jr, et al. Predominance of early endometrial cancers after long-term estrogen use. *JAMA.* 1980;244:2419–2422.

68. Collins J, Conner A, Allen LN. Oestrogen use and survival in endometrial cancer. *Lancet.* 1980;1:961–964.

69. Kelsey JL, LiVolsi VA, Holford TR, et al. A case-control study of cancer of the endometrium. *Am J Epidemiol.* 1982;116:333–342.

70. Robboy SJ, Bradley R. Changing trends and prognostic features in endometrial cancer associated with exogenous estrogen therapy. *Obstet Gynecol.* 1979;54:269–277.

71. Chu J, Schweid AI, Weiss NS. Survival among women with endometrial cancer: A comparison of estrogen users and nonusers. *Am J Obstet Gynecol.* 1982;143:569–573.

72. Ewertz M, Schou G, Boice JD Jr. The joint effect of risk factors on endometrial cancer. *Eur J Cancer Clin Oncol.* 1988;24:189–194.

73. Rubin GL, Peterson HB, Lee NC, et al. Estrogen replacement therapy and the risk of endometrial cancer: Remaining controversies. *Am J Obstet Gynecol.* 1990;162:148–154.

74. Ettinger B, Golditch IM, Friedman G. Gynecologic consequences of long-term, unopposed estrogen replacement therapy. *Maturitas.* 1988;10:271–282.

75. Gambrell RD Jr, Massey FM, Castaneda TA, et al. Use of the progestogen challenge test to reduce the risk of endometrial cancer. *Obstet Gynecol.* 1980;55:732–738.

76. DuPont WD, Page DL. Menopausal estrogen replacement therapy and breast cancer. *Arch Intern Med.* 1991;151:67–72.

77. Steinberg KK, Thacker SB, Smith SJ, et al. A meta-analysis of the effect of

estrogen replacement therapy on the risk of breast cancer. *JAMA.* 1991;265:1985–1990.

78. Ross RK, Paganini-Hill A, Gerkins VR, et al. A case-control study of menopausal estrogen therapy and breast cancer. *JAMA.* 1980;243:1635–1639.

79. Hoover R, Glass A, Finkle WD, et al. Conjugated estrogens and breast cancer risk in women. *J Natl Cancer Inst.* 1981;67:815–820.

80. Kelsey JL, Fischer DB, Holford TR, et al. Exogenous estrogens and other factors in the epidemiology of breast cancer. *J. Natl Cancer Inst.* 1981;67:327–333.

81. Hulka BS, Chambless LE, Deubner DC, et al. Breast cancer and estrogen replacement therapy. *Am J Obstet Gynecol.* 1982;143:638–644.

82. Kaufman DW, Miller DR, Rosenberg L, et al. Noncontraceptive estrogen use and the risk of breast cancer. *JAMA.* 1984;252:63–67.

83. Brinton LA, Hoover R, Fraumeni JF Jr. Menopausal oestrogens and breast cancer risk: An expanded case-control study. *Br J Cancer.* 1986;54:825–832.

84. Wingo PA, Layde PM, Lee NC, et al. The risk of breast cancer in postmenopausal women who have used estrogen replacement therapy. *JAMA.* 1987;257:209–215.

85. LaVecchia C, Decarli A, Parazzini F, et al. Non-contraceptive oestrogens and the risk of breast cancer in women. *Int J Cancer.* 1986;38:853–858.

86. Ewertz M. Influence of non-contraceptive exogenous and endogenous sex hormones on breast cancer risk in Denmark. *Int J Cancer.* 1988;42:832–838.

87. Bergkvist L, Adami HO, Persson I, et al. The risk of breast cancer after estrogen and estrogen-progestin replacement. *N Engl J Med.* 1989;321:293–297.

88. Mills PI, Beeson WL, Phillips RL, et al. Prospective study of exogenous hormone use and breast cancer in Seventh-Day Adventists. *Cancer.* 1989;64:591–597.

89. Colditz GA, Stampfer MJ, Willett WC, et al. Prospective study of estrogen replacement therapy and risk of breast cancer in postmenopausal women. *JAMA.* 1990;264:2648–2653.

90. Sartwell PE, Arthes FG, Tonascia JA. Exogenous hormones, reproductive history, and breast cancer. *J Natl Cancer Inst.* 1977;59:1589–1592.

91. Hiatt RA, Bawol R, Friedman GD, et al. Exogenous estrogen and breast cancer after bilateral oophorectomy. *Cancer.* 1984;54:139–144.

92. McDonald JA, Weiss NS, Daling JR, et al. Menopausal estrogen use and the risk of breast cancer. *Breast Cancer Res Treat.* 1986;7:193–199.

93. Nomura AM, Kolonel LN, Hirohata T, et al. The association of replacement estrogens with breast cancer. *Int J Cancer.* 1986;37:49–53.

94. Rohan TE, McMichael AJ. Non-contraceptive exogenous oestrogen therapy and breast cancer. *Med J Aust.* 198;148:217–221.

95. Grady D, Ernster V. Does postmenopausal hormone therapy cause breast cancer? *Am J Epidemiol.* 1991;134:1396–1400.

96. Byrd BF Jr, Burch JC, Vaughn WK. The impact of long-term estrogen support after hysterectomy. A report of 1016 cases. *Ann Surg.* 1977;185:574–580.

97. Vakil DV, Morgan RW, Halliday M. Exogenous estrogens and development of breast and endometrial cancer. *Cancer Detect Prevent.* 1983;6:415–424.

98. Gambrell RD Jr, Maier RC, Sanders BI. Decreased incidence of breast cancer in postmenopausal estrogen-progestogen users. *Obstet Gynecol.* 1983;62:435–443.

99. Ernster VL, Cummings SR. Progesterone and breast cancer. *Obstet Gynecol.* 1986;68:715–717.

100. Key TJ, Pike MC. The role of oestrogens and progestagens in the epidemiology and prevention of breast cancer. *Eur J Cancer Clin Oncol.* 1988;24:29–43.

101. Kaufman DW, Palmer JR, De Mouzon J, et al. Estrogen replacement therapy and the risk of breast cancer: Results from the case-control surveillance study. *Am J Epidemiol.* 1991;134:1375–1385.

102. Palmer JR, Rosenberg L, Clarke EA, et al. Breast cancer risk after estrogen replacement therapy: Results from the Toronto breast cancer study. *Am J Epidemiol.* 1991;134:1386–1395.

103. Voigt LF, Weiss NS, Chu JR, et al. Progestagen supplementation of exogenous oestrogens and risk of endometrial cancer. *Lancet.* 1991;338:274–277.

104. Whitehead MI, Fraser D. The effects of estrogens and progestogens on the endometrium. *Obstet Gynecol Clin North Am.* 1987;14:299–320.

105. Gelfand MM, Ferenczy A. A prospective 1-year study of estrogen and progestin in postmenopausal women: Effects on the endometrium. *Obstet Gynecol.* 1989;74:398–402.

106. Gambrell RD Jr, Castaneda TA, Ricci CA. Management of postmenopausal bleeding to prevent endometrial cancer. *Maturitas.* 1978;1:99–106.

107. Ferenczy A. How progestogens effect endometrial hyperplasia and neoplasia. *Contemp Obstet Gynecol.* 1978;11:137–143.

108. Thom MH, White PJ, Williams RM, et al. Prevention and treatment of endometrial disease in climacteric women receiving estrogen therapy. *Lancet.* 1979;2:455–457.

109. Armstrong BK. Oestrogen therapy after the menopause—boon or bane? *Med J Aust.* 1988;148:213–214.

110. Speroff L, Gelfand M, Gibbons WA, et al. Symposium: Adding progestogen to estrogen replacement therapy. *Contemp OB/GYN.* 1985;26:225–243.

111. Beck RP. Pelvic relaxation prolapse. In: Kase NG, Weingold AB, eds. *Principles and Practice of Clinical Gynecology.* New York: John Wiley & Sons; 1983:677–685.

112. Cardozo L. The causes, diagnosis, and treatment of prolapse. *Midwife, Health Visitor and Community Nurse (London).* 1988;24:207–210.

113. Lewis AL. Major gynecological surgery in the elderly. *Journal of the International Federation of Gynaecology and Obstetrics.* 1968;6:244–258.

114. Schreiter F, Fuchs D, Stockamp K. Estrogenic sensitivity of alpha-receptors in the urethra musculature. *Urol Int.* 1976;31:13–16.

115. Iosif MD, Batra S, Ek A, et al. Estrogen receptors in the human female lower urinary tract. *Am J Obstet Gynecol.* 1981;141:817–820.

116. Smith P, Heimer G, Norgren A, et al. Steroid hormone receptors in pelvic muscles and ligaments in women. *Gynecol Obstet Invest.* 1990;30:27–30.

117. Haadem K, Lennart L, Marten F, et al. Estrogen receptors in the external anal sphincter. *Am J Obstet Gynecol.* 1991;164:609–610.

118. Batra SC, Iosef CS. Effect of estrogen treatment on the perioxidase activity and estrogen receptors in the female rabbit urogenital tissues. *J Urol.* 1992;148:935–938.

119. Norton PA. Histological and biochemical studies. In: Benson JT, ed. *Female Pelvic Floor Disorders.* New York: WW Norton; 1992:166–175.

120. Prockop D, Kivirikko K, Tuderman L, et al. The biosynthesis of collagen and its disorders. *N Engl J Med.* 1979;301:13–24.

121. Braverman I, Fonfuko E. Studies in cutaneous aging. I. The elastic fiber network. *J Invest Dermatol.* 1972;58:347–361.

122. Brincat M, Moniz CJ, Studd JWW, et al. Long-term effects of the menopause and sex hormones on skin thickness. *Br J Obstet Gynecol.* 1985;92:256–259.

123. Brincat M, Versi E, Moniz CF, et al. Skin collagen changes in postmenopausal women receiving different regimens of estrogen therapy. *Obstet Gynecol.* 1987;70:123–127.

124. Alberts B, Bray D, Lewis J, et al. Cell-cell adhesions and the extra-cellular matrix. In: Alberts B, ed. *Molecular Biology of the Cell.* New York: Garland Publishers; 1983:673–715.

125. Brincat M, Moniz CJ, Studd JWW, et al. Sex hormones and skin collagen context in postmenopausal women. *Br Med J.* 1983;287:1337–1338.

126. Savvas M, Bishop J, Laurent G, et al. Type III collagen content in the skin of postmenopausal women receiving oestradiol and testosterone implants. *Br J Obstet Gynaecol.* 1991;100:154–156.

127. Thomas TM, Plymat KR, Blannin J, et al. Prevalence of urinary incontinence. *Br Med J.* 1980;281:1243–1245.

128. Einhorning G. Simultaneous recording of intravesical and intraurethral pressure. A study on urethral closure in normal and stress incontinent women. *Acta Chir Scand.* 1961;276(suppl).1–68.

129. Gosling JA. The structure of the bladder and urethra in relation to function. *Urol Clin North Am.* 1979;6:31–38.

130. Ulmsten U, Ekman G, Fiertz G, et al. Different biochemical composition of connective tissue in continent and stress incontinent women. *Acta Obstet Gynecol Scand.* 1987;66:455–457.

131. Versi E, Cardozo L, Brincat M, et al. Correlation of urethral physiology and skin collagen in postmenopausal women. *Br J Obstet Gynecol.* 1988;95:147–152.

132. Taber P, Heidenreich J. Treatment of stress incontinence with estrogen in postmenopausal women. *Urol Int.* 1977;32:221–223.

133. Walters S, Wolf H, Barlebo H, et al. Urinary incontinence in postmenopausal women treated with estrogens. A double blind clinical trial. *Urol Int.* 1978;33:136–143.

134. Rud T. The effects of estrogens and gestagens on the urethral pressure profile in urinary continent and stress incontinent women. *Acta Obstet Gynecol Scand.* 1980a;59:265–1270.

135. Rud T. Urethral pressure profile in continent women from childhood to old age. *Acta Obstet Gynecol Scand.* 1980b;59:331–335.

136. Hilton P, Stanton SL. The use of intravaginal oestrogen cream in genuine stress incontinence. *Br J Obstet Gynecol.* 1983;90:940–944.

137. Beisland HO, Fossberg E, Moer A, et al. Urethral sphincter insufficiency in postmenopausal females: Treatments with phenylprophanolamine and estriol separately and in combination. *Urol Int.* 1984;39:211–216.

138. Larsson B, Andersson KE, Batra S, et al. Effects of estradiol on norepinephrine-induced contraction, alpha-adrenoceptor number and norepinephrine content in the female rabbit urethra. *J Pharmacol Exp Ther.* 1984;229:557–563.

139. Versi E, Cardozo LD, Studd JWW, et al. Internal urinary sphincter in maintenance of female incontinence. *Br Med J.* 1986;292:166–167.

140. Brincat M, Versi E, Moniz CF, et al. Skin collagen changes in postmenopausal women receiving different regimens of estrogen therapy. *Obstet Gynecol.* 1987;70:123–127.

141. Baron JA, LaVecchia C, Levi F. The centiestrogenic effect of cigarette smoking in women. *Am J Obstet Gynecol.* 1990;162:502–514.

142. Mishnovicz JJ, Hershcopf RJ, Naganuma H, et al. Increased 2-hydroxylation of estradiol as a possible mechanism for the anti-estrogenic effect of cigarette smoking. *N Engl J Med.* 1986;315:1305–1309.

143. Mishnovicz JJ, Naganuma H, Hershcopf RJ. Increased urinary catechol estrogen excretion in female smokers. *Steroids.* July-August 1988:69–83.

144. Barbieri RL, York CM, Cherry ML, et al. The effects of nicotine, cotinine, and anabasine on rat adrenal 11B-hydroxylase and 21-hydroxylase. *J Steroid Biochem.* 1987;24:1–14.

145. Greenblatt RB. The use of androgens in the menopause and other gynecologic disorders. *Obstet Gynecol Clin North Am.* 1987;14:251–268.

146. Longcope C, Johnston CC Jr. Androgen and estrogen dynamics in pre- and postmenopausal women: A comparison between smokers and non-smokers. *J Clin Endocrinol Metab.* 1988;67:379–383.

147. Grodin JM, Siiteri PK, MacDonald PC. Source of estrogen production in post-menopausal women. *J Clin Endocrinol Metab.* 1973;36:207–214.

148. Siiteri PK. Extraglandular oestrogen formation and serum binding of oestradiol: Relationship to cancer. *J Endocrinol.* 1981;89:119–129.

149. Barbieri RL, Gochberg J, Ryan KJ. Nicotine, cotinine and anabasine inhibit aromatase in human trophoblast in vitro. *J Clin Invest.* 1986;77:1727–1733.

150. Barbieri RL, McShane PM, Ryan KJ. Constituents of cigarette smoke inhibit human granulosa cell aromatase. *Fertil Steril.* 1986;46:232–236.

151. MacMahon B, Trichopoulos D, Cole P, et al. Cigarette smoking and urinary estrogens. *N Engl J Med.* 1982;307:1062–1065.

152. Jensen J, Christiansen C, Rodbro P. Cigarette smoking, serum estrogens, and bone loss during hormone replacement therapy early after menopause. *N Engl J Med.* 1985;313:973–975.

153. Jensen J, Christiansen C. Effects of smoking on serum lipoproteins and bone mineral content during post-menopausal hormone replacement therapy. *Am J Obstet Gynecol.* 1988;159:820–825.

154. Mattison DR. The effects of smoking on fertility from gametogenesis to implantation. *Environ Res.* 1982;28:410–433.

155. Balfour DJK. The effects of nicotine on brain neurotransmitter systems. *Pharmacol Ther.* 1982;16:269–282.

156. Mattison DR. Morphology of oocyte and follicle destruction by polycyclic aromatic hydrocarbons in mice. *Toxicol Appl Pharmacol.* 1980;53:249–259.

157. Schmiterlow CG, Hansson E, Andersson G, et al. Distribution of nicotine in the central nervous system. *Ann N Y Acad Sci.* 1967;142:2–14.

158. Sershen H, Lajtha A. Cerebral uptake of nicotine and of amino acids. *J Neurosci Res.* 1979;4:85–91.

159. Benowitz NL, Jacob P III. Metabolism, pharmacokinetics, and pharmacodynamics of nicotine in man. In: Martin WR, Van Leon GR, Iwamoto ET, Davis L, eds. *Tobacco and Smoking and Nicotine: A Neurobiological Approach.* New York: Plenum Press; 1987.

160. Schwartz RD, McGee R Jr, Kellar K. Nicotinic cholinergic receptors labeled by [^{3}II] acetylcholine in rat brain. *Mol Pharmacol.* 1982;22:56–62.

161. Morley BJ. The properties of brain nicotine receptors. In: Balfour DJK, ed. *Nicotine and the Tobacco Smoking Habit.* Oxford: Pergamon Press; 1984.

162. Kellar KJ, Schwartz RD, Martino AM. Nicotinic cholinergic receptor recognition sites in brain. In: Martin WR, Van Loon GR, Iwamoto ET, Davis L, eds. *Tobacco Smoking and Nicotine: A Neurobiological Approach.* New York: Plenum Press; 1987:467–479.

163. Balfour DJK. The effects of nicotine on brain neurotransmitter systems. *Pharmacol Ther.* 1982;16:269–282.

164. Rowell PP. Current concepts on the effects of nicotine on neurotransmitter release in the central nervous system. In: Martin WR, Van Loon GR, Iwamoto ET, Davis L, eds. *Tobacco Smoking and Nicotine: A Neurobiological Approach.* New York: Plenum Press; 1987:191–208.

165. Andersen AN, Ronn B, Tjonneland, et al. Low maternal but normal fetal prolactin levels in cigarette smoking pregnant women. *Acta Obstet Gynecol Scand.* 1984;63:237–239.

166. Andersen AN, Lund-Anderson C, Larsen JF, et al. Suppressed prolactin but normal neurophysin levels in cigarette smoking breast-feeding women. *Clin Endocrinol.* 1982;17:363–368.

167. Anderson AN, Schioler V. Influence of breast-feeding pattern on pituitary-ovarian axis of women in an industrialized community. *Am J Obstet Gynecol.* 1982;143:673–677.

168. Andersen AN, Semczuk M, Tabor A. Prolactin and pituitary-gonadal function in cigarette smoking infertile patients. *Andrologia.* 1984;16:391–396.

169. Baron JA, Bulbrook RD, Wang DY, et al. Cigarette smoking and prolactin in women. *Br Med J.* 1986;293:482–483.

170. Baron JA. Cigarette smoking and Parkinson's disease. *Neurology.* 1986;36:1490–1496.

171. Blake CA, Scaramuzzi RJ, Norman RL, et al. Nicotine delays the ovulatory surge

of luteinizing hormone in the rat (36922). *Proc Soc Exp Biol Med.* 1972;141:1014–1016.

172. Kanematsu S, Sawyer CH. Inhibition of the progesterone-advanced LH surge at proestrus by nicotine. *Proc Soc Exp Biol Med.* 1973;143:1183–1186.

173. Fuxe K, Andersson K, Eneroth P, et al. Neuroendocrine actions of nicotine and of exposure to cigarette smoke: Medical implications. *Psychoneuroendocrinology.* 1989;14:19–41.

174. Tachi N, Aoyama M. Effects of cigarette smoke exposure on estrous cycles and mating behavior in female rats. *Bull Environ Contam Toxicol.* 1988;40:584–589.

175. Hiatt RA, Fireman BH. Smoking, menopause, and breast cancer. *J Clin Invest.* 1986;77:833–838.

176. Baron JA. Smoking and estrogen related disease. *Am J Epidemiol.* 1984;119:9–22.

177. Hammond EC. Smoking in relation to physical complaints. *Arch Environ Health.* 1961;3:28–164.

178. Jick H, Porter J, Morrison AS. Relation between smoking and age at natural menopause. *Lancet.* 1977;2:1354–1355.

179. Bailey A, Robinson D, Vessey M. Smoking and age at natural menopause. *Lancet.* 1977;2:722. Letter.

180. McNamara PM, Hjortland MC, Gordon T, et al. Natural history of menopause: The Framingham study. *J Contemp Ed Obstet Gynecol.* 1978;20:27–35.

181. Lindquist O, Bengtsson C. Menopausal age in relation to smoking. *Acta Med Scand.* 1979;205:73–77.

182. Kaufman DW, Stone D, Rosenberg L, et al. Cigarette smoking and age at natural menopause. *Am J Public Health.* 1980;70:420–422.

183. Adena MA, Gallagher HG. Cigarette smoking and the age at menopause. *Ann Hum Biol.* 1982;9:121–130.

184. Anderson FS, Transbol I, Christiansen C. Is cigarette smoking a promoter of the menopause? *Acta Med Scand.* 1982;212:137–139.

185. Willett W, Stampfer MJ, Bain C, et al. Cigarette smoking, relative weight, and menopause. *Am J Epidemiol.* 1983;117:651–658.

186. McKinlay SM, Bifano NL, McKinlay JB. Smoking and age at menopause in women. *Ann Intern Med.* 1985;103:350–356.

187. Stanford JL, Hartge P, Brinton LA, et al. Factors influencing age at natural menopause. *J Chronic Dis.* 1987;40:995–1002.

188. Schottenfeld D, Fraumeni JT Jr. *Cancer Epidemiology and Prevention.* Philadelphia: WB Saunders; 1982.

189. Thomas DB. Do hormones cause breast cancer? *Cancer.* 1984;53:595–604.

190. Kay TJA, Pike MC. The role of oestrogens and progestogens in the epidemiology and prevention of breast cancer. *Eur J Cancer Clin Oncol.* 1988;24:29–43.

191. Smith EM, Sowers MF, Burns TL. Effects of smoking on the development of female reproductive cancers. *J Clin Invest.* 1984;73:371–376.

192. Baron JA, Byers T, Greenberg ER, et al. Cigarette smoking in women with cancers of the breast and reproductive organs. *J Clin Invest.* 1986;77:677–680.

193. Stockwell HG, Lyman GH. Cigarette smoking and the risk of female reproductive cancer. *Am J Obstet Gynecol.* 1987;157:35–40.

194. Lawrence C, Tessaro I, Durgerian S, et al. Smoking, body weight, and early-stage endometrial cancer. *Cancer.* 1987;59:1665–1669.

195. Ramcharan S, Pellegrin FA, Ray R, et al. *The Walnut Creek contraceptive drug study.* Vol 3. Washington: Department of Health and Human Services; 1981.

196. Parazzini F, La Vecchia C, Negri E, et al. Epidemiological characteristics of women with uterine fibroids: A case-control study. *Obstet Gynecol.* 1988;72:853–857.

197. Ross RK, Pike MC, Vessey MP, et al. Risk factors for uterine fibroids: reduced risk associated with oral contraceptives. *Br Med J.* 1986;293:359–362.

198. Wyshak G, Frish RE, Albright NL, et al. Lower prevalence of benign diseases of the breast and benign tumors of the reproductive system among former college athletes compared to non-athletes. *Br J Cancer.* 1986;58:841–845.

199. Cramer DW, Wilson E, Stillman RJ, et al. The relation of endometriosis to menstrual characteristics, smoking and exercise. *JAMA.* 1986;255:1904–1908.

200. Hiller JE, Liang KY, Polk BF, et al. The protective effect of smoking on endometriosis. In: Program supplement of the forty-third annual meeting of the American Fertility Society. American Fertility Society; 1987:56.

201. Stillman RJ, Rosenberg MJ, Sachs BP. Smoking and reproduction. *Fertil Steril.* 1986;46:5454–566.

202. Mattison DR. The effects of smoking on fertility from gametogenesis to implantation. *Environ Res.* 1982;28:410–433.

203. Bernhard VP. Sichere Scheden des Zigarettenrauchen bei der Frau. *Med Monatsschr.* 1949;3:58–60.

204. Hammond EC. Smoking in relation to physical complaints. *Arch Environ Health.* 1961;3:28–164.

205. Kauramiemi T. Gynecologic health screening by means of a questionnaire. *Acta Obstet Gynecol Scand.* 1964;48(suppl 4):114–121.

206. Drac VP, Kopecny J. Sterilitaet bei raucherinnen unt nichtraucherinnen. *Zentralbl Gynakol.* 1970;27:865–869.

207. Procope BJ, Timonen S. The premenstrual syndrome in relation to sport, gymnastics and smoking. *Acta Obstet Gynecol Scand.* 1971;50(suppl 9):77.

208. Pettersson F, Fries H, Nillius SJ. Epidemiology of secondary amenorrhea. *Am J Obstet Gynecol.* 1973;117:80–86.

209. Wood C. The association of psycho-social factors and gynecological symptoms. *Aust Fam Physician.* 1978;28:471–478.

210. Wood C, Larsen L, Williams R. Social and psychological factors in relation to premenstrual tension and menstrual pain. *Aust N Z J Obstet Gynaecol.* 1979;19:111–115.

211. Andersch B, Milson I. An epidemiologic study of young women with dysmenorrhea. *Am J Obstet Gynecol.* 1982;144:655–660.

212. Sloss EM, Freirichs RR. Smoking and menstrual disorders. *Int J Epidemiol.* 1983;12:107–109.

213. Greenberg G, Thompson SG, Meade TW. Relation between cigarette smoking and use of hormonal replacement therapy for menopausal symptoms. *J Epidemiol Community Health.* 1987;41:26–29.

214. Hartz AJ, Kelber S, Borkowf H, et al. The association of smoking with clinical indicators of altered sex steroids—a study of 50,145 women. *Public Health Rep.* 1987;102:254–259.

215. Brown S, Vessey M, Stratton I. The influence of method of contraception and cigarette smoking of menstrual patterns. *Br J Obstet Gynaecol.* 1988;95:905–910.

216. Daniell HW. Osteoporosis and smoking. *JAMA.* 1972;221:509.

217. Daniell HW. Osteoporosis of the slender smoker. *Arch Intern Med.* 1976;136:298–304.

218. Williams AR, Weiss NS, Ure CL, et al. Effect of weight, smoking, and estrogen use on the risk of hip and forearm fractures in postmenopausal women. *Obstet Gynecol.* 1982;60:695–699.

219. Aloia JF, Cohn SH, Vaswani A, et al. Risk factors for postmenopausal osteoporosis. *Am J Med.* 1985;78:95–100.

220. Kreiger N, Hildreth S. Re: cigarette smoking and estrogen-dependent diseases. *Am J Epidemiol.* 1986;123:200.

221. Jensen GF. Osteoporosis of the slender smoker revisited by epidemiologic approach. *Eur J Clin Invest.* 1986;6:239–242.

222. Nelson DT, Kiel DP, Anderson JJ, et al. Alcohol consumption and hip fractures: The Framingham study. *Am J Epidemiol.* 1988;128:1102–1110.

223. Holbrook TL, Barrett-Connor E, Wingard EL. Dietary calcium and risk of hip fracture: 14-year prospective population study. *Lancet.* 1988;2:1046–1049.

224. Lau E, Donnan S, Barker DJP, et al. Physical activity and calcium intake in fracture of the proximal femur in Hong Kong. *Br Med J.* 1988;297:1441–1443.

225. Cooper C, Barker DJP, Wickham C. Physical activity, muscle strength, and calcium intake in fracture of the proximal femur in Britain. *Br Med J.* 1988;297:1443–1446.

226. Kiel DP, Baron JA, Anderson JJ, et al. Smoking eliminates the protective effect of oral estrogens on the risk of hip fracture among women. *Ann Intern Med.* 1992;116:716–721.

227. Zacharin RT. Abdominoperineal urethral suspension in the management of recurrent stress incontinence of urine—a 15 year experience. *Obstet Gynecol.* 1983;62:644–654.

228. Last JA, King TE, Nerlich AG, et al. Collagen cross-linking in adult patients with acute and chronic fibrotic lung disease. *Am Rev Respir Dis.* 1990;141:307–313.

229. Swash M. The neurogenic hypothesis of stress incontinence. In: Bock G, Whelan J, eds. *Ciba Foundation Symposium 151: Neurobiology of Incontinence.* New York: John Wiley & Sons; 1990;156–170.

230. Bump RC, McClish DK. Cigarette smoking and urinary incontinence in women. *Am J Obstet Gynecol.* 1992;167:1213–1218.

231. Gilpin SA, Gosling JA, Smith ARB, et al. The pathogenesis of genitourinary

prolapse and stress incontinence of urine: a histological and histochemical study. *Br J Obstet Gynaecol.* 1989;96:15–23.

232. Smith ARB, Hosker GL, Warrell DW. The role of partial denervation of the pelvic floor in the aetiology of genitourinary prolapse and stress incontinence of urine. A neurophysiological study. *Br J Obstet Gynaecol.* 1989;96:23–28.

233. Snooks SJ, Badenoch DF, Tiptaft RC, et al. Perineal nerve damage in genuine stress incontinence: An electrophysiological study. *Br J Urol.* 1985;57:422–426.

234. Young RL, Goepfert AR, Goldzeiher HW. Estrogen replacement therapy is not conducive of venous thromboembolism. *Maturitas.* 1991;13:189–192.

235. Devor M, Barrett-Connor E, Renvall M, et al. Estrogen replacement therapy and the risk of venous thrombosis. *Am J Med.* 1992;92:275–282.

236. The Boston Collaborative Drug Surveillance Program. Surgically confirmed gall-bladder disease, venous thromboembolism and breast tumors in relation to post-menopausal estrogen therapy. *N Engl J Med.* 1974;290:15–19.

237. Natchigall LE, Natchigall RH, Natchigall RD, et al. Estrogen replacement therapy II: A prospective study in the relationship to carcinoma and cardiovascular and metabolic problems. *Obstet Gynecol.* 1979;54:74–79.

238. Petitti DB, Wingerd J, Pellegrin F, et al. Oral contraceptives, smoking, and other factors in relation to risk of venous thromboembolic disease. *Am J Epidemiol.* 1978;108:480–485.

239. Petitti DB, Wingerd J, Pellegrin F, et al. Risk of vascular disease in women. *JAMA.* 1979;242:1150–1154.

240. Astedt B, Bernstein K, Cassien B, et al. Estrogens and postoperative thrombosis evaluated by the radioactive iodine method. *Surg Gynecol Obstet.* 1980;151:372–374.

241. Notelovitz M, Ware M. Coagulation risks with postmenopausal oestrogen therapy. In: Studd J, ed. *Progress in Obstetrics and Gynecology.* Edinburgh: Churchill Livingstone; 1982:228–240.

242. Astedt B. Does estrogen replacement therapy predispose to thrombosis? *Acta Obstet Gynecol Scand.* 1985;130(suppl):71–74.

243. Nilsson K, Heimer G. Low-dose oestradiol in the treatment of urogenital oestrogen deficiency—a pharmacokinetic and pharmacodynamic study. *Maturitas.* 1992;15:121–126.

244. Stalborg E, Thiele B. Motor unit fibre density in the exterior digitorum communis muscle. *J Neuro Neurosurg Psych.* 1976;38:874–880.

245. Anderson RS. A neurogenic element to genuine stress incontinence. *Br J Obstet Gynaecol.* 1984;91:41–45.

246. Smith ARB, Hosker GL, Warrell DW. The role of partial denervation of the pelvic floor in the etiology of genitourinary prolapse and stress incontinence: A neuro-physiological study. *Br J Obstet Gynaecol.* 1989;96:24–28.

247. Warrell DW. Pelvic floor neuropathy: Partial denervation in pelvic floor prolapse. In: Benson JT, ed. *Female Pelvic Floor Disorders.* New York: WW Norton; 1992:153–156.

248. Snooks SJ, Swash M, Henry MM, et al. Risk factors in childbirth causing damage to the pelvic floor innervation. *Int J Colorectal Dis.* 1986;1:20–24.

248. Snooks SJ, Swash M, Henry MM, et al. Risk factors in childbirth causing damage to the pelvic floor innervation. *Int J Colorectal Dis.* 1986;1:20–24.

249. Snooks SJ, Swash M, Mathers SE, et al. Effect of vaginal delivery on the pelvic floor: A 5-year followup. *Br J Surg.* 1990;70:1258–1360.

250. Allen RE, Hosker GL, Smith ARB, et al. Pelvic floor damage and childbirth: a neurophysiological study. *Br J Obstet Gynaecol.* 1990;97:770–779.

251. Smith PH, Balentine B. The neuroanatomical basis for denervation of the urinary bladder following major pelvic surgery. *Br J Surg.* 1968;55:929–932.

252. Mundy AR. Anatomical explanation for bladder dysfunction following rectal and uterine surgery. *Br J Urol.* 1982;54:501–504.

253. Benson JT, McClellan E. The effect of vaginal dissection on the pudendal nerve. *Obstet Gynecol.* 1993;82:387–389.

The Anatomy of Pelvic Relaxation and Stress Urinary Incontinence

Bob L. Shull

In gynecologic surgery for pelvic support defects, abnormal bladder or bowel function, and sexual dysfunction, the skilled surgeon must be able to integrate history, physical findings, and tests of function to design an effective management plan. Knowing how to perform and interpret the pelvic examination and how to identify supporting tissues and support defects is essential. The intraoperative confirmation of the support defects allows execution of an objective surgical procedure specifically designed for that patient.

Many excellent references deal with comparative as well as surgical anatomy.[1–3] Few, however, emphasize the importance of understanding normal pelvic anatomy as a prerequisite to recognizing abnormal anatomy.[4] It is trite, but true, to say that one cannot recognize what is abnormal without having a firm understanding of normal, whether affect, appearance, or anatomy.

NORMAL PELVIC ANATOMY

Two major approaches for learning normal gross anatomy are physical examination and operative dissection, preferably in the living patient. First, let us define the anatomic landmarks and physical findings in women who have no complaints of pelvic relaxation and who have a "normal" pelvic examination. Later we will review how these findings change in women with anatomic loss of support.

Experienced gynecologists see many women who have "normal" examinations but the physicians cannot describe objectively the specific landmarks used to determine normal. The stationary points of reference in the pelvis are the two innominate bones, including ischial spines, ischial tuberosities, pubic rami, and symphysis; the sacrum; and the coccyx. All of the soft tissue structures are suspended or attached directly or indirectly to one or more of these bones. Consider the vagina to be a flexible tube with an external epithelial lining and an inner musculofascial layer of tissue forming a sheath between the epithelium and the adjacent viscera, specifically the urethra, bladder, and rectum. At the apex of this tube, the cervix penetrates the sheath but does not rely on the sheath for support. The vaginal epithelium is unimportant for support; however, the underlying musculofascial tissue provides support for the pelvic viscera and is itself attached to the bony pelvis, muscles, and uterus. The cervix and uterus are suspended supravaginally by the uterosacral and cardinal ligament complexes, which maintain normal apical vaginal as well as uterine support.[5]

On pelvic examination, topographical landmarks provide clues regarding support for the following sites: the urethra, bladder, cervix (or vaginal cuff), cul-de-sac, rectum, and perineum. How do you determine when these sites are normally supported? First, standardize the conditions of the examination and objectively describe specific sites in the vagina. Examine the patient in the dorsal lithotomy position, using the split blade of a Grave's speculum to visualize each site individually. Because findings in the resting lithotomy position do not reproduce the findings of a woman standing erect, the patient must bear down maximally as each site is evaluated.

Normal must be defined before abnormal can be described. Assume an imaginary line from mid-hymen extending posteriorly to the midpoint of the vaginal apex—the mid-vaginal axis (Figure 2-1). Women who have normal pelvic support can strain maximally, and the urethra, bladder, cul-de-sac, and rectum will not sag past this mid-vaginal axis. The cervix or cuff has normal support when it is suspended at or above the level of the ischial spines. The perineum is normal when there are no lacerations. To facilitate organization of the examination and our subsequent discussion, divide the vagina into three segments: anterior (the urethra and bladder), superior (the cervix or cuff and cul-de-sac), and posterior (the rectum and perineum). The key to accurate physical examination is to identify which, if any, of these sites has abnormal support, and where the abnormalities (defects) exist.

SUSPENDING AND SUPPORTING STRUCTURE

What are the specific suspending and supporting structures that maintain normal findings? The bony pelvis provides a symmetrical scaffolding for muscular, fascial,

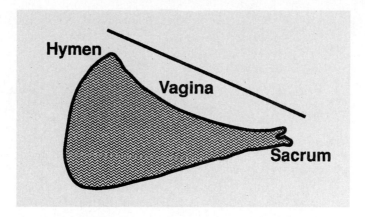

Figure 2-1 Mid-vaginal axis.

and ligamentous structures. A sagittal view illustrates key landmarks: symphysis pubis, superior ramus of pubis, obturator internus muscle and fascia, pubococcygeus muscle and fascia, levator ani muscle and fascia, the ischial spine, and fascial condensations known generally as the "white line" but specifically as the arcus tendinous levator ani (ATLA), the junction of ileococcygeus and its fascia to obturator internus muscle and fascia, and the arcus tendinous fascia pelvis (ATFP), a fascial condensation between obturator internus and levator ani extending from the ischial spine to the posterior margin of the pubis (Figure 2-2). The pubocervical fascia, which supports the anterior vaginal segment, attaches laterally to the ATLA and ATFP, superiorly to the cervix or vaginal cuff, and distally fuses with the perineal membrane. In addition, the pubourethral ligament complex, which attaches to the urethra anteriorly and laterally, has anterior and posterior urethral divisions that are noted on pelvic examination by the appearance of the anterior urethral crease, mid-urethra bulge, and posterior urethral fold. The bladder and urethra rest on the pubocervical fascia. The anterior vaginal epithelium forms a lateral vaginal groove, or sulcus, at the lateral points of attachment of pubocervical fascia to the ATFP, or white line.

The uterosacral ligaments originate along S2 to S4 and insert posteriorly on the uterus, suspending it from the bony pelvis. The cardinal ligament complex has a more lateral origin, starting from fascia over piriformis muscle and following the vascular and neural sheaths along the uterine vessels, attaching not only to the cervix laterally but also to the upper 2 to 3 cm of the vagina, suspending the uterus posteriorly and laterally. In the patient who has previously had hysterectomy, the attachment of uterosacral cardinal ligament complex to the vaginal cuff should be visible as dimples at approximately 3 o'clock and 9 o'clock in the cuff. Intrafascial hysterectomy helps to preserve the cardinal ligament attachment to the upper

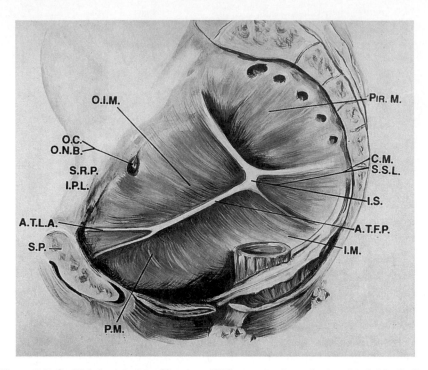

Figure 2-2 Sagittal view of retropubic space. ATFP, arcus tendineus fascia pelvis "white line"; ATLA, arcus tendineus levator ani; CM, coccygeus muscle; IM, ileococcygeus muscle; IPL, iliopectineal line; IS, ischial spine; OC, obturator canal; OIM, obturator internus muscle; ONB, obturator neurovascular bundle; PIRM, piriformis muscle; PM, pubococcygeus muscle; SP, symphysis pubis; SRP, superior ramus of pubis; SSL, sacrospinous ligament.

vagina, thereby maintaining support to the vaginal apex. The cul-de-sac provides the only serosal covering adjacent to the vagina and is bounded laterally by the uterosacral ligaments and distally by the attachment of the rectovaginal fascia along the posterior and superior vagina.

The rectovaginal fascia covers the anterior rectum and is attached laterally to the superior fascia of levator ani posterior to the ATFP; superiorly to the cardinal-uterosacral ligament complex and posterior vaginal wall; and distally is fused to the overlying vaginal epithelium and perineal body.

The apex of the vaginal canal is directed posteriorly into the hollow of the sacrum when the patient is lying in the dorsal lithotomy position. The anterior vaginal wall is approximately 7 to 9 cm deep and 2 to 3 cm shorter than the posterior wall because the cervix sits in the anterior wall. The vaginal epithelium normally has more rugae anteriorly than posteriorly and less around the cervix or cuff.

ABNORMAL SUPPORT: DEFECTS

Abnormal support can be specifically located in single, multiple, or all sites in the vagina. Anterior vaginal segment loss of support may result from defects in the pubocervical fascia beneath the urethra or bladder, *midline defects*; from loss of lateral attachment of the fascia to the pelvic sidewall, *paravaginal defects*; or loss of support of the superior portion of the fascia to the cervix or cuff, *superior defects or avulsions.* The superior segment has poor support when the uterosacral ligaments or cardinal ligaments (or both) elongate or are avulsed. In the case of uterine prolapse, some portion of the uterosacral ligament usually can be identified by palpation along the posterior cervix and cul-de-sac. In women with post-hysterectomy vaginal vault prolapse, the ligament remnants may be seen at the site of dimples at 3 o'clock and 9 o'clock. Occasionally they may only be identified following surgical entry into the posterior cul-de-sac and clamping intraperito-neally near the vaginal cuff at 4 o'clock and 8 o'clock, stretching and palpating medially and posteriorly toward the sacrum. Transabdominally, the uterosacral ligaments stand out in relief with upward traction on the rectum. The other superior segment defect, enterocele, occurs when the cul-de-sac peritoneum dissects be-tween the rectovaginal fascia and the posterior vaginal epithelium.

Posterior segment defects can be related to several factors. Rectocele occurs either when the rectovaginal fascia is deficient in its midportion as it covers the anterior rectum, a so-called *midline defect*; when the rectovaginal fascia is detached from the perineal body or upper vagina, a *transverse defect*; or when the recto-vaginal fascia is detached from the superior surface of the levator ani fascia, a *lateral defect.* Perineal defects result from lacerations, usually obstetric in origin, and may involve bulbocavernosus and transverse perineal muscles, the perineal body, or the anal sphincter and mucosa, or all of these structures.

Analysis and Localization of Defects

To use specific reparative techniques tailored to the patient's needs, all support defects must be identified preoperatively and confirmed during the intraoperative dissection. The examination is performed as earlier described, assessing the site and origin of each defect. An easy way to quantitate the loss of support is the "halfway system," described by Baden and Walker.[4] Any site may descend past the mid-vaginal axis halfway to the hymen, to the hymen, halfway outside the hymen, or fully outside the hymen (Figure 2-3). Perineal defects are described in the same manner as obstetric lacerations with a fourth degree laceration extending entirely through the anal sphincter. Once the defects have been identified, localized, and quantified, longitudinal evaluation can begin and objective pre- and postoperative

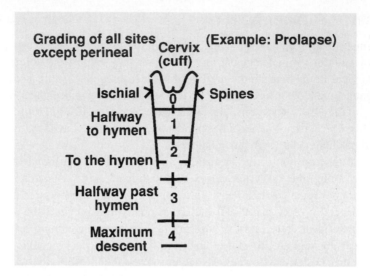

Figure 2-3 Grading of prolapse.

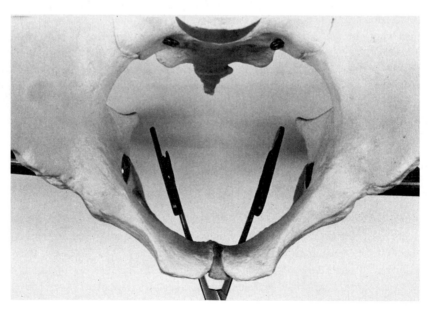

Figure 2-4 Baden analyzer. (Reproduced with permission from Baden and Walker.[4])

comparisons can be made.[6] Unfortunately, few reports in our literature give precise pre- and postoperative descriptions of pelvic support for patients who have had pelvic reconstruction. We have used this approach extensively to assess the efficacy of our repairs and to modify surgical techniques based on our findings.

Anterior Segment

The location of anterior segment defects is identified by using the Baden analyzer, or a curved ringed sponge forceps. The split blade of the speculum depresses the posterior vagina. The open forceps are placed lateral to the urethra and bladder with the curve pointing toward the ischial spines (Figure 2-4), elevating the anterior segment to its normal point of attachment laterally as the patient strains. If lateral elevation corrects the support loss, the defect is at the lateral attachment of the periurethral and perivesical fascia to the pelvic sidewall. When the patient strains and a bulge continues to protrude through the open arms of the forceps, a midline loss of fascial support exists. Anterior, superior defects are associated with a "high cystocele," an elongated anterior vaginal wall, and loss of rugation of the vaginal epithelium over the defect, indicating lack of fascia beneath the epithelium. These defects occur when the pubocervical fascia is not properly attached to the cervix or vaginal cuff. They must be confirmed intraoperatively and specifically repaired to ensure long-term surgical success. Combined lateral, midline, and superior defects may occur, each requiring specific identification and repair (Figures 2-5, 2-6, and 2-7). In my practice, the most challenging patients are those with anterior loss of support in all three areas: midline, lateral, and superior. I learned by longitudinal evaluation of my own postoperative patients that successful anatomic reconstruction occurs only when all three sites are individually repaired. The superior loss of support for pubocervical fascia is the defect that more often escapes detection and repair because many surgeons are not aware of its presence. As shown in Figure 2-7, these defects should be closed by using nonabsorbable suture material to approximate the superior portion of pubocervical fascia to the undersurface of the vaginal cuff.

Almost all urethral support defects are lateral, requiring reattachment of pubocervical fascia or shortening and plication of pubourethral ligaments for best results. Urethral support defects occur in women with or without genuine urinary incontinence. In patients with a primary complaint of genuine urinary incontinence and urethral hypermobility, I prefer the retropubic paravaginal defect repair because I know it provides not only excellent anatomic restoration but also excellent results for relief of incontinence. However, the vaginal approach has advantages in women who have other support defects that must be repaired vaginally. In patients who present primarily with complaints of pelvic relaxation, I prefer the vaginal

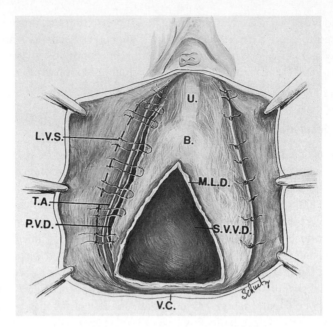

Figure 2-5 Anterior segment (bladder and urethra) defects show loss of support in the midline, laterally, and superiorly. Sutures are placed for the repair of the right lateral defect. B, bladder; LVS, lateral vaginal sulcus; MLD, midline defect; PVD, paravaginal defect; SVVD, superior vesicovaginal defect; TA, "tendinous" arch; U, urethra; VC, vaginal cuff. (Reproduced with permission from Baden and Walker.[4])

route for complete anatomic restoration, including the vaginal reattachment of periurethral and perivesical fascia to the white line. Such a repair requires a wide dissection into the retropubic space with specific identification of the white line, ischial spine, and obturator fascia. Unless the surgeon has a thorough knowledge of retropubic space anatomy, such a vaginal approach is potentially hazardous. The skilled reconstructive surgeon should possess the versatility to use this approach.

Superior Segment

Superior segment defects are identified by noting whether the cervix or vaginal cuff prolapses past its point of normal suspension at or above the ischial spines. An entcrocele may be identified by direct palpation of small bowel in the rectovaginal epithelium. An enterocele can be more accurately identified preoperatively by examining the patient in the standing position as described in the text by Nichols and Randall.[2]

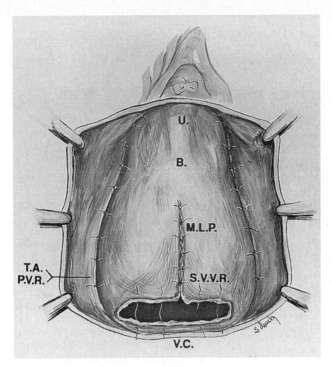

Figure 2-6 Both lateral defects have been repaired by reattachment to the white line and the midline defect has been plicated as in the traditional cystocele repair. B, bladder; MLP, midline plication; PVR, paravaginal reattachment; SVVR, superior vesicovaginal reattachment; TA, "tendinous" arch; U, urethra; VC, vaginal cuff. (Reproduced with permission from Baden and Walker.[4])

Posterior Segment

Rectoceles are usually almost midline but may be lateral or transverse. Using the ringed sponge forceps, reapproximate the lateral vaginal tissue posteriorly toward the ischial spines and have the patient bear down. If a bulge continues to appear through the open arms of the forceps, a midline defect exists. If lateral replacement corrects the defect, a lateral loss of support exists. If a bulge remains near the hymen or high in the rectovaginal septum, a transverse loss of support exists. Once the vaginal epithelium has been reflected away from the rectum, identify the rectovaginal fascia and confirm the site of the fascia defect by direct inspection.

The perineal defects are usually less extensive than those in other sites; however, some women will present primarily with abnormal bowel function directly related to perineal defects involving the anal sphincter.

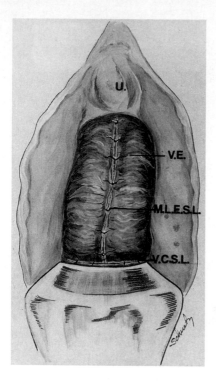

Figure 2-7 The superior portion of pubocervical fascia has been closed and attached to the vaginal cuff. MLESL, midline epithelial suture line; U, urethra; VCSL, vaginal cuff suture line; VE, vaginal epithelium. (Reproduced with permission from Baden and Walker.[4])

RETROPUBIC SPACE ANATOMY

Although all the clues for pelvic support defects are seen on vaginal examination, the operative confirmation and surgical therapy may require a retropubic approach, particularly for the anterior or superior segments. In my practice, most of the anterior paravaginal defects are repaired retropubically, as are some cuff prolapses and enteroceles.[7] Whether you choose a vaginal or retropubic approach, a thorough knowledge of retropubic space anatomy is essential to the skilled reconstructive surgeon (Figure 2-8).

The dissection can be approached through either a vertical or transverse incision. Transversalis fascia is entered posterior to the rectus muscles and the loose areolar tissue gently dissected away from the bony pelvis. Several landmarks can be identified by palpation. The symphysis is almost always convex, located in the anterior midline. The superior rami of the pubic bones mark the boundary of the bony inlet. A set of circumflex veins, which are easily traumatized by retractors, courses along the inner aspect of the superior rami. Electrocautery effectively stops bleeding in this area. The loose areolar tissue adjacent to the bladder and urethra often covers the anterior vagina and the pelvic sidewalls. It can easily be dissected off the sidewalls, allowing direct visualization of the white line, obturator fascia,

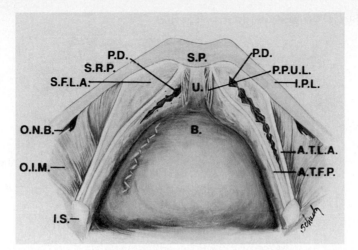

Figure 2-8 A view into the retropubic space shows all the key landmarks as well as paravaginal defects lateral to the urethra and bladder. ATFP, arcus tendineus fascia pelvis "white line"; ATLA, arcus tendineus levator ani; B, bladder; IPL, iliopectineal line; IS, ischial spine; OIM, obturator internus muscle; ONB, obturator neurovascular bundle; PD, paravaginal defect; PPUL, posterior pubourethral ligament; SFLA, superficial fascia levator ani; SP, symphysis pubis; SRP, superior ramus of pubis; U, urethra. (Reproduced with permission from Baden and Walker.[4])

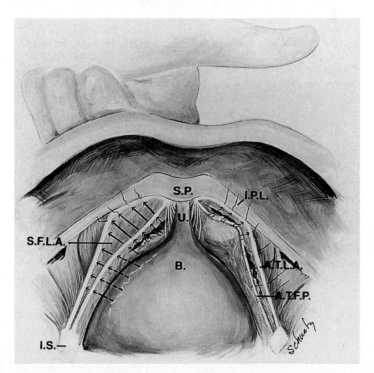

Figure 2-9 Interrupted nonabsorbable sutures are used to repair each defect in much the same way you would close fascial edges in an incision. ATFP, arcus tendineus fascia pelvis "white line"; ATLA, arcus tendineus levator ani; B, bladder; IPL, iliopectineal line; IS, ischial spine; SFLA, superficial fascia levator ani; SP, symphysis pubis; U, urethra. (Reproduced with permission from Baden and Walker.[4])

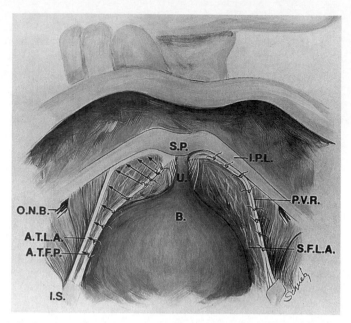

Figure 2-10 Both sides have been repaired. The left side used ATFP because the defect was medial to it. The right side used ATLA because the defect was lateral to ATFP. ATFP, arcus tendineus fascia pelvis "white line"; ATLA, arcus tendineus levator ani; B, bladder; IPL, iliopectineal line; IS, ischial spine; ONB, obturator neurovascular bundle; PVR, paravaginal reattachment; SFLA, superficial fascia levator ani; SP, symphysis pubis; U, urethra. (Reproduced with permission from Baden and Walker.[4])

and posterior pubourethral ligament complex. The anterior vagina may be quite vascular. Vessels in the vaginal fascia generally run front to back and can be safely included in sutures used to reattach the vagina to the white line, Cooper's ligament, or symphysis. Bleeding from them is minimal if the sutures are securely tied. Vessels in the bladder run side to side and should not be included in any repair for support defects. Bleeding from the pelvic sidewall is uncommon except near the posterior border of symphysis as the pubocervical fascia attaches to the perineal membrane and white line.

The repair is performed using nonabsorbable suture material to approximate the anterior vagina to the white line (Figure 2-9). I prefer to place the stitch near the ischial spine first, establishing support for the perivesical tissue high in the vagina. Next, I place the stitch from the pubourethral ligament to the white line to elevate the distal urethra. After the two stitches are tied and cut, I place interrupted sutures approximately 1 cm apart until the repair is complete from back of the symphysis to a point near the ischial spine (Figure 2-10).

A thorough knowledge of retropubic space anatomy provides the surgeon with flexibility in choosing the right procedure for the patient with urinary stress incontinence; however, retropubic elevation of the urethrovesical junction by any means will not correct coexisting midline or superior defects in pubocervical fascia support. These defects, as well as defects in support for the cuff, cul-de-sac, and rectum, require their own specific repairs to complete total pelvic reconstruction.

REFERENCES

1. Thompson JD, Rock JA. *TeLinde's Operative Gynecology.* 7th ed. Philadelphia: Lippincott; 1992.

2. Nichols DH, Randall CL. *Vaginal Surgery.* 3d ed. Baltimore: Williams & Wilkins; 1989.

3. Masterson BJ. *Manual of Gynecologic Surgery.* 2d ed. New York: Springer-Verlag; 1986.

4. Baden WF, Walker T. *Surgical Repair of Vaginal Defects.* Philadelphia: Lippincott; 1992.

5. DeLancey JOL. Anatomic causes of vaginal eversion after hysterectomy. *Am J Obstet Gynecol.* 1992;166:1717–1728.

6. Shull BL, Capen CV, Riggs MW, Kuehl TJ. Pre- and postoperative analysis of site-specific pelvic support defects in 81 women treated by sacrospinous ligament suspension and pelvic reconstruction. *Am J Obstet Gynecol.* 1992;166:1764–1771.

7. Shull BL, Baden WF. A six-year experience with paravaginal defect repair for stress urinary incontinence. *Am J Obstet Gynecol.* 1989;160:1432–1440.

Preoperative
Evaluation
and Management

Marvin H. Terry Grody

Overeagerness to operate on the older population may prove to be a deadly sin. What you can get away with in younger people is markedly diminished in seniors. In short, the standards are not equitable and, therefore, the care and caution that must be exercised with the older group on the path to the operating room is greater and more time-consuming. Recognizing the decreased margin of safety and acting accordingly can spell the difference between success and disaster. When all precautions have been exercised, coupled with appropriate timing, expressed concern, and common sense, older women tolerate anesthesia and pelvic surgery, particularly when performed vaginally, amazingly well.

Having endured the progressively disabling condition of uterine prolapse, genuine stress incontinence, or massive eversion, the patient will finally conclude that she can no longer dodge the issue and must do something about her condition. "I cannot go on living like this," she bluntly states to her often enthusiastic gynecologist who can hardly repress jubilation when she further demands, "I want to get this over with as soon as possible." Responding avidly, the operating room is telephoned at once and the case is on for next week; the trap is set for trouble. Does this happen often? Regrettably, it does—I see it all the time.

Why does this occur? In the mad rush to operate, common sense fades like the twilight sun. In 90 percent of the cases in which I am called on to participate, replacement estrogen has not entered anyone's thoughts. When a full urodynamics work-up is clearly indicated, often not even a Q-tip test is done "because the situation is so obvious it's not necessary." A one pack per day cigarette addiction goes unquestioned. An unbalanced diet, replete with snacks and ordered-in fast foods, remains undiscovered. An obese "couch potato" is not taught the necessity of a change in habits and a motivation to exercise. Autologous blood storage is not considered "because my cases don't need transfusions." No attempt is made to discuss the patient's problem with a caring relative.

Despite innumerable consultations and second opinions over many years, I have yet to find the patient destined for surgical repair of pelvic support defects, disabling while erect, who has been examined in anything but the lithotomy position. Certain laboratory tests are not ordered "because my hospital doesn't require them." Chart documentation by the doctor who has scheduled the surgery is almost invariably too sparse for current acceptability. Equally unacceptable, plans reveal that the patient will be tailored to a standard procedure rather than undergo surgery designed specifically to suit her particular condition. These are just some of the multitude of negligent factors that lead to intraoperative and postoperative trouble.

Preoperative preparation and management for the kind of surgery performed for nonmalignant problems of the postreproductive woman are as vital to long-term success as is the actual operation itself. Such planning is even more essential than it is for the surgically correctable conditions of the premenopausal woman, not just because the surgery is generally more involved and more apt to be related to structure rather than organs but because of the aging nature of postchildbearing pelvic tissue. Beyond localized concerns, obviously preoperative reassessment of overt and disclosure of subliminal systemic deficiencies, followed by correction and stabilization, must be far more intense in the older woman than in the younger.

THE SETTING FOR THE INITIAL INTERVIEW

Ideally, in the consideration of surgery of any kind in the older patient, the presence of a close relative, preferably husband or daughter, is mandatory. If not, the surgeon must be prepared to endure the agonies that noncompliance and misunderstanding may produce after surgery, which inevitably involve not just the patient herself but, perhaps worse, her relatives. No matter how thoroughly conscientious a physician may be, particularly a gynecologist, in dealing with this age group preoperatively, even though detailed descriptions in language absolutely comprehensible to the patient, accompanied by lucid illustrations, are included, if the patient is originally seen alone, the physician leaves himself or herself much more highly vulnerable to postoperative adversarial confrontation, despite an excellent outcome. Shocked and frightened by the final and inevitable decision for major surgery, she may well only half-listen to her doctor. Frequently, the patient may be too embarrassed to mention a hearing deficiency, sometimes compounded by inadequate education, increasing the incomprehensibility of the doctor's information. Therefore, when no family member is present for support and understanding, it is not surprising that the patient often brings home a markedly distorted version of what went on in the doctor's office. She may claim that no explanation was given to her, or that the doctor "used big medical words which I could not understand at all," or that "he was in a big rush with a lot of other patients waiting and he just told me to trust him." The days of blind faith are gone; a beclouded situation preoperatively can erupt into an avalanche of questions, suspicions, and doubts in the postoperative phase whether things go well or not.

For reasons not always easily explicable, many patients complain that "the doctor never once looked directly at me throughout the interview." I have had patients tell me that the previous doctor "turned completely around, talking away from me most of the time." The physician is literally talking to the wall. Eye-to-eye contact is a key to conveying compassion and concern, and confidence in the doctor is not likely to develop without it.

When a solitary appearance initially is unavoidable and major surgery is indicated and planned, the gynecologic surgeon should insist that the patient return, with her family, for an office visit at the earliest convenient time. A meeting to explain and clarify is most successful when scheduled at the end of office hours, when the waiting room is empty. An appropriate fee should be charged for the extra time involved. The payoff for both the doctor and the patient will ultimately prove enormous through the atmosphere of confidence, understanding, trust, and cooperation thereby established.

The importance of bringing her spouse and offspring into such a sphere of participation cannot be overemphasized not just because of revelation concerning the condition and its planned correction but for two other basic reasons. First, stern discipline in patient compliance, both preoperatively and postoperatively, is basic to sustained success in most procedures performed in this age category. When the family acts as a watchdog group, the doctor's job is always easier and results, too often tenuous at best, are guaranteed to be better than without family cooperation.

Second, all the major and minor events that might happen postoperatively, ranging from an initial inability to void spontaneously, or fever, to ultimate need for a later small additional suprapubic procedure to correct genuine stress incontinence, whether or not it preexisted the surgery, can be explained in advance, as well as the risks of the surgery itself. Antagonism and confrontation can thus be averted and all energies will be concentrated on improving the patient's condition.

Questionnaires presented to the patient to fill in while sitting in the waiting room are of uncertain value. Proponents claim that they save time and give the patient a chance to think more accurately regarding her medical problems. Opponents say that questions cannot be intelligently addressed until the patient is first interviewed to learn the nature of her particular complaints. Psychologically, patients prefer a subjective start, directly with the doctor, not with a piece of paper that creates immediately an impression of "cold" objectivity. Even questions posed in advance by a paramedical aide, designed to save time, may in the end be misdirective because the doctor, in a hurry, may be pulled off course and miss the primary problem. I do not use questionnaires. There is always time later for the patient to check out the medications she is taking or to recall better her previous medical experiences, or whatever.

I also tend not to give out printed material because often it is too general, composed to cover multiple abnormalities. This can be misleading, confusing, and frightening to the patient, even when only those parts directly pertinent to the patient are circled. However, carefully composed, precisely written instructions and expectations, including risks and possible shortcomings, may be helpful if given at the end of the visit.

My principal explanatory approach, to educate both the patient and her family, is visual. The use of photographs, accurate drawings in color, and sketches can explain in moments the nature of the lesions and the intention of surgical correction in ways far superior to any images conjured through graphically verbal and simplified oral communication.

Finally, to endear the patient and her family to yourself forever and create a truly heroic image, offer two "specials," one a privilege, the other a promise. First, disclose your home telephone number to be used only if unusual interferences prevent contact through the office telephone in situations of an urgent or emergency nature. The usual retort is "No doctor ever did this for me (us) before." I have always made known my telephone number at home, even having it published in the local directory. No patient has ever abused the privilege of this knowledge, and it has helped to build a warm atmosphere regarding good care and concern.

Second, promise that you will not go on vacation while the patient is still in the hospital recovering, that only when she is safely at home would you consider further temporary coverage of her care, if needed, by partners or colleagues. If you are a dedicated physician, you will not schedule an elective case in which the anticipated hospital recovery time will overlap the start of a vacation.

GENERAL PERTINENT INFORMATION

Because the patient is primarily interested in ridding herself of the symptoms that brought her to the doctor, exploratory questioning must be incisive and persistent, with frequent interjections by the doctor asking, "What else?" Obviously, the doctor wishes to accomplish all that is necessary to render the patient as symptom free as possible postoperatively. So, this approach in this age group is crucial to overall surgical success because the patient often forgets to mention ancillary but important symptoms. How upsetting it becomes when the patient tells her doctor as she is being wheeled toward the operating room, "I forgot to tell you that...." or, much worse, when she utters the same statement after the surgery has been completed. The amount of information a patient can forget to tell you, especially such things as a previous operation or a crucial medication, is often unbelievable. Again, help from the family and persistent interrogation cannot be emphasized enough. Additional probing by the physician must cover questions concerning nutrition, exercise, endurance, estrogen replacement, drugs, previous oral contraceptives, urinary habits, bowel habits, current or prior cigarette smoking, any habits that increase intra-abdominal pressure, systemic diseases, prior surgery of any kind, family history, occupational stresses (especially physical), and psychiatric disorders.

Because most of the benign problems in the postreproductive woman lie in the area of loss of tissue and organ support and suspension, my discussion of preoperative preparation will be weighted in that direction. For example, the elaboration on preparation for such cases as those with the unexpected finding of a lesion of the vulva or a pelvic mass in women being checked at their annual physical examination is more direct and concise than would be that for conditions of incontinence or uterine prolapse or massive vaginal eversion.

Rarely in this older age group are problems as simple as they seem initially. After the particular pertinent interrogation is satisfied, investigation of nutritional habits is a prime starting point to learn in general what lies below the surface to avoid compromising surprises. For a variety of reasons, the dietary habits of the retired segment of the population often fall far short of basic requirements. The principal deficiencies are those of protein, vitamins, especially ascorbic acid, and iron. Older people tend to emphasize starches, and snack foods may well predominate over regular planned meals. Indolence, earmarked by chronic television watching, directly reflects the absence of fresh foods in the household, especially fruits and vegetables. Canned and processed foods may be the rule. Undoubtedly, the attempt to live within the budgetary limitations of Social Security and low pension payments, if any, catalyzes the nutritional deficiency status. Also not to be forgotten as negative elements are socially confining abnormal states themselves, such as incontinence and severe prolapse. Vitamin C intake may be close to zero in a large number of these patients, and a chronic level of mild anemia reflects an inadequate intake of iron.

Any and all perceived or suspected nutritional insufficiencies must be corrected as best as possible preoperatively. Because a rush into surgery is rarely necessary, a delay of 1 to 3 months, as most likely will be required for other reasons also, can be used to correct this inadequate status with the help of an informed and caring family. The physician must emphasize the need for nutrition at a neverending high level to help produce and preserve the best healing and the best long-term result. Regrettably, I find this facet of preparation generally ignored.

Exercise induces anabolism, essential to good healing. The physician cannot expect a woman habitually addicted to an armchair to reverse her habits suddenly postoperatively by pleading with her, after the operation is over, to walk 2 to 3 miles per day. Despite inhibiting lesions of supportive attenuation, commonly used as an excuse by women to explain their chronic lassitude, improvised supports can effectively eliminate objections to a program of muscular activity that should be indoctrinated *at least 6 to 8 weeks before surgery* whenever possible. Even if walking is restricted, a regimen of intensive compatible aerobics will work almost as well. Not surprisingly, in today's world, many older women live in apartment or condominium complexes that include a swimming pool, thereby providing another medium for exercise. Without question, a routine initiated and accepted preoperatively is far more easily incorporated into a recovery agenda than one delayed until after the surgery. The patient must prove that she means business from the outset. The anabolic effects secondary to improved muscle tone and circulation from exercise alone cannot be denied.

Hand in hand with appropriate diet and exercise almost invariably lies the need for weight loss. Experience reveals an inordinately high percentage of obesity, sometimes overwhelming, in those in need of pelvic reconstructive surgery in any form. This should come as no surprise because the pelvic floor must support the weight of the superimposed torso and, in addition to the previous deleterious effects of childbirth, it is further weakened by fatty infiltration in association with obesity. Any doctor who rushes the truly corpulent patient into corrective surgery is destined to shoulder a high level of failure and recurrence. Almost without exception, monographs reporting results of surgery aimed at correction of pelvic support defects include only those patients under a certain upper weight limit. Obviously, the conscientious physician should postpone surgery until the patient establishes a track record of significant weight reduction. A corollary commitment to sustained weight loss postoperatively must be exacted from the patient with corresponding commitment by the family to see that the patient sticks to the rules. Emphasize the heightened postoperative failure rate accompanying failure to comply.

All experts agree that the most crucial element of insurance toward the achievement of the most effective surgery is preoperative estrogen replacement therapy (ERT). Estrogen deficiency, with its associated loss of connective tissue strength and elasticity, severe vascular depletion, and mucosal degeneration, is a major natural factor in the development of postmenopausal lesions. Obviously preoperative maximum efforts at reversal of these negative factors are vitally necessary and cannot be accomplished without adequate ERT. Experienced clinicians, including myself, feel that a daily oral dose of 0.625 mg natural conjugated estrogens (Premarin) for 5 weeks is the very minimum prerequisite. A longer term of preparation, when possible, is most desirable because 13 to 14 months of replacement is thought to be needed for maximum restoration of tissue maturity and integrity. A commitment by the patient, in the presence of family members, with accompanying emphasis by the physician, to lifetime ERT must be obtained before surgery is undertaken. Vaginal estrogenic administration is unquestionably effective but often impractical until after surgery because of external protrusion of organs.

Many operators discontinue ERT preoperatively on the erroneous supposition that ERT enhances the potential for vascular thrombosis. At the current treatment doses, no supportive evidence for this notion appears anywhere in the literature, and objectively it seems silly because the dosage levels are so minimal compared to the markedly higher normal natural standards of the premenopausal woman. Rather, clinical studies reveal no effect of standard ERT on the incidence of thromboembolic phenomena.[1,2] Some physicians, even when recognizing the need for estrogen support, foolishly stop the replacement routine weeks before the surgery for fear of initiating thromboembolism. False assumption of risks of venous thrombosis are based on anecdotal remarks and vapid superstition. Even if it were true, routine use of sequential compression devices or heparin, as will be discussed, should dissolve unfounded fears of unusual incidents of thrombotic occurrences from this source.

If ovaries have not been removed in previous surgery, then certainly the physician should raise the subject for discussion with the patient. If hysterectomy is involved in the surgical plan, the indications for oophorectomy are the same regardless of abdominal or vaginal route. Because the patients under consideration in this book are all postreproductive, then ovaries should be removed, when possible and practical, in all hysterectomies in this age group. In planned pelvic surgery using a suprapubic entry, bilateral oophorectomy should be performed, almost uniformly, with or without the presence of a uterus.

Having made these statements, even in the knowledge that statistically a ridiculously and unacceptably low number of oophorectomies are performed in association with vaginal hysterectomy in the perimenopausal and menopausal woman, I must enter some modifications. Quite often, in patients aged 65 to 70 and older, atrophic ovaries are retracted and relatively fixed high on the sidewalls of the pelvis. In these cases, the difficulties and risks of hemorrhage and possible urethral or bowel damage might render attempts at removal as unreasonable from the vaginal approach. Also, in cases of extensive repair, both anteriorly and posteriorly in association with vaginal hysterectomy, wherein anesthesia and operative time may be prolonged, and unusual blood loss might occur, unless both ovaries flop directly into the visual field, oophorectomy should not be included, especially if the ovaries seem normal, if any difficulty in removal is perceived. When posthysterectomy pulsion enterocoeles are under excision in patients holding residual ovaries, rarely do the ovaries come close enough to the operative field to be removed unless they have been trapped in the vault hysterectomy scar.

Considering all the publicity in recent years via the various media on the malignant potential of ovaries, in most cases the physician probably should discuss this matter, along the lines noted above, with both the patient and her family before the surgery is performed.

Concentrated discussion on any circumstance that increases intra-abdominal pressure should be included in the approach to surgery. The pelvic diaphragm, the weakest major support in the entire human structure, paradoxically performs one of the body's most major ongoing physical functions—holding up not just the pelvic organs but also the weight of the entire torso from its bottom position. It is totally subservient to intra-abdominal pressure, and any increases of a chronic nature in this pressure will promote herniations in the pelvis.

In this regard, habitual cigarette smoking is perhaps the worst offending factor. Despite vociferous contrary remonstrations by the patient who smokes, all smokers cough. Persistent repetitive coughing translates into a staccato of increases in intra-abdominal pressure. Coughing not only contributes to the development of supportive lesions but is a prescription to recurrence after repair. It is an accepted fact additionally that "ever smokers," including those who have quit sometime previously, heal more poorly than "never smokers."[3] Full explanation to the patient of the terribly deterrent effect of smoking is mandatory. I will not perform corrective surgery on any patient without her pledge, witnessed by one or more family members, to absolute lifetime smoking restriction. Because guilt often masks the truth, I never ask the patient if she smokes. I startle them, as though catching them red-handed, by asking, "How much do you smoke? One or more packs per day?" The nonsmoker instantly retorts, "I have never smoked!" but the nicotine offender, caught off-guard, after initial hesitation, tells all, especially if her family is present. Coughing is but one of the interfering evils of cigarette smoking. Interference with the healing mechanism from cigarette smoke inhalation and absorption is just as important as the repetitive pressure effects of coughing. This negative healing influence is mediated directly by barrier action on collagen synthesis and indirectly by impeding the beneficial influence of estrogen on connective tissue revitalization.[4] Amplification of these issues can be found in Chapters 1 and 16.

Some women are accustomed to wearing girdles. These abdominally constrictive devices literally eliminate all natural expansive capacity of the abdominal muscles and force increased pressure downward onto the pelvis. This ill effect is exaggerated in obese women, a negative situation in itself, as already discussed. Girdles and similar apparel must be forbidden without compromise forever.

In today's world a significant number of retired women occupy themselves in baby-sitting and child care capacities. In such situations they are prone to considerable lifting activity, especially with heavier children, a most undesirable form of exertion. Except for prewalking infants, they can easily learn how to avoid lifting and still keep this kind of job. Children at a very early age learn how to climb into laps, with help, without being lifted. Preoperatively the patient must accept the prohibition of heavy lifting forever.

Constipation, whether a lifetime bad habit or an acquired one in association with pelvic lesions, not only is an ancillary factor in creating pelvic defects but can quickly destroy a good repair. Instruction in overcoming this major deleterious contributor to chronic increased intra-abdominal pressure should begin preoperatively with the creation of sensible bowel habits correlated with appropriate diet, stool softeners, and laxatives. Postoperative implementation of such a regimen, after surgical elimination of posterior pelvic imperfections, becomes remarkably effective in the already indoctrinated patient. Too often the physician mistakenly assumes correction of the defect automatically resolves the constipation; sadly, this assumption may be wrong and could jeopardize what may well be good work by negligence in instruction on developing good bowel habits in advance of the operation.

Never ignore or neglect to elicit information regarding severe reactions of nausea and vomiting that may have developed after previous operations. Such immediate postoperative occurrences may literally blow open the most meticulous restoration within hours of the conclusion of a procedure or they can predetermine a future massive vaginal eversion after a properly performed vaginal hysterectomy. Pertinent preoperative anesthesiologic consultation in prelude to precise postoperative prophylaxis can prevent such disaster. Dermal scopolamine patches placed behind the ear can be extremely effective as antiemetics.

Chronic pulmonary disorders predispose pelvic musculofascial deterioration secondary to the almost incessant downward force emanating from the chest via coughing or labored respiratory effort or both. Emphysema and asthma are such examples. Under the active influence of conditions like these, reparative attempts are doomed to failure and should not be undertaken. Alternative nonoperative methods serve the patient best in these circumstances. The zealous operator who ignores these warnings and proceeds surgically spawns grave injustice to the patient.

BLOOD STORAGE

Correctly performed wide and deep dissection, requisite to good pelvic reconstructive surgery, with or without hysterectomy, and particularly if both anterior and posterior pelvic compartments are involved, may provoke appreciable blood loss, even in the best hands. In instances of direct house staff participation, bleeding can reach alarming proportions, especially if prophylactic heparin is used. For several decades blood banks have been integral units of hospitals in modernized nations, perhaps most exemplified by the United States. Each unit would take blood from willing donors, check the blood for purity, and then appropriately store it for use in cases requiring replacement such as those we are discussing herein. Generally surgeons did not give much advance thought to blood loss; if the need suddenly arose, there seemingly was no problem, because "there's always plenty of blood in the bank."

During the 1980s, the pall of uniformly fatal acquired immunodeficiency syndrome (AIDS) and deadly strains of hepatitis was cast over the entire globe. Prior methods of processing blood for transfusion were inadequately screening out these lethal blood-borne diseases and were being passed on to innocent recipients via transfusion. Additionally, the danger of transmission of these catastrophic infections to blood bank workers by the slightest carelessness became alarmingly manifest. Suddenly patients were frightened beyond measure at the mere thought of receiving a transfusion, despite rapid technological screening developments to provide safe blood. Simultaneously both blood bank workers and hospitals progressively quit the business of taking blood from donors and processing and screening it within hospital confines. In 1985 and 1986, medically responsible authorities began advising physicians throughout the United States to encourage autologous blood donation by patients in anticipation of possible need during surgery.[5-9] Throughout the nation the American Red Cross essentially became the only receiving and storage center for donated transfusion blood and storage of it at its multitude of locations, with a new emphasis on autologous donation.[9] In the 1990s, despite excellent accurate screening methods for AIDS and hepatitis, patients generally demand the privilege of preoperative storage of their own blood, where feasible. It is also the indisputable moral responsibility of the physician in charge to encourage such action and to provide the mechanism to each patient to store autologous blood during a 5-week preoperative course, the usual storage period. When necessary, but generally not applicable to the kind of surgery under discussion in this book, blood can be frozen and held as long as 2 years in specially designated sites to be shipped to the patient's medical facility the day before surgery. The gynecologist of today cannot gamble on the chance that any major surgical procedure will not need blood. A callous and careless attitude about preoperative arrangements for blood storage by any physician, especially if the patient makes such a request, is utterly reprehensible. If in such cases the surgeon is forced to give general bank blood, such negligence should be considered immoral, unless the patient refused the privilege of self-donation when it was offered.

No matter how accurate and sophisticated a hospital laboratory may be, mistakes are still made, and the gravity of these blood-borne maladies leaves no margin for error. The fear of the patient alone is sufficient driving force to compel the surgeon to insist on storage of at least 1 U of autologous blood and, if possible, 2 U especially in cases of expected magnitude. During this 5-week presurgical time, the patient should be placed on an appropriate diet and daily ferrous sulfate therapy to help her rebuild her blood. When for whatever reason the patient cannot contribute her own blood, type-compatible trustworthy relatives can be solicited for donation.

ANCILLARY INVESTIGATION AND PREPARATION

Systemic review must incisively cover cardiovascular, pulmonary, urinary, and psychological areas. The aging patient has often been subjected to decades of duress of various kinds, which she may not readily recall, necessitating directed questioning by the physician to avoid omission. Investigation of the patient's general health involves evaluation and participation by her medical doctor. So many of the problems faced preoperatively involve the lower urinary system, directly or indirectly, that urogynecologic assessment, including urodynamics, is often indicated. A review of the patient's old medical and surgical records may uncover valuable information that might help prevent the development of hazardous situations.

Even though we may place preoperative cardiovascular clearance in the hands of a certified cardiologist rather than a medical generalist and then abide by those decisions, heart and blood vessel aberrations are so much more common than all others in the menopausal woman that they deserve some special attention. Obviously, previous myocardial infarction elevates surgical risk. Postoperatively such cases show a 6.6% chance of recurrence.[10,11] If silent infarctions are included, the perioperative incidence is 2%.[12] Perhaps the most sobering fact about heart disease to deter both physician and patient from rushing ahead with surgery, no matter how disabling a procidentia or urinary incontinence, is the odds-on chance of serious reinfarction if major surgery is performed within 6 months of the initial attack. Similarly, unstable angina pectoris of 3 months' duration or less absolutely signals postponement of elective surgery.

Sensibly speaking, when elective pelvic surgery is contemplated in the presence of established coronary artery disease, certainly appropriate bypass surgery becomes the primary consideration. The gynecologist can work later. However, experts state that there is not an increased surgical risk if angina pectoris is controlled and there is no history of previous myocardial infarction.[13] Compensated cardiac activity under therapeutic control after previous congestive heart failure also seems to present no increased risk under conditions of benign pelvic surgery.

Hypertension, either already under treatment or newly discovered, is present in 28% of postmenopausal candidates for gynecologic surgery.[14] Surgery must not be scheduled until the blood pressure is stabilized within or close to normal limits. However, oddly enough, the experts feel that surgery is tolerated without cardiac consequences very well if diastolic pressures are contained under 110 mm Hg.

A thorough drug study, both current and past, as to effects and side effects, and previous reactions, is integral in the work-up. I consider the *Physicians' Desk Reference* (PDR) invaluable in this regard; I keep a copy on my desk and refer to it in almost every case. I cannot trust myself to remember all the different pharmacologic impacts of the myriad of drugs used in other specialties, often new and unfamiliar, particularly those with autonomic nervous system effects and simulations. As we know, the older the patient, the more medications she is apt to be taking. Looking things up in the presence of the patient is equally invaluable in building her confidence.

The most commonly used medications in the older population can be classified as cardiovascular, diabetic, diuretic, steroid, tranquilizing, and rheumatic. The impact of particular drugs in any given case must be appreciated from all angles by the surgeon, the internist, and the anesthesiologist.

The desirability of a preoperative anesthesia consultation several days before admission of postmenopausal patients cannot be underestimated; delay of such evaluation until admission, when heretofore unnoticed factors may suddenly be brought to light, may necessitate postponement of the operation. Certainly an advance arrangement allows time for an anesthetic team to prepare for a special situation, so often the case with older patients, with special reference to drugs and taxing medical conditions, thereby avoiding possible last minute cancellation of surgery.

Antibacterial and antibiotic medications deserve special attention. The older the patient, the greater the probability that she has received such agents in the past, and, it follows, the more apt for her to have developed allergic reactions to one or more of them. Because this group of drugs generally plays such a key role in both prophylactic and therapeutic management in this age group, investigative omission could lead to anaphylactic disaster. Fortunately, we have such wide pharmaceutical choices available for ready substitution that such dilemmas, given an accurate history, should be avoided.

I have strong feelings, admittedly controversial, about the use of antibiotic medication in pelvic reconstructive, vaginal, and urogynecologic surgery in older patients for multiple reasons. Not the least of these are the greater pronicity to surgically associated infection because of negative medical conditions, general lower resistance to infection, older more fragile tissue, and a significant incidence of prior surgery that has failed to achieve its goals. Infection weakens and destroys surgical wounds and I consider it heresy, in situations disposed to infection (i.e., pelvic surgery), to sit by "and see what happens." I break the rules of established tradition and try to take no chances of my operation breaking down, especially if there has been previous failure. I assume preoperatively the great likelihood of infection and, as I will discuss in other chapters in this book, if fever develops postoperatively, I jump on it, so to speak. Therefore, countrary to some current opinions, even those on isolated postmenopausal vaginal hysterectomy, I advocate preoperative antibiotic prophylaxis in all cases of pelvic surgery, administered immediately on entry into the operating room, pragmatically the best time for adequate tissue deposition.

Although we necessarily depend greatly on collaboration with our medical and anesthesiologic colleagues for coverage of issues related to medications, a few final words, in anticipation of surgery, are relevant. The tradition of discontinuing most drugs preoperatively no longer applies. Especially referable are antihypertensive drugs which, under current anesthesiologic surveillance, are acceptable up to the moment of surgery with resumption soon afterward. Similarly thiazide diuretics, commonly used in hypertension and also in conjunction with ERT to counteract fluid retention, need not necessarily be stopped 5 to 7 days before surgery as we have routinely done in the past. Although some patients under this therapy may present with hypokalemia, most do not because of an intense awareness by both patient and physician for the constant replacement of potassium, principally through diet alone. Monitoring of patients taking diuretics regularly almost always reveals serum potassium levels well within the norm. The lifting of presurgical exogenous estrogen restriction has already been discussed earlier in this chapter.

In contrast, extreme caution must be exercised relative to aspirin and medications containing aspirin derivatives, used commonly in postreproductive women secondary to the prevalence of arthritis in this age group. Cessation of platelet function can last 10 days in the sphere of continuous aspirin ingestion. Nonsteroidal anti-inflammatory drugs, used for the same purpose, also inactivate platelets, as do phenothiazines and steroids. Treatment with steroids, used widely for a variety of reasons, presents a difficult problem of still another dimension. These medications significantly retard wound healing, as will be discussed in Chapter 16, and this ill effect is an absolute anathema in pelvic reconstructive surgery. Equally undesirable is the depression by steroids of host response to infection. An additional complication is adrenal suppression by continuous steroid administration, necessitating special supplementation during and after surgery to avoid catastrophe.

It goes almost without saying that insulin regimens must not only be continued without a break perioperatively, but insulin regulation at that time must be monitored with hawklike acuity. Alterations of glycogen blood levels under conditions of surgery, including the effects of anesthesia and certain drugs used conjunctively, are highly volatile; knowledgeable and persistent regulation is mandatory.

Drugs mimetic of action of the autonomic nervous system are commonly used on a daily basis not only for vascular ills but also for control of dysfunction in the lower urinary system in this patient group. Considering how common are the voiding problems, particularly incontinence, at the postmenopausal level, and the use of various medications to attempt to achieve regulation, gynecologic surgeons should not only have a working knowledge about these drugs but they should make certain that relevant contraindications and side effects are reasonably explained to the patient. Such informed discussion, both presurgically and postoperatively, can avert later distasteful situations. Preoperative orders should direct immediate resumption of all habitually necessary medications postoperatively, within reason. It is easier to list these before surgery than after when mental concentration is consumed in promoting surgical recovery and may be inattentive to habitually necessary medications.

The need, or lack of need, for an intravenous pyelogram (IVP) to be included at all in preoperative work-up in cases involving anterior compartment repair or pelvic reconstructive surgery of any nature is a subject guaranteed to stir up controversy. In essence, it has no place as part of routine preparation. It offers little information, it carries certain risks, and it adds to the costs.[15,16] In situations of previous surgery in the region of the lower urinary tract, one knows in advance that the ureters may be distorted and out of position, so the IVP is not an excuse from good surgical performance. It will not tell the surgeon where to find the ureters during the dynamics of the surgery and therefore does not protect them from injury secondary to operative carelessness. If one is truly concerned that a ureter may have become obstructed in previous surgery, an ultrasonogram will reveal the atrophy of the corresponding kidney. An IVP is not necessary.

Cardiac arrest and fatal respiratory occurrences are rare, but they can and do happen because of dye toxicity. However, the dye used in IVPs can cause generalized allergic reactions in 1 in 200 patients. It can be significantly nephrotoxic in 1 of

20 patients, particularly those with diabetes or underlying renal deficiency or dehydration.[15,16]

THE EXAMINATION

In all cases, but especially in the older patient, gentleness and deliberately slow manual movements offer the best opportunity for accurate evaluation. This becomes especially true in such situations as chronic senile vaginitis, or postmenopausal or postsurgical vaginal stricture, or edematous inflammatory organ protrusions. A single digit exploration of the introitus dictates what size speculum, which should be warm, can be used comfortably. Only gentle slow steadily increasing pressure, accompanied by soft reassuring words, allow for the best bimanual assessment of the entire pelvis to rule out an unsuspected asymptomatic mass. The rectal examination is most successful after the patient, on command, has been bearing down for some 10 seconds, thereby self-inducing a numbing effect. I have yet to find a young practitioner aware of this amelioration.

When prolapse or eversion is obvious, the tendency is to assume that nothing else is wrong, to forget that a silent coincidental mass might exist above. Replacement of protrusion followed by careful manual evaluation must apprise the presence or absence of a higher lesion. Whenever there is a question or suspicion, particularly if accompanied by a heavy or scarred lower abdominal wall, or voluntary nonabsolvable tension, an ultrasonogram can be helpful. The bidigital examination, with one finger in the rectum, may uncover a posterior lesion unnoticeable by vaginal examination alone. Certainly the only method for determination of the level of perineal body integrity demands a bidigital approach, not to mention rectocele and enterocele evaluation.

The ultimate precise technique in judgment of the quality of pelvic support is to examine the patient while she stands in the erect posture. Lithotomy assessment is usually adequate in a patient appearing for her annual checkup and who presents no complaints directly or indirectly referable to breakdown in tissue stability. However, if the patient presents symptoms that might even remotely suggest loss of support as a possible cause, then examination while she stands, which is minimally time-consuming, becomes obligatory. Properly executed, the patient stands on a stool elevated off the floor some 6 to 8 inches with her legs about 20 inches apart and the knees slightly bent to allow for access by the doctor. Awkwardness can be avoided if the physician kneels with the right knee on the floor. As examining fingers are positioned, the patient is requested to bear down to produce a Valsalva effect, thereby helping set the optimum stage for evaluation. Curiously, as women age, they undergo increasing difficulty in their ability to generate increased abdominal pressure voluntarily in the lithotomy position, but they seem to have no trouble while erect. Thus, the physician who neglects to use the standing position for examination may obtain limited information and pursue a correspondingly inadequate operative course. Even in the upright stance, bidigital examination, using only one hand, markedly limits the extent of exploration. However, insertion of the index finger of the right hand into the rectum and the first two fingers of the left hand intravaginally in opposition offers a remarkable opportunity to delineate perineal defects and rectocele. Usually, using this approach, if an enterocele is present, it too can be well outlined, especially if large enough to accommodate a palpable loop of small intestine and if, in conjunction with a rectocele, the vaginal fingers can demonstrate a "double-hump" configuration. In this type of presentation, the rectal finger can only enter the lower hump while the vaginal fingers outline a distinctly separate hump superior and anterior to the more external one. Finally, the vaginal fingers can easily be rotated 180 degrees to assess anterior defects relative to the urethra and bladder, implementing the findings and special test results (Q-tip and Baden) noted in the lithotomy examination. Illustrations of this evaluation in the erect posture can be found in Chapter 9.

If the interval between the determinant examination and the day of scheduled surgery is greater than 5 to 6 weeks, the doctor would be wise to reexamine the patient during the few days just before admission. Once pelvic lesions due to loss of support, with or without the presence of a uterus, become symptomatic, they frequently progress rapidly. This can lead to embarrassing situations of surprise and dismay to the surgeon in the operating room, especially if the patient is already anesthetized and if the doctor feels unqualified to tackle a large enterocele or a severely rotated urethra, for example, which "were not there when I first saw her only 3 months ago." I feel well qualified, yet I always reexamine under these circumstances. It could change the entire picture, involving operating time, extent of surgery, additional tests, and recovery time.

CONCLUDING DISCUSSIONS WITH THE PATIENT

It takes no real extra effort and consumes no additional time, and it certainly reassures the patient, if the doctor, during the examination, gives a running verbal description of what is being done and why, explaining also the findings during the examination. This builds confidence and avoids resentment "at being left in the dark." The "disease of silence" is all too prevalent among physicians, and speaking up during a gynecologic examination does wonders in helping to establish a good patient–doctor relationship. Such a scenario can be augmented immediately afterward, as mentioned earlier, by showing the patient and her accompanying family graphic illustrations of her lesions, whatever they may be. Then, continuing the pictorial display, the "complete" doctor outlines the operative intentions and anticipated results, much to the satisfaction of the patient and her family.

Following in sequence, this is the time to explain to the patient what she should expect immediately postoperatively. Let her know that pain relief will be available and all efforts will be made to keep her comfortable. Explain succinctly but clearly about intravenous fluids, vaginal packing, early ambulation, acceleration to normal diet, and the role of the urinary catheter, whether it be transurethral or suprapubic. Anticipate questions about length of hospital stay and time span until return to full normal activity. Discuss these issues before the questions are raised; your thoroughness will be impressive. Disguise annoyance and irritation over repetitive, inane, and nonrelevant questions.

Crucial to this initial planning are the goals and expectations of the particular projected surgical procedure. Physicians should offer no absolute guarantees but, in most cases, dealing with benign disease, they can reasonably volunteer the best results possible, all things considered, with especial reference to unknown extents of denervation and permanent atrophy. One specific area of marked trepidation lies in the realm of anterior pelvic reconstruction and the potential for postoperative urinary incontinence, whether or not it preexists the operation. The patient must be informed that this can be a postsurgical problem, most often of functional nature, destined to disappear within 4 months of the procedure. However, that it could be a genuine stress incontinence, as happens in a very small percentage of cases, requiring additional but limited surgery in the future, must be clearly stated, and documentation of such discourse should be entered in the patient's chart. Other possibilities must be mentioned to the patient and documented accordingly, noting always that, although nothing and no one achieves 100%, we all strive for it.

Extreme caution and care are urged particularly in situations already marked as previous failures, especially when augmented by patient (and family) anger and resentment. Beware the patient who seems preoccupied with beratings of other doctors, and supply no support directly that might nourish such ill will; it can backfire terribly, particularly because you are hearing only one side of the story and the outcome of your surgery is yet to be seen. The extreme case warranting the utmost prudence and apprehension for the doctor is that which is already involved in a malpractice suit. Others that demand wariness are those involving personal unhappiness and negative attitudes, psychiatric difficulties, overt displays of low confidence, and relative indifference. In the latter instance, if the patient is not absolutely convinced that surgery is her best pathway, beg off and postpone the operation. These are benign problems and one can wait until the patient concludes that the only way out is surgery. Such a posture is applicable to conditions of structural alteration, such as prolapse and organ protrusion, where one should never talk the patient into surgery, but is not applicable to those diseases of the cervix, uterus, ovary, vulva, and vagina related to cellular disturbance that, although currently benign, might become malignant. In these instances it behooves the physician to encourage therapeutic resolution of the abnormal process within the bounds of accepted standards of care, accompanied by chart documentation to this effect. Persuasion toward a second opinion is always good policy for the competent and self-confident physician.

THE LABORATORY WORK-UP

All hospitals require certain tests to be performed before or at admission on patients scheduled for surgery. These are standard and vary slightly from one institution to the next and from one case to the next depending on the peculiar nature of the diseased condition demanding surgery and any incidental medical problems that must be considered. The importance of this work-up is paramount to good care. Adequate discussion of this preparation can be found in multiple surgical and gynecologic textbooks and treatises and will not be included in this publication.

Instead certain tests will be pinpointed for their unique pertinence to benign pelvic surgery in older women. A preoperative urine culture is almost always essential, especially if anterior compartment repair is contemplated. The proximity of gynecologic surgery to the lower urinary tract, and so often the direct involvement of it in reconstructive and urogynecologic operations, signals a need to know in advance if the bladder is infected. Old tenets indicate that concern need be raised only when the bacterial count is at the 100,000 (10^5) per milliliter of urine level. However, many seasoned practitioners feel that quiescent situations of only 10^2 bacterial count can be agitated by adjacent surgery into active overt infection with high bacterial counts. I clear all preoperative positive cultures, no matter how minimal, before I embark on pelvic surgery in the elderly woman. A 1-week course of macrobid (Procter and Gamble) usually adequately does the job.

Poor nutrition is often reflected by the hematocrit, hemoglobin, and white blood cell count. Correction of low levels of these blood elements must be accomplished before the patient goes to the operating room. The hematocrit should be 35 mL/dL or over, the hemoglobin 11 g/dL or better, if possible, and the white cell count not below 4000/mm^3. When poor nutrition is strongly suspected, a serum albumin determination is necessary (see Chapter 16).

Two tests that are universally standard preoperatively demand mention here— the blood sugar and the blood urea nitrogen (BUN). Because statisticians estimate that 7 million women in this country are diabetics as yet undiagnosed, most of them over 55 years of age, and because diabetes is a known deterrent of good wound healing, a fasting value over 100 mg/dL might arouse suspicion. The BUN rises as a normal component of aging, but kidney problems may exist when the number reaches 30 mg/dL or more, indicating need for further investigation before surgery. A necessary corroborating test, particularly when operating so close to the ureters, is the creatinine level, which should not exceed 1.0 mg/dL as a preoperative value. A level any higher than that postoperatively may indicate ureteral obstruction or interference, something that can happen to even the best of surgeons. The need for early recognition is obvious.

Because hypertension is so common among the older population, and because diuretics are so commonly used in its treatment, it behooves the surgeon to check the patient's serum potassium level about 7 to 10 days before surgery, probably the best time for final assessment of all elements. In most cases this allows ample time for correction of deficiencies, such as a low potassium level, depleted by diuretic effects. Anything below 3.0 mEq/L is considered a deficiency, and some anesthesiologists express trepidation if the level is not at least up to 3.5 mEq/L.

This list has included those laboratory tests of special interest in all postreproductive women scheduled for elective pelvic surgery. The internist will pursue and evaluate fully, as necessary, the cardiovascular, pulmonary, renal, and hepatic systems to determine the patient's capabilities to tolerate anesthesia and medication, particularly if general anesthesia is used. Also in the reckoning process lies the element of approach, abdominal or vaginal, the latter much more easily tolerated than the former, particularly by the older patient. Such additional work-up, including ultimate classification under the standards of the American Society of Anesthesiologists, is adequately covered in other texts on surgery and anesthesiology.

Clinical incidental observation of asymptomatic but overt vaginitis, such as the leukorrhea of bacterial vaginosis, should not be ignored. The question of need for laboratory assessment with associated prophylactic treatment is covered in Chapter 16.

ADMISSION ROUTINES

With few exceptions, hospital entry for elective major surgery on the same day as the scheduled operation is currently the rule. Although it is difficult to argue against the benefits of well-supervised preoperative preparation in the hospital, starting in the late afternoon before the day of surgery, followed by a good night's sleep before being wheeled to the operating room in the morning, we hardly experience this sequence anymore. We have all made adjustments as dictated authoritatively to us in the interest of cost control, but it is not always easy for the patient.

For someone who lives a short distance from the hospital, the problems are considerably less than those of the patient who must travel for 1 to 4 hours to gain admission, as often happens in a referral center. Considering all the possible maloccurences that can happen on the way to the hospital, I advise and encourage the patient to spend the preentry night at a nearby hotel or friend's home. This allows for a decent restful night before surgery, avoiding the ungodly awakening at a wee hour followed by mad dashes spiced with frenzy if there is a detour, or a delaying accident, or the car breaking down, hardly acceptable overtures in the prelude to major surgery.

Important advantages have been realized as a direct result of same day admission and these should be mentioned to the distraught patient as a form of rationalization. Undergoing all the laboratory, x-ray, and electrocardiographic work-up, plus the medical, anesthesiologic, and other consultations 1 to 3 weeks before surgery can reveal unanticipated problems correctable in the time gap that would otherwise force last minute cancellation and postponement if squeezed into the presurgical late afternoon and evening as has happened in the past. These remarks are obviously more relevant to the postmenopausal woman than to the younger patient. Equally obviously, these new rules are not applicable to patients encumbered with serious medical problems that demand close hospital surveillance and regulation in the approach to surgery; these cases still require admission in the afternoon of the day before surgery. Cost control should not obviate good medical practice.

A clear bowel is considered an essential to good pelvic surgery. The sluggish peristalsis, so often including progressive constipation, that we are more apt to see in older women, must be reckoned with to avoid mechanical impediments to good surgical performance, whether done from above or below, but especially the latter. To avoid this interference, I advise patients to discontinue oral iron therapy 2 days before surgery and to eat a normal breakfast and lunch on the day before admission, including a piece of fresh fruit with each meal. Supper or dinner of the preadmission evening, in my regimen, should consist of clear fluid and should be followed by the use of a simple Fleet enema at bedtime, then nothing orally afterward. Not only does the resultant empty bowel allow for full operative leeway, but fecal contamination is reduced if the bowel is unexpectedly opened during surgery. Carried still further, an empty rectum postoperatively is far less conducive than a full one to constipation, anathema in cases of meticulous posterior repairs. Some physicians insist on more extensive bowel preparation, but incidental rectal entry, if recognized, in posterior compartment repair, should not present a problem, as discussed in Chapter 11.

Preoperative douching is discussed more thoroughly in Chapter 16. Douching, regardless of the agent used, does not sterilize the vagina. Iodine-containing solutions are questionably more effective than water because the best that can be hoped for is appreciable dilution of the vaginal bacterial population. However, the psychological effects on the patient implied by apparent measures of cleanliness are generally positive and not to be ignored. I routinely instruct the use of betadine or iodochlor douche at bedtime after the Fleet enema. Certainly such a routine in situations of marked prolapse or massive vaginal eversion, because the vagina is literally inside out, becomes ridiculous and is not applicable.

The standard preoperative order, "Nothing PO after midnight," is routine for all of us. Although implemented in the past when patients were admitted to the hospital the afternoon of the day before surgery, such a rule might not be taken seriously by same day admission patients. English-speaking educated patients generally are made to understand quickly the dangers of food or fluid in the stomach when general anesthesia is administered, but do not count on it. Less educated women and those with an expected low level of compliance, as well as those who only half-listen to instructions, particularly older women without physically present family support, frequently ignore the rule. Whenever the slightest suspicion arises regarding the potential for oral ingestion within hours of impending surgery, the patient should be told blatantly, "You can *die* if you eat or drink and then undergo anesthesia." Buffer this strong statement by telling her how well you expect things to go if this danger is averted.

Once admitted, the question of prophylaxis against venous thromboembolism in these highly vulnerable older patients must be addressed. The consensus conference orchestrated by the National Institutes of Health in 1986 on the broad subject of prevention of venous thrombosis and pulmonary embolus left no doubt about not just the advisability but the absolute necessity for preoperative and postoperative administration of prophylactic heparin in major pelvic surgery, particularly applicable to the elderly. Well-designed studies, including one major multicenter report, have unquestionably shown a statistically significant reduction in the incidence of thromboembolic phenomena when prophylactic heparin is used.[17,18] These investigations also reveal no increase in intraoperative bleeding. A recent report, directed specifically at the question of the effect of protective heparin on bleeding in extensive pelvic surgery, concludes that intraoperative blood loss is not augmented appreciably but that significant postoperative bleeding, measured objectively by hematocrit, does occur.[19]

Over 10 years, until 2 years before the publication of this book, I steadfastly and routinely adhered to a heparin regimen similar to that outlined in the consensus bulletin. In those days when we still were allowed to admit patients late in the day before surgery, they received an initial 5000-U dose subcutaneously during the evening, and this was repeated 1 to 2 hours before surgery began the next morning. The same-day patients received the 5000-U dose immediately on hospital entry in the morning.

Over and over again I listened to my friends and colleagues, most well-known professors at institutions of high repute, complain about the excessive bleeding they were encountering in association with prophylactic heparin in the recommended doses. I invariably countered with evidence from the scientific literature that said this could not be so and that I was not experiencing the same hemorrhagic effects despite wide and deep dissections. I finally came to the acceptance, some 2 years before this publication, that I was fooling myself, that I really had been seeing too much bleeding in most cases. For 2 years now I have not been using heparin and I am convinced, despite the absence of any scientific method, that bleeding has been markedly reduced. I am much the happier for this and so are the patients. Certainly my need to give back autologous blood has been reduced to half what it was before, including the long drawn-out cases with large front and back dissected surfaces.

Fortunately, a completely satisfactory and reputedly equally effective alternative to heparain began coming into general use perioperatively in 1988 and 1989. This progressive popularity of a new method followed on the heels of a classic monograph by Scurr and colleagues on the use of intermittent pneumatic compression to the lower extremities through envelopment with synthetic pneumatic sleeves.[20] They are identified by the letters SCD (Kendall Healthcare Products), standing for sequential compression devices. Placing the patients' legs into thromboembolic disease (TED) antiembolism elastic stockings first, which most of us have been using for years anyhow, and which are recommended for greatest effectiveness of pneumatic compression, the SCDs are then applied in the operating room and set into action before the surgery begins. At first I used these pneumatic sleeves in conjunction with heparin, but I stopped the heparin, as noted above, 2 years ago. Today the SCDs coupled with the TED stockings should be considered obligatory for protection against thromboembolism in major gynecologic surgery in all postreproductive women, and probably in premenopausal women also.

The routine use of preoperative prophylactic antibiotics has been discussed earlier in this chapter and will be referred to again in later chapters. I routinely use them in every case in the postreproductive woman without exception. If the operation takes longer than 2.5 hours, I administer a second dose intraoperatively. The latter is probably not necessary when the substance has a half-life of 12 hours. I have learned that the only pragmatic timing for antibiotic administration is simultaneous with the moment of entry into the operating room itself. Even under the most rigid scheduling conditions, an order to give the antibiotic on call to the operating room or 1 hour before scheduled surgery, the ideal time, results either in negligence of administration at all or in giving it much too early because of the prevalence of late starts.

SETTING UP IN THE OPERATING ROOM

Arrangements for abdominal cases require nothing special from a purely operative viewpoint other than the placement of a catheter for constant bladder drainage and cleansing of the vagina, discussed already to be of questionable value.

Vaginal cases demand particular care. The older the patient, the more the attention required in setting up for surgery. Positioning and general exposure must be at a maximum for the best benefits for patient, surgeon, assistants, and nursing staff. Nonetheless, in this age group, adequate allowances must be made for compromising arthritic and orthopedic conditions as the patient is positioned while she is under anesthesia, unable to voice a complaint if you are hurting her. Similarly, while anesthetized, these patients are far more prone to injury than younger women from improper stresses, strains, and pressures on skin, tendons, nerves, joints, and blood vessels of the lower extremities. In my visits to widely disparate medical centers, it is always surprising to me to see multiple inadequacies in the methods of setting up vaginal cases. The resulting mechanical awkwardness is not good for anybody involved, especially the patient.

The best type of leg supports for vaginal surgery, whether the patient is old or young, are those that elevate the legs so that the feet are at the highest points, slightly lateral to the body, and in the same vertical plane as the buttocks. These supports are metal and, because of their special shape, are commonly known as "candy canes," as seen in Chapter 4. They allow for multiple adjustments to suit the individual patient, referable primarily to leg length. Also, the most common restricted hip movement in the elderly, lateral extension, is bypassed because the legs are rotated upward, not laterally, as they would be in any type of device in which the popliteal space rests on a right-angled metal support. This latter type of contrivance angles the legs out laterally from the body, cramping the assistants against the surgeon if they stand inside the legs or taking them visually away from the field if they stand outside the legs. In either case, too often the assistants may lean or rest on the knee, inviting popliteal nerve damage or significant vascular compression in long procedures.

Allen stirrups, which are highly maneuverable and support the feet and legs of the patient, are excellent for use in cases involving suprapubic urethral suspension types of surgery and also for abdominal sacrocolpopexy. These stirrups allow an assistant to stand most usefully between the patient's legs and also create ready accessibility into the vagina, a necessity for these types of cases.

In instances of arthritis of the hip or knee, or of previous artificial replacement of either joint, I will test the involved areas positionally before surgery on an outpatient basis to learn the limits of positional tolerance while the patient is awake. This prudence can help to avoid overextension or overflexion when the patient is asleep later in the operating room.

Before the feet are elevated, I place them in protective foam rubber boots (Bareskin Products Foot Protector, Devon Industries, Inc., Chatsworth, CA), held in position by Velcro bands. When the feet are then lifted into the straps comprising the stirrups, there is a comfortable cushion between foot and strap. Even then, the uppermost strap is placed under the heel, not under the Achilles tendon, which might be dangerously weakened from direct compression after prolonged procedures. The curved tops of the candy cane rods are then rotated outward and cephalad to move the feet away from the heads of the surgical assistants, again as pictured in Chapter 4.

The next step is the elongation of the candy cane rods so that the thighs will not be too acutely flexed on the abdomen. If flexion is overdone for long periods of time, the femoral nerve can be overstretched, directly affecting the adductor muscles of the thighs, thereby impeding walking for as much as 2 weeks. Rarely, permanent nerve damage can be sustained.

At this point, an interjection regarding possible nerve compression and damage in abdominal procedures on older women should be mentioned. In these patients abdominal wall tissues are often quite attenuated, offering minimal resistance to vigorously applied retracting devices. Care must be exercised to avoid injury to the inguinal and obturator nerves from pressure by overstretching self-retaining retractors.

With the legs in position, the nursing team must then drop the bottom leaf of the table, rotating it down and back on itself to the absolute maximum to allow the operator's knees the most forward room possible. When this is done, and the patient's buttocks have been moved down to overlap the edge of the table by 3 cm, the sitting operator can, without having to overreach, work in comfortable proximity to the operative field. This is most essential for surgeons of short or medium height.

How often I have heard gynecologists preparing for vaginal surgery command the charge nurse to roll the stool down as low as possible. How backbreaking this becomes for the tall or even medium height assistant in major cases, obviously decreasing operational efficiency! Conversely, when the sitting stool is rotated to its highest point, all participants can enjoy comfort, the need for bending over having been eliminated. The shorter assistants can stand on foot stools, which are also to be placed under the operator's feet so they will not dangle freely, at the same time creating a lap on which an emesis basin (not a cumbersome tray) can hold instruments.

Some operators prefer to stand while doing vaginal surgery. The great majority, including myself, however, find this uncomfortable and awkward for many reasons and prefer to sit. Similarly some surgeons use a head lamp for light into the operative field. Admittedly, this can illuminate the deeper corners of the vaginal entry without readjustment of overhead lighting. However, when I have tried the head lamp, I have found myself so busy constantly adjusting my head that the surgery seems almost secondary to good lighting. Besides, modern operating rooms are equipped with fluidly moving wide-scope overhead lights with available sterile handle adjusters. If this is not quite enough, the new Vital-Vue tip (Davis and Geck) more than compensates because of its bright bulb alongside its suction and lavaging apertures. It easily lights up the deepest recesses and, because it is so narrow, does not crowd the operative field. Simultaneously this multipurpose instrument can retract.

In addition to easier surgical access, as already mentioned, the overhanging buttocks overcomes the chagrin of the surgeon who, thinking the position of the patient is adequate without having her bottom quite at the edge of the table break, sees the vulva slide away when "Trendelenburg, please" is uttered. Not only does surgery become more difficult, working at a greater distance, but often the weighted speculum no longer has room to hang down. Such a dilemma is avoided when the patient is pulled down lower than seems necessary at the outset.

Correct operative field preparation is covered in the discussion of wound healing in this publication. However, it is worth mentioning again that, in vaginal cases, whether young or old, (1) the anal region should be cleansed last and (2) if an antiseptic-carrying sponge contacts this area, it should be discarded after use there and not applied anywhere else. Care should later be taken during the draping of the patient to cover the anus adequately before surgery begins. The advice of this paragraph may seem totally redundant, but I see these errors of contamination, by ignorant aides, over and over wherever I go.

A common error in draping patients in the lithotomy position occurs in the

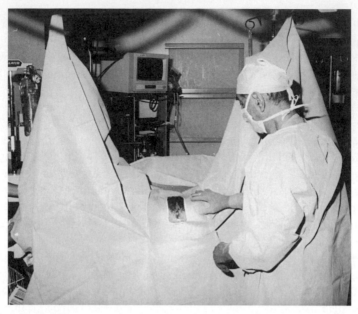

Figure 3-1 Single full coverage paper drape for vaginal surgery. The patient is fully covered. Only the operative field is exposed through the aperture in the drape.

application of the pockets that cover the lower extremities. I have seen not merely students and new residents but veteran physicians bring the leading edge of the leg drape, while slipping it on, repeatedly into contact with unprepared leg and thigh areas until this now grossly contaminated portion of the drape is finally dropped directly onto the fully prepared operative area. All likely contamination can be averted, however, by using the new packaged one-piece sterile paper drapes that also save time and money (Figure 3-1).

And now, before I say "Let the operation begin," a few final comments. I always position the patient myself, with the help of residents. While scrubbing, I most attentively observe the antiseptic preparation of the operative field by looking through the window over the sink, and I actively participate in and direct the draping of the patient. Sounds picayune, but it is the best way I know to start a case off on the right foot.

REFERENCES

1. Devon M, Barrett-Connor E, Renvall M, et al. Estrogen replacement therapy and the risk of venous thrombosis. *Am J Med.* 1992;92:275–282.
2. Young RL, Goekfert AR, Goldzieher HW. Estrogen replacement therapy is not conducive of venous thromboembolism. *Maturitas.* 1991;13:189–92.

3. Bump RC, McGlish DK. Cigarette smoking and urinary incontinence in women. *Am J Obstet Gynecol.* 1992;167:1213–1218.

4. Baron JA, LaVecchia C, Levi F. The antiestrogenic effect of cigarette smoking in women. *Am J Obstet Gynecol.* 1990;162:502–514.

5. Goodnough LT, Shuck J. Risks, options and informed consent for blood transfusion in elective surgery. *Am J Surg.* 1990;159:602–608.

6. Council on Scientific Affairs. Autologous blood transfusions. *JAMA.* 1986;256:2378–2382.

7. Surgenor DM. The patient's blood is the safest blood (editorial). *N Engl J Med.* 1987;316:542–543.

8. Toy PT, Strauss RG, Stehling LC, et al. Predeposit autologous blood for elective surgery: a national multicenter study. *N Engl J Med.* 1987;316:517–522.

9. Goodnough LT. Autologous donation—a safe transfusion alternative. *Contemp OB/GYN.* 1993;April:27–37.

10. Tarhan S, Moffitt EA, Taylor WF, et al. Myocardial infarction after general anesthesia. *JAMA.* 1972;220:1451–1455.

11. Steen PA, Tenker JH, Tarhan S. Myocardial reinfarction after anesthesia and surgery. *JAMA.* 1978;239:2566–2570.

12. Driscoll AC, Hobika JH, Etsten BE, et al. Clinically unrecognized myocardial infarction following surgery. *N Engl J Med.* 1961;264:633–639.

13. Goldman L, Caldera DL, Southwick FS, et al. Cardiac risk factors and complications in non-cardiac surgery. *Medicine.* 1978;57:357–366.

14. Goldman L, Caldera DL. Risks of general anesthesia and elective operation in the hypertensive patient. *Anesthesiology.* 1979;50:285–289.

15. Byrd L, Sherman RL. Radiocontrast-induced acute renal failure: a clinical and pathophysiologic review. *Medicine.* 1979;58:270–274.

16. Harkonen S, Kjellestrand CM. Exacerbation of diabetic renal failure following intravenous pyelography. *Am J Med.* 1977;63:939–945.

17. Multicenter Trial Committee. Dihydroergotamine-heparin prophylaxis of postoperative deep vein thrombosis. *JAMA.* 1984;251:2960–2966.

18. Koppenhagen K, Haring R. Zuhlke HV, et al. Efficiency and risk of thromboembolism prophylaxis in surgery: clinicoexperimental results in 1,434 general surgery patients. *Thromb Haemost.* 1979;179:249–256.

19. Clarke-Pearson DL, Synan IS, Doge R, et al. A randomized trial of low-dose heparin and intermittent pneumatic calf compression for the prevention of deep venous thrombosis after gynecologic oncology surgery. *Am J Obstet Gynecol.* 1993;168:1146–1154.

20. Scurr JH, Coleridge-Smith PD, Hasty JH. Regimen for improved effectiveness of intermittent pneumatic compression in deep venous thrombosis prophylaxis. *Surgery.* 1987;102:816–820.

Prolapse
and Vaginal
Hysterectomy

Robert E. Rogers

Marvin H. Terry Grody

HISTORY

Uterine prolapse has been a problem for as long as medical history has been recorded. The Kahun papyri, which reflected medical thought approximately 2000 years before Christ, had three references to uterine prolapse. Uterine prolapse concerned Hippocrates who used numerous medical treatments, all nonsurgical. Following Hippocrates, physicians of the day advised a procedure called succussion, by which the legs of the patient were tied together and the body elevated on a ladderlike device with the patient's head down. The procedure was used widely and described as highly successful. Massage, irrigation, fumigation, diet therapy, sitz baths, numerous drugs, and phlebotomy were all used. Surgical methods were suggested on a number of occasions, but the technique was never described. Soranus, who lived in Rome from 98 AD to 138 AD, suggested that a uterus should be partially or completely removed in the event that it prolapsed and became black. Albucasias, who practiced in Spain in 1100 AD, advised excision for uterine prolapse but did not explain how to do it. According to Ricci, a prolapsed uterus was removed in the 1300s by Marcus Gatinaria of Pavia, but no details were given.[1] A vaginal hysterectomy was attributed to Berengario da Carpi in 1521. The procedure evidently involved tying off the prolapsed uterus and gradually tightening the ligature over a period of days until the organ fell off. Christobal de Vega described the removal of a prolapsed, gangrenous uterus in a 34-year-old woman in 1575. According to his report, the patient was believed to have survived for 10 years.

History recognizes, as reported by Willouby in 1670, that perhaps the first deliberately intended, and successful, vaginal hysterectomy for prolapse was performed not by a doctor but by Faith Raworth, a peasant woman. A regularly recurring uterine prolapse, whenever she carried heavy loads, allegedly so aggravated her that she finally was driven to drastic measures. Simply stated, she lifted her skirts, pulled down on the cervix with all her might, and slashed off the protrusion with a sharp blade. Despite initial heavy bleeding, this indomitable woman survived many years, tolerating incessant loss of urine.

One of the very first hysterectomies documented in the medical literature of the day was performed by Lagenbeck of Gottingen, Germany, in 1813. The primary indication for the procedure was a cervical cancer, but uterine prolapse made it possible. The operation was accomplished without any knowledge of anesthesia or antisepsis. While he performed it, the doctor was faced with severe hemorrhage and the impending death of his patient. He grasped the uterus and compressed it while he sutured bleeding pedicles with his free hand. Near the termination of the procedure the patient was rejuvenated by dashing cold water in her face. The patient apparently lived for 26 years afterward, and the operation was confirmed by autopsy at the time of her death.

With the development of anesthesia and an understanding of the importance of asepsis, many surgical techniques were developed for the treatment of uterine prolapse. Before the acceptance of vaginal hysterectomy as a primary operative procedure for uterine prolapse, physicians practiced denudation of the vaginal mucosa, closure of tissues of the vulvar and vaginal orifice, and high perineal repairs. It appears that the first professionally performed vaginal hysterectomy specifically for prolapse was accomplished in 1861 by Choppin in New Orleans. Dr. Choppin had the opportunity to present his patient to a medical class, holding her uterus in his hand to prove that she had survived.

In 1877, Le Fort described vaginal occlusion, or colpocleisis. The procedure is still in use today. In 1888, Donald of Manchester, England, performed an operation for uterine prolapse consisting of anterior-posterior vaginal repair, perineorrhaphy, amputation of the cervix, and transposition of the cardinal ligaments. This operation was the basis for Fothergill's procedure, which he reported in 1908. It became extremely popular as the Manchester-Fothergill procedure.

Fruend, in 1895, described an operation wherein the uterine fundus was pulled downward and sutured under the vaginal mucosa. Schauta improved on this in a procedure he called the interposition operation in which the uterus was pulled anteriorly and sutured in place under the bladder.

At the turn of the century a number of operations were developed to correct prolapse. Gilliam reported a uterine suspension operation using the round ligaments. Crile described an abdominal hysterectomy with suspension of the vagina to the anterior undersurface of the abdominal wall. In 1915, Mayo described his technique for the correction of uterine prolapse.[2] In 1919, Young described an operation in which he suspended the uterus to the sacrum using linen sutures for both uterine and vaginal prolapse.

Spaulding described an operation that was improved by Richardson in 1937. The Spaulding-Richardson composite operation involved cervical amputation followed by supravaginal hysterectomy to preserve the cervical isthmus to maintain vaginal support.

In 1934, Heaney reported 565 vaginal hysterectomies for benign prolapse and described a technique for hysterectomy that is still in use today.[3] Heaney was the first to delineate a method that would significantly reduce surgical mortality and provide lasting correction of uterine prolapse. In the last half of the 20th century, refinements in our knowledge of pelvic anatomy, anesthesia, sutures, antibiotics, and blood transfusion have made the operation a primary resource for the treatment of uterine prolapse.

UTERINE PROLAPSE IN OLDER WOMEN

Prolapse of pelvic organs due to relaxation of supportive and suspensory mechanisms is the most common reason for removal of the benign postreproductive uterus, with or without associated repair.[2] In 1964, Quinlivan evaluated data on 600 women over 60 years of age and found that 25% had significant uterovaginal relaxation.[4] Secondary to the marked increase in life expectancy and in numbers of women seeking specific or maintenance health care over the intervening 30 years, the percentage of women with these defects is thought to be quite substantially higher today. In 1956, Folsome and colleagues published a survey evaluating data on 680 elderly institutionalized women and found cystoceles in 23%, uterine protrusion in 3%, rectoceles in 43%, and an enterocele in one patient.[5] Because only half of these patients with protrusions actually complained of a "mass" in the perineal area, it was difficult to assess the impact on quality of life. Forty to 50 years ago people accepted as "natural" occurrences in life such anatomic defects that today, in a more educated and assertive female population, would be found distinctly objectionable.

Procidentia of the uterus is overwhelmingly the most common benign reason for hysterectomy in the postreproductive woman. Its occurrence is multifactorial, beginning with genetically acquired poor supporting structures and deficiencies in collagen metabolism. Certainly such causes must be considered primary in the very uncommon cases of prolapse in nulliparous women.

However, despite such inheritances, general agreement accuses one or more elements of traumatic insult as the trigger mechanism in prolapse. Foremost and most obvious is childbirth with its attendant stress on the cardinal-uterosacral complex, the vaginal walls, and the pelvic diaphragm. Additional commonly occurring negative forces are chronic pulmonary disease and heavy duty occupations. The atrophy of aging, smoking, poor nutrition, and hypoestrogenism play vitally important contributory roles in the pathogenesis of uterine prolapse.

The degree of lasting surgical success, namely avoiding posthysterectomy prolapse, is as contingent on the elimination of as many causative factors preoperatively in uterine procidentia as it is in any herniation repair, pelvic or otherwise. For example, preoperative induction of an ongoing obesity reduction program is mandatory as is lifetime commitment to estrogen replacement and smoking abstinence. A perpetual focus on control of abnormal pulmonary conditions, such as asthma and chronic bronchitis, is obligatory. Too many physicians, attentive to such requirements in instances of correction of cystocele, rectocele, enterocele, and hypermotile urethra, are far less stringent when uterine prolapse exists alone and thereby, in time, may well live to regret such neglect. The demands are the same. In situations of poor genetic heritage, one must consider surgical overcorrection and ancillary compensation to give the best guarantees for the future.

SYMPTOMS OF UTERINE PROLAPSE

Patient complaints and associated disability because of prolapse often are related to the rate of development of the condition. A slow progression over years may be much worse by the time of declared discomfort than those cases of sudden or abrupt onset from a single traumatic event, the "straw that breaks the camel's back." A precipitous fall from a height, as on stairs, or a speeding automobile accident can be recalled by many patients as the precise moment when symptoms began.

As the abnormality evolves, the patient may experience a dragging or pulling sensation in the lower pelvic or perineal area, with or without low backache. Just as frequently she may first become discontent when the descending cervix protrudes through the introitus. Usually she will note its presence when she is up and about but not when sitting or lying down. The bulging cervix may first be noted when straining at stool, while practicing aerobics, or while playing tennis. The lower the uterine descent exists and the greater it becomes, the more it will affect urinary and rectal function. Often manual replacement upward is necessary for excretory action.

DIAGNOSIS OF UTERINE PROLAPSE

Prolapse is most simply diagnosed by placing the patient in a lithotomy position, asking her to strain as if she were trying to have a bowel movement, and observing the descent of the uterus. Patients who are unable to cooperate in this regard can be

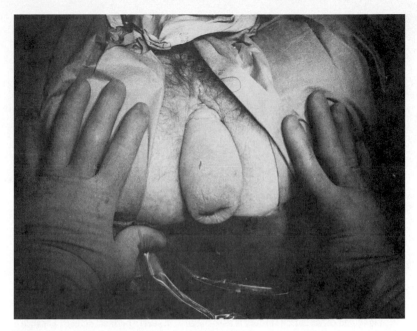

Figure 4-1. Severe prolapse of an elongated cervix.

studied by placing a tenaculum on the cervix and gently pulling it toward the vaginal introitus. This test is valid only in the awake patient. In the anesthetized patient, traction on the cervix will almost always allow descent far beyond that which would be possible in the conscious patient. Uterine prolapse is best studied with the patient standing with her feet separated, leaning forward, and resting on an examining table or chair back. The examiner stands behind the patient and spreads the labia with the examining fingers to observe the descent of the cervix through the introitus. Valsalva exertion by the erect patient reveals the true extent of attenuated uterine supports.

Uterine descensus has been classified in many ways. The simplest system is as follows: first degree, the cervix prolapses to the level of the ischial spines; second degree, the uterus prolapses to the introitus; third degree, the cervix prolapses through the vaginal introitus. This is a somewhat simplistic grouping because it ignores anatomic variables such as the length of the cervix, the size of the uterus itself, and introital thickness. An associated cystocele, enterocele, or rectocele should be described at the time that the prolapse is categorized because additional repairs of these defects must by accomplished simultaneously.

Not infrequently one encounters a cervix that is prolapsed through the introitus primarily because of its elongation by as much as 3 to 6 inches with accompanying minimal, if any, true prolapse of the uterus (Figure 4-1). There is no gynecologist who has not been fooled on more than one occasion by this combination, which is

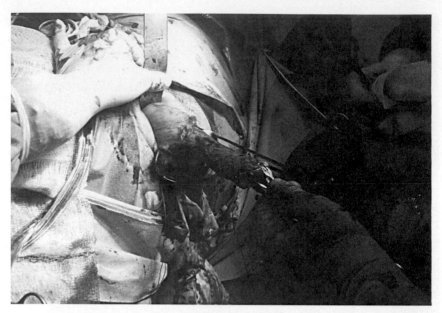

Figure 4-2. Elongated cervix during surgery is associated with severe perineal defects, absence of vaginal axis, and a markedly tilted levator plate.

particularly difficult to pick up when a heavy or tense abdomen precludes accurate palpation of uterine fundus or corpus. Thus, because of a false assumption that the uterus has prolapsed with the cervix accompanied by inadequate examination and assessment preoperatively of cervical dimensions, the discovery of this unwelcome organ arrangement frequently occurs as a startling surprise during the surgery itself (Figure 4-2). Such a situation may present technical problems to the inexperienced operator.

The etiology of the isolated elongation-protrusion of the cervix is explained by the singular deterioration of pelvic floor support with angulation of the levator plate in the absence of upper cardinal-uterosacral disruption at the level of the isthmus uteri but defective at its lower levels of cervical support. In these circumstances, the cervix, with no levator plate to rest on and weakened suspension from above, slowly slides downward and lengthens, progressive over time, while the corpus uteri remains fixed. The most common situation, in which the cervix is not longer than expected, or only minimally so, reflects more or less temporally incidental attenuation of both full cardinal-uterosacral tissues and pelvic floor. However, to keep the record straight, it is not totally uncommon to experience prolapse of the complete uterus secondary to full cardinal complex disruption in association with minimal or no levator support defects.

The prolapsed uterus has been commonly conceived for many decades, even to the present time, as the "hanger," or the "resident's case," because of dangerously false illusions about ease of vaginal removal just because it protrudes. In truth, the opposite view must be taken, that hysterectomy performed on uterine procidentia presents much greater technical difficulty and potential for harm than does surgery on the uterus that presents negligible or no descensus. In the latter, the planes are clearly defined, without the muddling effect of edema, and the anatomic situation of adjacent organs is undisturbed, i.e., things lie just where you expect them. In uterine prolapse, particularly if other pelvic organs have simultaneously descended, connective tissue supports are all abnormally stretched and overstretched, throwing organs out of position and distorting geographic interrelationships. Compounding this annoying state, and perhaps a much more ominous factor, is the inevitable ubiquitous edema accompanying the "fallen womb," and the greater the drop, the worse is the swelling. Natural planes, to vision and palpation, become essentially nonexistent. Inexperience, fear, carelessness, and a touch of recklessness can lead one not just into uterine substance, throwing off all sense of direction, but into major vessels, bladder, rectum, and ureters. Hysterectomy to cure procidentia, in a word, requires expert technique and supervision. It demands the ultimate respect of the surgeon.

CONTRAINDICATIONS TO VAGINAL HYSTERECTOMY

Possible roadblocks and distinct contraindications to vaginal hysterectomy for prolapse are essentially the same as those for vaginal hysterectomy for any other indication. They fall in the following categories: (1) medical and surgical conditions that might contraindicate any surgery; (2) orthopedic and medical conditions that preclude use of the lithotomy position; (3) surgical problems requiring intraperitoneal operation, i.e., adnexal masses of possible malignant potential; (4) old adhesive disease involving the uterine fundus or cul-de-sac; (5) residua from endometriosis obliterating the cul-de-sac; and (6) all but the earliest stages of cervical or endometrial cancer.

The size of the prolapsed uterus is seldom a contraindication to vaginal hysterectomy in view of the fact that uterine prolapse is prevented by more than minor degrees of fundal enlargement. However, the usual cause of benign fundal enlargement, fibromyomata, is not generally a factor because of the remarkable atrophy of such lesions within a short period of time after entry into the climacteric.

PREPARATIONS FOR SURGERY

In assessing and preparing for treatment of uterine prolapse, several questions must be answered:

1. Will the quality of the patient's life be improved by operative correction?
2. Is the patient a suitable risk for surgery, and do the anticipated benefits exceed the risk?
3. Is surgery the simplest effective option, as determined by inclusion of the patient in full discussion and decision-making?

An in-depth history must always be taken, with particular attention to past medical and surgical experiences. The physical evaluation should be a joint effort involving the gynecologist, internist, and anesthesiologist. Older patients often require a comprehensive cardiovascular evaluation. In the absence of pulmonary findings, or a history of pulmonary complaints, a chest x-ray will suffice for the evaluation of pulmonary status. Cervical cytology should be recent. An abnormal history of postmenopausal bleeding will mandate some type of endometrial sampling, either an endometrial biopsy or a dilatation and curettage before hysterectomy, not at the time of actual surgery. Some practitioners do a dilatation and curettage at the time of hysterectomy as a routine, but this does not allow time for thorough histologic study and certainly the naked eye is not capable of detecting early cellular changes.

Complete details for preparation for operative intervention have been thoroughly discussed in the preceding chapter. Nonetheless it is still worth emphasizing, before one embarks on vaginal hysterectomy, that intensive history-taking must unearth preoperatively any symptomatology of the lower urinary and lowermost digestive tracts. If such exist and explanatory anatomic surgically corrective defects are present, any operation must also repair these abnormalities at the same time as the hysterectomy.

Again, although previously discussed in Chapter 3, the necessity for preoperative storage of autologous blood, when feasible, for hysterectomy of any type, must be stressed to the patient. Also to be emphasized is the administration of appropriate intravenous prophylactic antibiotic medication before the surgery begins, usually most practically administered on entry into the operating room. As an anti-infection measure, as explained in Chapter 16, the patient is not shaved.

SURGICAL TECHNIQUE

Depending on preferences and special circumstances, the operation may be performed under general or regional anesthesia. Once anesthetized, the patient is placed in the lithotomy position, using either high orthopedic stirrups or Allen stirrups with provisions for avoiding pressure on any area of the lower extremity. Care must be taken to avoid extremes of flexion or extension and, as ascertained preoperatively, arthritic joints must be respected. Excessive abduction can cause

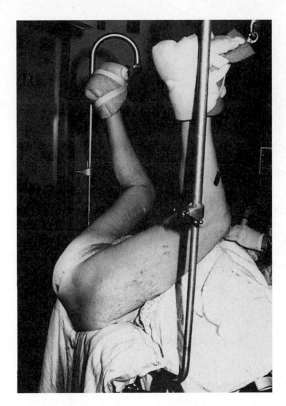

Figure 4-3. Correct lithotomy position in the operating room.

nerve damage. With judicious positioning of the patient, including low enough placement of the hips on the table, good visualization and access to the perineal area and comfortable room for assistant participation should be provided (Figure 4-3).

After appropriate antiseptic application and draping, catheterization is performed, using a metal catheter, with cradling between two fingers placed in the vagina to guide it to avoid injury (Figure 4-4). A small amount of urine can be left in the bladder so as to provide a signal in the event cystotomy occurs during anterior dissection of the bladder from the uterus. Some doctors insert a small amount of dye or sterile milk into the bladder if difficult anterior dissection is anticipated. Reexamination is then performed to confirm the preoperative findings and especially to rule out again, under better conditions of relaxation (anesthesia), any adnexal lesions that might make a vaginal approach imprudent. It also provides the best opportunity to ensure freedom of movement of the cervix with no fixations that might interfere with well-directed surgery.

A weighted vaginal speculum is placed in the vagina and the cervix is visualized and grasped with two tenacula, one on the anterior and one on the posterior lip (Figure 4-5). The uterus is moved backward and forward to observe the reflections of vaginal mucosa and to help to determine the location of the peritoneal reflection

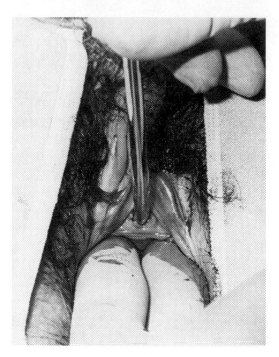

Figure 4-4. Metal catheter, cradled by fingers, is inserted into bladder at outset of surgery.

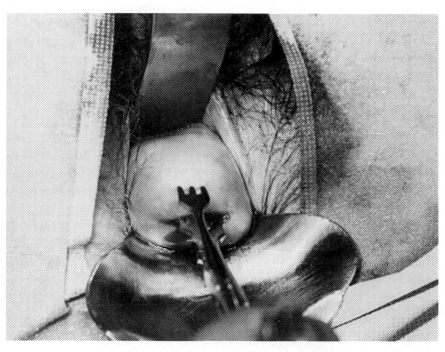

Figure 4-5. Thyroid tenacula are applied on anterior and posterior cervical lips just outside the transformation zone.

of the posterior cul-de-sac. An Allis clamp is applied to the mucosa of the posterior vaginal fornix 1 cm away from the point that has been chosen for entry into the posterior cul-de-sac. The cul-de-sac is entered with a snip of the Mayo scissors; this incision is sharply widened, a rather standard procedure at the Indiana University Medical Center (IUMC) and one advocated widely.[6]

Frequently, there is considerable concern over preservation of vaginal length, particularly when prolapse of the uterus is accompanied by significant posterior pelvic compartment defects that demand simultaneous repair. Thus, to ensure an adequate vaginal axis and associated adequate vaginal dimensions in such situations, some operators, as performed at the Temple University Hospital (TUH), initiate the hysterectomy by circumcising the cervix just outside the transformation zone (Figure 4-6). The experienced operator, maintaining traction on the cervix and using the Mayo scissors in semiparallel position, with scissor points firmly against the cervix, can then deftly strip away anterior and posterior cervical and forniceal mucosa (Figure 4-7) in preparation for anterior and posterior entries into the peritoneal cavity. Some surgeons advocate submucosal saline injections before the start of any dissection in an effort to facilitate delineation of tissue planes and to avoid bladder intrusion. The inclusion of vasoconstrictive agents in the saline is advocated in some institutions to decrease bleeding. However, proficient operators can dissect quickly and keep blood loss at a minimum, thereby avoiding the disadvantages of the vasoconstrictives. These agents can alter cardiovascular stability, much to the chagrin of the anesthesiologist, and they can produce prolonged tissue anoxia in the region, leading to both increased vault infection[7] and to loss of tissue quality at the vaginal vault.

In the cervical circumcision approach, as at TUH, the posterior rather than the anterior peritoneal opening is made first as is also done at IUMC. The peritoneal fold generally comes readily into view and then is snipped open and widened bilaterally.

At this point a discussion of so-called excess vaginal mucosa is germaine. A common erroneous presumption seems to exist, in cases of uterine prolapse, that the protruding organ has automatically produced overabundant vaginal mucosa through imagined stretching and that the greater the projection, the more the excess mucosa. Consequently, but illogically, the operator feels compelled, at the time of cervical circumcision, to excise some vaginal mucosa, usually in the form of triangles, off both the anterior and posterior vaginal walls. The greater the procidentia, the greater the externally visible vagina, of course, so the greater the amount of vagina removed. Although admittedly in cases of severe prolapse, a true vaginal overstretching and resultant excess of mucosa does exist, generally it is the same square surface of vagina whether inverted or everted and there is no real surplus. Thus, as illustrated in Figure 4-8, literally, the more it sticks out, the more mucosa removed. As the sketches demonstrate, it is the same hypothetical 14 cm from introitus to cervix no matter how one measures. Thus, in removing any of this surface, and the more removed, the worse, the vagina accordingly becomes fore-

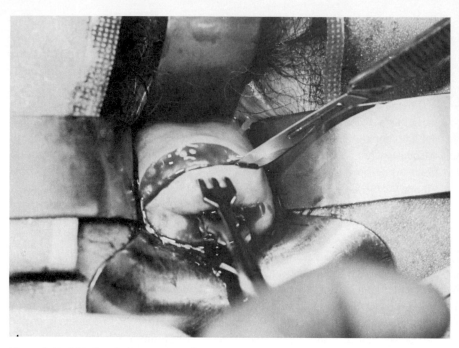

Figure 4-6. Initiating the hysterectomy. Incision is designed to conserve mucosal surface to ensure vaginal length.

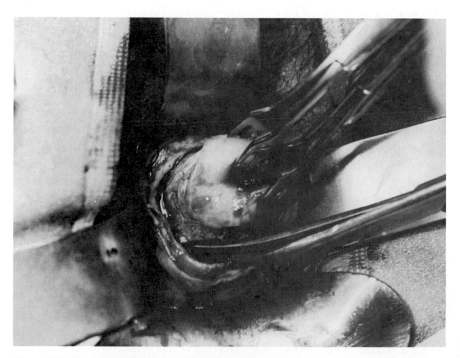

Figure 4-7. The posterior fornix is easily freed from the cervix directly up to the cul-de-sac.

shortened and thereby dysfunctional. Regrettably, it will also set the stage for future enterocele because of the resultant loss of vaginal axis. This is more thoroughly discussed in Chapters 10 and 11.

In most facilities, "fixed" retractors, such as the popular right-angled Heaney and the Deaver, are standard in vaginal hysterectomy. However, there is a trend toward the use of malleable ribbon retractors (see Figures 4-6 and 4-7) to allow for adjustment to accommodate for dimensional differences from one case to another and for changes during the progression of each operation. Additionally, by appropriate bending of the ribbons, their tips will be kept from dislodging sutures on stumps, a potential menace with the unadjustable inserting arms of Heaney and Deaver retractors.

Once the pouch of Douglas has been entered, the operator should inspect the posterior surface of the uterus with one or two fingers, feeling for adhesions and to ensure that the fundus is mobile and free.[8] Further examination will determine the presence of an enterocele by placing a finger into the depths of the cul-de-sac and searching for a space between the posterior vaginal wall and the rectum.[9] Occasionally, with marked prolapse, it is easy to enter the wrong vaginal mucosal plane and the mucosal incision does not enter the cul-de-sac. In these cases, a finger inserted through the mucosal wound will palpate peritoneum to detect the location of the posterior cul-de-sac. Once the peritoneum is felt, it can be grasped with an Allis clamp and the cul-de-sac entered with the scissors.

An identifying suture is passed through the edge of the opened cul-de-sac peritoneum and the vaginal mucosa at the midpoint. Traction on this suture facilitates insertion of the long-lipped weighted Steiner-Auvard speculum (Figure 4-9) and exposure of the posterior peritoneal surface later in obliteration of the cul-de-sac or excision of enterocele peritoneum. Some surgeons place this labeling stitch only through the peritoneal edge because of less restriction in outward pull for better exposure of retrouterine peritoneum up to the "yellow line" of fat demarcating the border between abdominal and cul-de-sac peritoneum.

In the IUMC technique, the most common type of approach, after the posterior peritoneal entry, circumcision of the cervix is extended sharply anteriorly bilaterally and completed in the groovelike depression just below the bladder. The incision should be carried through the full thickness of the vaginal mucosa with care to avoid excessive depth laterally so as to prevent bleeding from large descending blood vessels.

Regardless of the starting incision level anteriorly, if the proper tissue plane is attained, dissection of the bladder off the upper cervix and isthmus uteri should proceed with ease. Finding the correct plane is crucial to averting bladder intrusion on the one hand and digging into cervical substance on the other. Experience is the positive catalyst in this dissection. If there is any history of cesarean section, sharp dissection is mandatory.

Although it can be considered academic if correct surgical principles are applied, in cases of considerable prolapse, after cervical circumcision and dissection

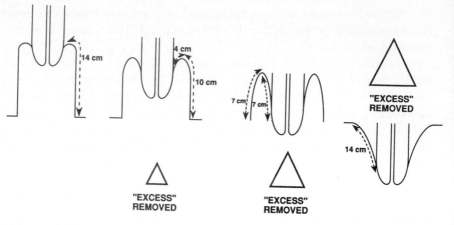

Figure 4-8. Illustration of wanton excision of presumed "excess" vaginal mucosa. False illusion: the greater the protrusion, the more surface to remove. Truth: vaginal length remains the same, except for the extreme case.

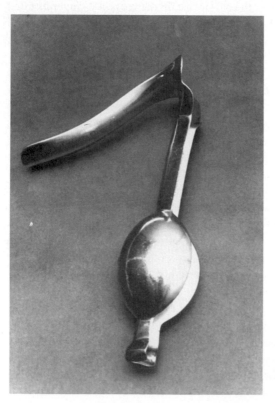

Figure 4-9. Long-lipped weighted posterior Steiner-Auvard speculum.

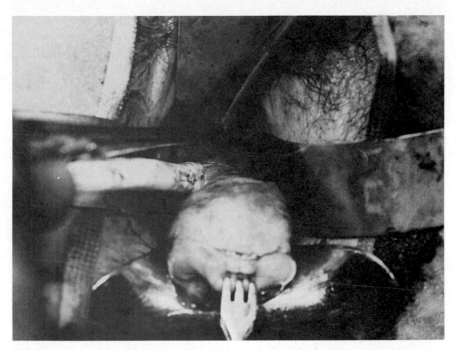

Figure 4-10. Anterior peritoneal fold is being elevated by forceps and pierced by scissors posterior to bladder.

of anterior and posterior fornices off the cervix, the ureters can often be palpated. This is considerably more difficult to do in vaginal hysterectomy without procidentia. In benign cases, assuming careful technique, there is generally no need to expose the ureters surgically because they lie 1.5 to 2 cm lateral to the uterus.[10,11] However, a word of caution is appropriate at this point. Because of urethral displacement and distortion in association with prolapse, the ureters are more prone to injury if the slightest deviation in good technique occurs than they would be without prolapse. Recent work describes a seemingly simple method of identifying and exposing the ureters at vaginal hysterectomy.[12] This study reveals conclusively that combined retractor elevation of the bladder, well dissected off the uterus, together with strong downward traction on the cervix, usually displaces the ureters cephalad out of reach of the first clamp placed on the cardinal-uterosacral complex. When these pedicles are cut and tied, and the bladder elevation and downward traction are continued, the ureters will flare out laterally, well away from danger.

The anterior peritoneal cavity may be entered either at this time or after the first bite on both sides has been completed. It makes little difference so long as the bladder has been cleared and elevated. Once the peritoneum has been identified and stretched between the elevated bladder and the anterior uterine surface, it can be grasped with forceps or an Allis clamp and pierced with the snip of a scissors (Figure 4-10). This anterior peritoneal opening is bilaterally extended. Then a suture tag is placed centrally in the peritoneal edge under the bladder, which is well retracted safely out of the way. The tag proves useful later in closure.

If unintended bladder intrusion becomes apparent by a gush of urine, closure should be postponed until dissection is completed or until after the uterus is removed. The repair is easily accomplished in two layers using rapidly absorbable polyfilament synthetic suture. Such a mishap is not a major problem so long as it is recognized and repaired.

When peritoneal entry anteriorly is difficult, it can be simplified sometimes by the insertion of a finger through the posterior opening and then over the top of the uterus. Also, a metal catheter or uterine sound can be inserted into the bladder through the urethral meatus to reveal the most posterior extent of the bladder. In either instance, the locale of the anterior peritoneal site for puncture can then be easily realized. Either a Deaver retractor or a malleable ribbon inserted through the incised peritoneum can then afford further adequate exposure in combination with that already supplied by the posterior weighted speculum. An additional comment on difficult peritoneal entry is pertinent to correct surgery. Altogether too much concern in penetrating into the abdominal cavity often preoccupies the surgeon so that he or she prolongs surgical and anesthesia time and frequently increases blood loss by entering into uterine substance because the correct plane is lost. If entry does not come easily and quickly, so long as the bladder and cul-de-sac are dissected freely from the uterus, the hysterectomy should be continued extraperitoneally. In time, a peritoneal fold will appear and entry will be made easily.[13–15]

Although a wide variety of clamps are used in vaginal hysterectomy, obviously the best, especially because of the limited operative field, are those least apt to slip. Thus, those with longitudinal grooves or striations, such as Heaney-Ballantine, Zeppelin, or Masterson clamps, are the most suitable (Figure 4-11).

At this point, traction on the cervix brings the cardinal-uterosacral complex into surgical range. The entire ligament composite is then clamped with the toe of the clamp in direct contact with the uterus and the heel at the vaginal edge (Figure 4-12). Such a placement, after the pedicle has been cut free, when tied, fortunately shortens the already attenuated cardinal complex by 3 to 4 cm. Detractors of this clamping technique claim that it will displace and kink the ureters. In truth, the knot moves upward to the uterine vessels as it is tied and the ureters remain undisturbed. Many operators, as at IUMC, doubly clamp and doubly suture at this level of security because these sutures, usually tagged, might be pulled off, despite transfixion, causing slipping, a potentially serious problem not likely to occur with double ligation. However, the wider tissue involvement brings sutures closer to ureters and also creates more necrotic tissue left behind. In either case, when the patient's history has revealed any previous anterior pelvic compartment repair, technique must be modified to avoid ureters that may be scarred down far from their natural positions.

Some operators prefer to ligate the uterosacral and cardinal ligaments separately. In the end, it probably makes no difference. When done in one bite, time is

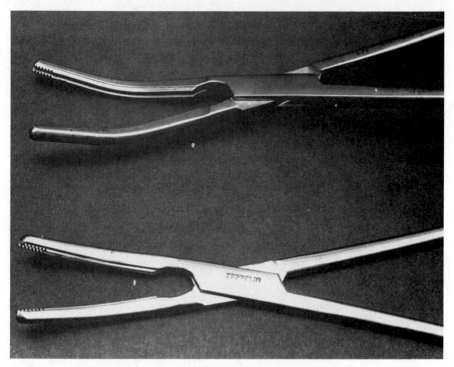

Figure 4-11. Zeppelin (ZSI) clamp has narrower width but less dependable tips on heavy bites.

saved and there is less suture and one less knot. When kept separate, slippage is less apt to occur. In instances of elongated cervix, the cardinal-uterosacral complex is often so spread out so that one may have no choice but to take as many as three bites on each side before reaching the level of the uterine blood vessels.

Clamping, cutting, and ligating proceeds in separate bites on each side until the uterus is completely detached and removed. Almost universal agreement exists regarding transfixion sutures of the Heaney type on each stump except for ligation of the major vessels. Many feel a single needle pierce well above the vessels followed by adequate inclusion in the tie of the whole pedicle is best because it avoids accidental penetration of the uterine artery or vein by the second needle thrust of the Heaney suture. Others contend that transfixion is vital in the prevention of disastrous suture slipping in this area. They claim that puncture of the uterine vessels is easily avoided because they are visible in the cut stump (Figure 4-13). Regardless, it is wisely suggested that the cut ends of the sutures on the pedicle containing the vessels be left long for easy identification in the event of heavy bleeding.

Clamps must be placed always immediately adjacent to the previous pedicle, and they must embrace the peritoneal surfaces on either side of the broad ligament,

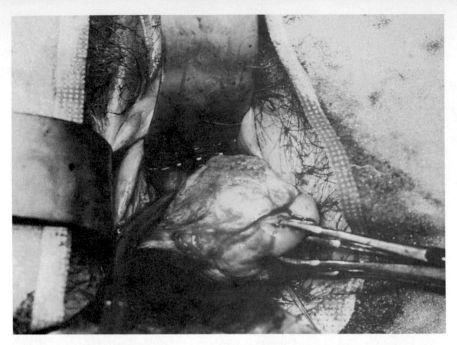

Figure 4-12. Placement of clamp on entire left cardinal-uterosacral complex in one initial bite. Toe of clamp is on cervix while heel of clamp is at vaginal mucosal edge. On tying, ligament shortens by 3 cm as pedicle moves upward and ureters flare laterally.

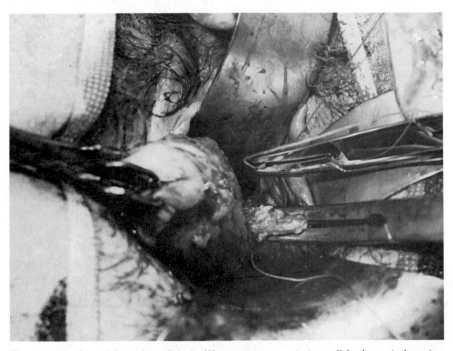

Figure 4-13. Second thrust (transfixion) of Heaney suture penetrates pedicle above uterine artery and vein, thus creating a double suture loop around them.

making certain that the toes of the clamp are immediately adjacent to the uterus. A variation of preference for single or double ligation of stumps throughout the operation exists. Advantages and disadvantages have already been discussed. The steps of uterine severance can advance in orderly fashion from the external cervix to the top of the fundus. However, as is most popular today, after the uterine circulation has been secured, the fundus is delivered, most usually posteriorly (Figure 4-14), and the Fallopian tube, utero-ovarian ligament, and round ligament are grasped in one bite. A special stitch can be used for this large, usually final, bite. The suture is first passed 2 to 3 mm from the tissue edge at the toe of the clamp (Figure 4-15). Then it is passed again, in reverse, at the heel of the clamp, also 2 to 3 mm from the tissue edge back to the starting side of the stump (Figure 4-16). Then the same working suture end is looped around the entire pedicle, capturing the free tissue edges not already enclosed, completing the circuit to be tied finally to the stationary counterpart suture end. These suture lengths are usually kept as tags to help locate the lateral corners when the peritoneum is closed. At this point they are gently held without tension as are the lowermost suture tags on the cardinal-uterosacral pedicles, and the space between the two on each side is carefully inspected for bleeding. If any is found, ligation is performed at a very superficial depth so as to remain clear of the ureters.

At this point, consideration of oophorectomy becomes paramount. The indications for oophorectomy are the same whether the approach is abdominal or vaginal.[16] Yet, in the United States, it is well known that oophorectomy accompanies 75% of abdominal hysterectomies and only 2% of those performed vaginally. There is no good excuse for this situation and the only explanations are unwarranted fear and inexperience. In a very few instances, usually only in women who are very elderly, the ovaries have retracted well out to the pelvic sidewalls. Also, uncommonly, one or the other adnexal areas may be tightly bound in local adhesions. In restrictive cases of this nature it might be foolhardy to attempt ovarian extrication. However, in general, the procedure is not at all difficult.

Placing gentle steady traction on the fundal ligament tag, accompanied by the effective use of retractors, the ovary will come into view and it should then be lightly held in a Babcock clamp (Figure 4-17). Simple sutures around the pedicle then allow it to be removed.

Obliteration of the cul-de-sac at this point becomes of prime importance. Most gynecologic surgeons today believe that such a closure should be performed in all hysterectomies, but especially in association with prolapse, as a choice prophylaxis against future enterocele. When there is negligible depth to the pouch of Douglas, then a standard purse-string closure, used both at IUMC and TUH, exteriorizing all stumps outside the peritoneal cavity, is adequate. The same goal can be accomplished in a side-to-side continuous closure. In each case the closure must include peritoneum behind the bladder base to prevent anterior enterocele as well as peritoneum at the "yellow line" posteriorly. When considerable cul-de-sac depth is present, a McCall type of elimination,[17] consisting of a series of connecting sutures

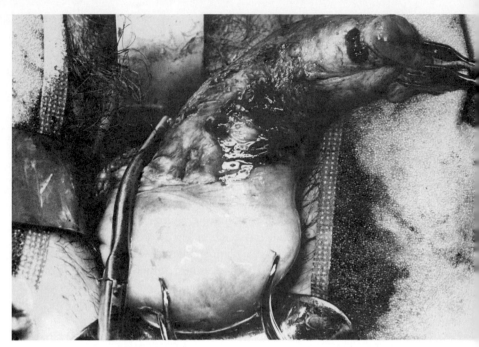

Figure 4-14. Posterior delivery of fundus. One grasp of clamp includes Fallopian tube, utero-ovarian ligament, and round ligament.

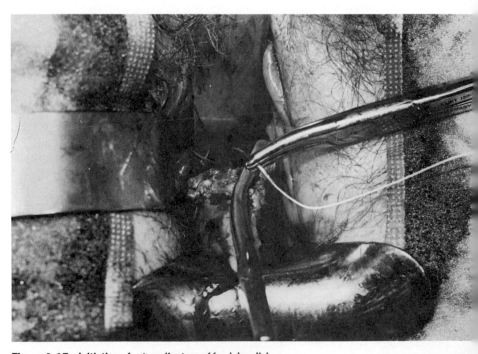

Figure 4-15. Initiation of suture-ligature of fundal pedicle.

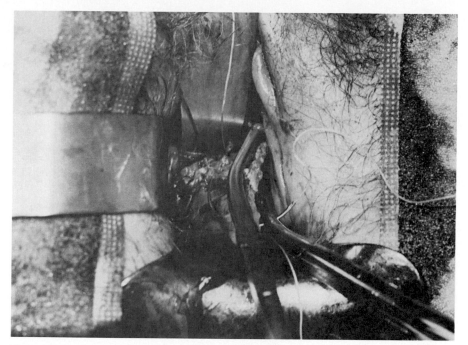

Figure 4-16. Second (reverse) puncture in horizontal mattress arrangement in ligation of fundal pedicle, to be followed by full encirclement of pedicle by needle end of suture, then tying.

involving uterosacral ligaments, sac peritoneum, and posterior cuff, may often be used. Care must be taken to avoid ureteral entrapment with this method. A simple type of effective closure, especially if the hysterectomy is to be accompanied by a deep posterior colpoperineorrhapy, is the Halban technique. This consists of a series of three to five sutures placed vertically in succession between the uterosacral ligaments, each running from the yellow line to the cuff, each taking three to four peritoneal bites. After all these stitches are in position, they are tied at once, dramatically eliminating the cul-de-sac without danger to the ureters.

When the pouch of Douglas is so deep as to be considered an enterocele, probably the best approach is excision of all the peritoneum comprising the enterocele sac. This is followed by suture closure of the raw surfaces, one to the other. Instead of peeling the peritoneum, some operators use a Moskowitz technic, requiring a succession of circular purse-strings into the peritoneum, but this is not deemed as prophylactically effective as the stripping of the entire sac.

Although peritoneal closure in pelvic laparotomy done abdominally is no longer widely performed, almost universally such closure is effected in vaginal hysterectomy. The reason for this is assurance that, if postoperative hemorrhage should occur, it will be extraperitoneal and visible rather than intraperitoneal.

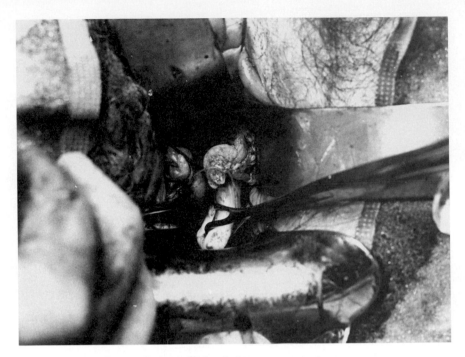

Figure 4-17. Ovary in gentle grasp of Babcock clamp.

The most essential prophylactic step against future vault (cuff) prolapse is the anchoring of the now shortened and unburdened cardinal-uterosacral pedicles to their respective posterolateral cuff corners, the natural location especially effective if significant rectovaginal septum fibers remain intact at the cuff level. As healing progresses and scar retraction develops, the upper vagina will then be drawn over the levator plate back toward the sacral hollow.

As for cuff closure, most surgeons make certain that at least a portion, if not all, of the vault area is left open for drainage. At IUMC, a running locking stitch is used around the entire cuff whereas at TUH, a similar stitch is used posteriorly but the anterior edges are sewn together in an anterior-posterior direction to the cardinal ligament anchorage.

Perhaps the best suture material for hysterectomy today is Dexon II-0 because it has a coating material that obviates the need for a surgeon's knot. It slides easily into place, and if the first throw loosens a bit, even when tying under tension, the second throw will slide the whole knot firmly down on the pedicle. Dexon II is a relatively rapidly absorbable essentially nonreactive polyfilament material.

At completion of the operation, the vaginal vault area should be dry. Any cuff bleeding may be controlled by oversewing bleeding edges. A vaginal pack, in the absence of any repair, is generally not necessary.

Postoperative care is covered in detail in Chapter 16. Ambulation is almost immediate and, when hysterectomy is not accompanied by repair, if there are no unexpected developments, patients will go home on average in 1 or 2 days. They are encouraged to return to normal activity as soon as possible.

Complications are thoroughly discussed in Chapter 17. However, it must be stated that straightforward vaginal hysterectomy, even in the elderly, conducted intelligently, skillfully, and responsibly from beginning to end, carries a very low morbidity and mortality rate.

REFERENCES

1. Folsome CE, Napp EE, Tanz A. Pelvic findings in the elderly institutionalized patient. *JAMA*. 1956;161:1447–1454.

2. Mayo CH. Uterine prolapse with associated pelvic relaxation. *Surg Gynecol Obstet*. 1915;20:253–260.

3. Heaney NS. A report of 565 vaginal hysterectomies performed for benign pelvic disease. *Am J Obstet Gynecol*. 1934;28:751–756.

4. Quinlivan LG. The gynecological findings in elderly women. *Geriatrics*. 1964;19:654–657.

5. Ricci JV. *The Development of Gynecological Surgery and Instruments*. San Francisco: Norman; 1990:270–274.

6. Nichols DH, Randall CL. *Vaginal Surgery*. 3rd ed. Baltimore: Williams & Wilkins; 1989:191.

7. England GT, Randall HW, Graves WL. Impairment of tissue defenses by vasoconstrictors in vaginal hysterectomies. *Obstet Gynecol*. 1983;61:271–274.

8. Nichols DH, Randall CL. *Vaginal Surgery*. 3rd ed. Baltimore: Williams & Wilkins; 1989:193.

9. Nichols DH, Randall CL. *Vaginal Surgery*. 3rd ed. Baltimore: Williams & Wilkins; 1989:217.

10. Mattingly RF, Thompson JD. *Te Lindes Operative Gynecology*. 6th ed. Philadelphia: J B Lippincott; 1985:325.

11. Nichols DH, Randall CL. *Vaginal Surgery*. 3rd ed. Baltimore: Williams & Wilkins; 1989:182.

12. Cruikshank SH. Surgical method of identifying the ureters during total vaginal hysterectomy. *Obstet Gynecol*. 1986;67:277–281.

13. Gary LA. *Vaginal Hysterectomy*. 3rd ed. Springfield, Ill: Charles C Thomas; 1983:36–41.

14. Käser O, Iklé A, Hirsch HH. *Atlas of Gynecologic Surgery*. 2nd ed. New York: Thieme-Stratton; 1985:1220.

15. Krige CF. *Vaginal Hysterectomy and Genital Prolapse Repair*. Johannesburg: Witwatersrand University Press; 1965:59.

16. Capen CV, Irwin H, Magrina J, et al. Vaginal removal of the ovaries in association with vaginal hysterectomy. *J Reprod Med.* 1983;28:589–591.

17. McCall ML. Posterior culdeplasty: surgical correction of enterocoele during vaginal hysterectomy: a preliminary report. *Obstet Gynecol.* 1957;10:595–598.

Investigating the Elderly Incontinent Woman

Richard J. Scotti

Although age changes occur at different rates in different people, they are universal, intrinsic, progressive, and eventually deleterious.[1]

The above statement graphically portrays the stark truth about aging and its associated degenerative changes. It is particularly true when one considers the changes that occur in the lower urinary tract as a consequence of aging.

Population dynamics and the demography of aging have significantly altered over the last few centuries and even more drastically over the last five decades. In 1700, 28% of women survived to menopause. Currently, 95% of women can be expected to reach menopause.[2,3] This change alone has altered the approach that gynecologists must take in respect to the concept of total care in patients entrusted to them.

Since 1950 we have seen what has been called a "rectangularization" of the population, depicted in Figure 5-1. The "baby-boom" has resulted in a large segment of the population now entering menopause. This large number of post-menopausal women has had several consequences including, but not limited to, potential bankruptcy of the Social Security system and, in a more practical vein for gynecologists, the need to have a thorough knowledge of menopause and its management. Included in this total management scheme is the recognition and satisfactory treatment of urinary and fecal incontinence.

The incidence of incontinence in community-dwelling women over 65 years of age has been reported to be between 15% and 38% according to a recent consensus

DEMOGRAPHIC CHANGES

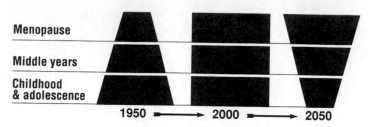

Figure 5-1 Dramatic demographic changes have occurred and will continue to occur. While the number of surviving women in the middle years will remain unchanged, the number of girls in childhood and adolescence and women surviving past menopause will essentially swap by the year 2050.

conference sponsored by the National Institutes of Health.[4] It has also been estimated that 50% of women who are institutionalized are incontinent (Table 5-1). In fact, the most frequent reason for committing a family member to a nursing home in the United States is incontinence.[5]

In the United Kingdom the incidence of incontinence is similar. Milne estimated between 16% and 42% of elderly patients to be incontinent, basing his data on a review of seven separate studies.[6] He estimated the incidence of incontinence in institutionalized postmenopausal patients to be between 21.9% and 47%.[7] Moreover, about 25% of nursing time in elderly care facilities is devoted to incontinence.[8]

One can speculate about the magnitude of the problems that deficient urinary control poses to the population by a cursory perusal of the aisles of supermarkets and drug stores displaying incontinence-related products. A dramatic proliferation in the type and kind of such items has occurred in the last decade alone. In short, the problem of urinary incontinence in the elderly has reached proportions such that federal and other agencies are acutely concerned about its impact on the health care of American citizens.[4]

TABLE 5-1 Incidence of Incontinence

United States
   15–38% of community-dwelling women over age 65
   50% of institutionalized women over age 65

United Kingdom
   16–42% of elderly women
   21.9–47% of institutionalized elderly women
   25% of nursing time devoted to incontinence

AGE-RELATED CHANGES AND SYMPTOMS IN THE URINARY TRACT

Many age-related changes may cause symptoms in the lower urinary tract. We will divide these changes into several categories to have a better understanding as to how aging has direct and often deleterious effects on urinary tract functioning.

General Age-Related Changes

Several general conditions can cause urinary tract symptoms. Poor locomotion can contribute to or worsen incontinence. Patients who are unable to transfer from bed to commode or from a sitting position to commode without assistance, particularly in nursing homes, may be incontinent even though they have no lower urinary tract dysfunction. This is simply a function of the inability to transfer at a time when urgency occurs. Orthopedic fracture is a common amplifier of incontinence as a result of inability to ambulate in a timely manner.

Congestive heart failure can also be a cause for urinary symptoms because it results in nocturia as well as daytime frequency. Medications given for heart failure, particularly diuretics, may also cause urinary frequency and may confuse the clinical picture. Psychiatric disturbances and inadequate mentation may also be causes for lower urinary tract symptoms. Psychogenic urgency may be related to feelings of helplessness in older people. Patients may void frequently to reinforce to themselves that they function normally.

Chronic constipation may also contribute to urinary frequency and possibly to genuine stress incontinence, particularly if fecal impaction is present. Moreover, straining to defecate or urinate may accentuate pelvic relaxation and cause enlargement of previously existing cystoceles, rectoceles, and enteroceles.

Diabetes may magnify urinary frequency and nocturia and will aggravate other urinary symptoms, particularly in older people whose bladder already has a low storage capacity. The increased frequency of urinary tract infections in diabetic patients further complicates the picture.

The postmenopausal decline of estrogen and associated loss of connective tissue throughout the body affects the lower urinary tract directly, causing decreased bladder compliance and contractility and concomitant decreased urethral resistance. These factors may promote urinary retention as well as low urethral pressure, thereby leading to genuine stress incontinence.

Acute urinary tract infections are more common in elderly people. Infections and their effects on the bladder and urethra may mimic both stress and urge incontinence.

Medications, including α and β agonists and antagonists, antidepressants, diuretics, tranquilizers, and hypnotics, may all alter urinary tract function. α-Blockers used in hypertension may cause significant urethral relaxation, promoting urinary incontinence due to low urethral pressure. Additionally, certain medications can cause chronic constipation with resultant detrimental straining. Fecal

TABLE 5-2 General Age-Related Changes

Poor locomotion
Orthopedic degeneration
Bone fractures
Cardiovascular disease
Hypertensive disease
Mental decline
Psychiatric crises
Hypoestrogenism
Diabetes onset or progression
Infection diathesis
Constipation
Central nervous system diseases
   Parkinsonism
   Multiple sclerosis
   Cerebral atherosclerosis
   Alzheimer's disease

Medication side effects
   Diuretics
   Antihypertensives
   Tranquilizers
   Hypnotics
     ↓
Predispose for
     ↓
Genuine stress incontinence
Detrusor instability
Overflow incontinence
General pelvic relaxation

---

impaction resulting from this constipation may contribute further to urinary retention or incontinence.

Various nervous system disorders can induce incontinence. Parkinsonism, cerebral atherosclerosis, and multiple sclerosis are all frequent causes of urge incontinence and detrusor instability. Table 5-2 lists most of these changes with respect to symptomatic effects on the lower urinary tract.

Vaginal Alterations

Several adverse changes in the vagina may also be responsible for symptomatic alterations in the lower urinary tract. The loss of mucosal integrity with the resulting increase in pH and unfavorable modifications in bacterial flora may predispose to recurrent vaginitis and to urinary tract infection because symptomatic infection

TABLE 5-3 Vaginal Age-Related Changes

Loss of mucosal integrity
Increased pH
Decreased *Lactobacillus* population
Connective tissue atrophy
Decreased elasticity
↓
Predispose for
↓
Vaginitis
Cystitis
Irritation
Cystocele
Rectocele
Enterocele

of the vagina is the most common precursor of lower urinary tract infection. This vaginal inversion also mirrors changes in the urethra with respect to estrogen status. Urethral hypoestrogenism often causes dysuria and urinary frequency, components of the "urethral syndrome." (see Section 2, Chapter 1).

Additionally, loss of connective tissue supporting the vagina can contribute to the development or progression of cystoceles, rectoceles, and enteroceles. A cystocele may be symptomatic and can be a cause for urinary frequency or retention with accompanying straining to void. These changes are summarized in Table 5-3.

Urethral Aging

The urethra undergoes age-related decline and this radiates adversely on the bladder. Urethral mucosa thins and the thickness and number of collagen fibers in its wall diminishes. Simultaneously, urethral flexibility decreases and its lumen widens. Vascularity is compromised as some blood vessels disappear while the walls thicken, narrowing the diameter of those remaining. This can be seen by comparing Figure 5-2A with 5-2B. The urethra may also undergo distal stenosis as another consequence of estrogen diminution. Hypoestrogenic changes are clearly evident during urethroscopy. The atrophic mucosa at the external meatus tends to create a stenotic band. The entire length of urethra appears pale and thin, revealing vessels close to the mucosal surface. As an additional consequence of all these negative reverses, urethral closure pressure drops and anatomic support weakens.

Symptomatically such urethral failure predisposes to dysuria, urgency, and frequency as the urethral syndrome in the hypoestrogenic woman develops. Decreased urethral compliance and distal stenosis can cause both prolonged flow and urinary retention (Figure 5-3). Trabeculations can be seen in patients who have

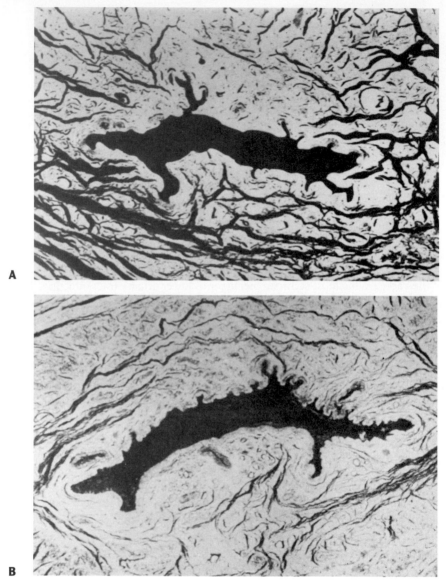

Figure 5-2 A, Premenstrual urethra. B, Postmenopausal urethra. (Reproduced with permission from Huisman, AB. 1979 Morphologie Van Der Vrouwelijke, Urethra, MD Thesis. Gronningen, the Netherlands. In: Stanton SL. *Clinical Gynecologic Urology.* St. Louis: CV Mosby; 1984:346-347.)

obstructive flow or vesical instability. There is also bleeding and easy friability during the examination because of the thinned mucosal lining in close proximity to the underlying blood vessels. These patients also strain to void because of urethral stenosis and difficulty in emptying the bladder. Straining further exaggerates pelvic floor relaxation. Urinary tract infections also result as a consequence of impaired emptying and thin mucosa because of reduction in normal urethral defense mecha-

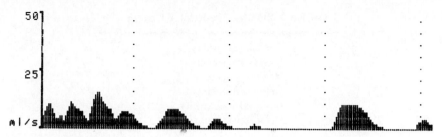

Figure 5-3 Prolonged obstructive uroflowmetry. Multiple peaks usually indicate successive attempts to void by straining.

nisms. Genuine stress incontinence, caused by a low pressure urethra (type III), may occur because of decreased urethral closure pressure. Detrusor instability may also appear as a consequence of weak support causing funneling of the proximal urethra, thereby significantly enlarging the bladder neck. It has been theorized that such funneling, abnormally allowing urine to rest in contact with urethral mucosa, can elicit detrusor contractions.[9] Table 5-4 presents the urethral changes.

Bladder Age-Related Changes

Brocklehurst and Dillane studied various bladder parameters in continent elderly women.[10] They found that approximately 40% of women over age 65 have less than 250 mL maximum bladder capacity. They also noted that 38% of such women had detrusor instability on cystometry; 50% of their study group had greater than 50

TABLE 5-4 Urethral Age-Related Changes

Thin epithelium
Collagen dimunition
Decreased vascularity
Muscular atrophy
Dilated lumen
Lower closure pressure
Distal urethral stenosis
Relaxed supports
↓
Predispose for
↓

Dysuria	Frequency
Prolonged flow	Retention
Obstructive flow	Inadequate emptying
Friability	Bleeding
Funneling	Infection

Genuine stress incontinence
Detrusor instability

TABLE 5-5 Bladder Age-Related Changes

Decreased capacity
Increased residuals
Neuromyopathy
Detrusor instability
Impaired contractility
Decreased compliance

Diverticula

Carcinoma in situ
Invasive carcinoma
↓
Predispose for
↓
Frequency
Urge incontinence
Overflow incontinence
Infection

mL of residual urine. These changes certainly can be associated with urinary frequency as well as urgency and urge incontinence. Moreover, bladder trabeculation due to difficulty in voiding was viewed as much more common in elderly than in younger women. Bladder diverticula are also more common in older patients, and this predisposes to urinary tract infections.

Resnick, Yalla, and Laureno have also described the combination of detrusor instability with impaired detrusor contractility in postmenopausal women.[11] Detrusor instability results in uninhibited contractions and involuntary urine loss, while impaired contractility promotes urinary retention. This combination, seemingly paradoxical, is nonetheless present in 30% of elderly patients according to these authors. Their study group, however, was composed of institutionalized women who may have had more significant degrees of urinary problems.

Decreased compliance is also common in this group of patients and is a normal consequence of bladder aging. Elderly women also have an increase in the incidence of carcinoma in situ and frank true carcinoma of the bladder. There is a fourfold increase in carcinoma of the bladder in women over age 65.

In summary, the bladder-related changes noted above predispose to frequency, urge incontinence, detrusor instability, urinary tract infection as a result of retention, and overflow incontinence (Table 5-5). The work-up will be remiss if it neglects suspicion and detection of any of these conditions.

Kidney Age-Related Changes

Many deteriorations occur in the kidney as a result of aging. There is an approximate nephron loss of 50% with resultant loss of concentrating ability[12] and declin-

TABLE 5-6 Kidney Age-Related Changes

Nephron numbers decreased
Glomeruli numbers halved
Concentrating capacity diminished
Vascular atrophy
Tubular endothelial hypertrophy
   Luminal occlusion
   Nephron diminution
Diverticula in renal pelvis
Medullary fibrosis
Kidney mass shrinkage
Diurnal/nocturnal rhythm disruption
Alkaline urine
↓
Predispose for
↓
Nocturia
Nephrodialysis
Sepsis

ing renal function. It appears that nephron dropout is accentuated by high-protein diets.[12] There are also numerous changes in the microvasculature, plus hypertrophy of tubular epithelium leading to luminal occlusion. Diverticula in the renal pelvis, medullary fibrosis, and shrinking kidneys are also consequences of old age. Patients also seem to have more frequent episodes of nocturia in association with alteration in the normal diurnal/nocturnal rhythm of voiding. This may be related to the kidney but is more likely related to changes in the cardiovascular system; with more sluggish circulation, buildup of fluid in the extremities occurs with elimination of this fluid at night when the patient is supine.

These kidney age-related changes may also promote urinary tract infections (secondary to alkaline urine and poor concentrating ability), urinary stones, and frank urosepsis. These are summarized in Table 5-6.

BASIC DEFINITIONS

Before considering the evaluation of the elderly incontinent patient, it is helpful to review the various types of urinary incontinence. The following definitions conform to the standards of the International Continence Society.[13] *Urinary incontinence* is involuntary urine loss that is objectively demonstrable and is a social or hygienic problem. Loss of urine through channels other than the urethra is *extraurethral incontinence* (i.e., fistula). The term urinary incontinence denotes a symptom, a sign, and a condition. The symptom indicates the patient's statement of involuntary urine loss. The sign is the objective demonstration of urine loss. The condition is the urodynamic demonstration of urine loss.

The sign and symptom of stress incontinence are easily understandable. The urodynamic diagnosis of *genuine stress incontinence* is the involuntary loss of urine occurring when, in the absence of a detrusor contraction, the intravesical pressure exceeds the maximum urethral pressure. To make this diagnosis, some measurement must be made at least of the bladder pressure to rule out bladder contractions. If there is urine loss through the urethra in the absence of detrusor contractions, one must therefore assume that, at the time of urine loss, the intra-urethral pressure momentarily drops below vesical pressure.

The symptom of *urge incontinence* is the involuntary loss of urine associated with a strong desire to void. Urgency may be associated with two types of dysfunction: (1) overactive detrusor function or "motor urgency" and (2) hypersensitivity or "sensory urgency." An overactive detrusor is synonymous with the term unstable bladder or detrusor dyssynergia. Detrusor overactivity is characterized by involuntary detrusor contractions during filling which may be spontaneous or provoked, and which the patient cannot completely suppress. Involuntary detrusor contractions may be incited by rapid filling, alterations of posture, coughing, walking, jumping, and similar stimulations when the bladder is hypersensitive. Some of these triggering events or activities might also increase intra-abdominal pressure and thus be confused with stress incontinence. It is for this reason that urodynamic evaluation is essential in identifying the type of incontinence the patient is experiencing.

Other common types of incontinence are detrusor hyperreflexia and overflow incontinence. *Detrusor hyperreflexia* is overactivity due to disturbance of the nervous control mechanisms. This term should be used only when objective evidence indicates a relevant neurologic disorder. *Overflow incontinence* is any involuntary loss of urine associated with overdistention of the bladder. It is common in diabetic and postmenopausal states.

Reflex incontinence is the loss of urine due to detrusor hyperreflexia or involuntary urethral relaxation (or both) in the absence of the sensation usually associated with the desire to micturate. This condition is seen in patients with neuropathic bladder or urethral disorders. It differs from urge incontinence simply by the absence of the symptom of urgency. It is also known as an automatic bladder.

The above definitions are those that have now been standardized. The use of conceptual and underdefined terms such as hypertonic, uninhibited, spastic, automatic, and neurogenic bladder should be avoided.

The most common forms of postreproductive incontinence are genuine stress incontinence, detrusor instability, and overflow incontinence. The investigation for diagnostic differentiation of these three conditions is somewhat similar to that used for women with lower urinary tract symptoms in general, with some exceptions. One must always be aware of problems unique to the older woman and tailor the work-up accordingly. We have conveniently divided the process into several phases, proceeding from simplified methods to more complex urodynamic techniques.

TABLE 5-7 Evaluation—Phase I:
Initial Urine Screening

Urinalysis
Culture and sensitivity
Cytology

EVALUATION—PHASE I: INITIAL URINE SCREENING

The first phase of urogynecologic investigation is urinalysis and urine culture and sensitivity. Urine cytology may also be useful in smokers and women over age 65 because these two factors pose higher risks for the development of bladder carcinoma.[14] We have singled out these simple studies into one phase of the analysis to underscore the importance of ruling out urinary tract infection or malignancy at the outset (Table 5-7).

Infection in the urinary tract can mimic both genuine stress incontinence as well as vesical instability. Moreover, continuing any invasive part of the work-up in the face of urinary tract infection may worsen the infection or the diagnostic testing may yield inaccurate results. If a culture is positive, the patient should be treated before the investigation continues. If she develops reinfections, she may require maintenance on a suppressive antibacterial regimen. If persistence of one pathogen is observed, an intravenous urogram is indicated to rule out renal stones or anatomic abnormalities of the urinary tract which may continually harbor pathogens. Once urinary tract infections are adequately treated or suppressed, the study may continue.

Urine in women at risk for bladder or renal cancer must always be screened by cytologic means. This includes patients who have been exposed to azo or aniline dye, those who have ever smoked, women with a history of schistosomiasis or exposure to it, and those revealing a record of recurrent urinary tract infections or renal or vesical lithiasis, as well as patients with histories of phenacetin abuse, pelvic irradiation, or cyclophosphamide treatment. A family history of bladder or renal transitional cell carcinoma or carcinoma in situ should arouse suspicion. In general, urine cytology as a screening method for the general population is not warranted.[14]

EVALUATION—PHASE II: HISTORY, PHYSICAL EXAMINATION, AND SIMPLE CLINICAL TESTS

History

A urogynecologic history poses several important key questions in the assessment of women with lower urinary tract symptoms. Major historical points are outlined

TABLE 5-8 Evaluation—Phase II:
Important Historical Points

Questionnaire
Quantitation of urine loss
Fluid intake habits
Use of pads
Daily activities
Voiding diary (urolog)
Vaginal bleeding
Menopausal status
Hormone replacement therapy
Breast disease (mammography)
Symptoms of pelvic relaxation
Previous urinary infections
Diabetes
Other medical conditions
Previous pelvic surgery
Other surgery
Medications
Status of sexual function
Mental status

in Table 5-8. A questionnaire is most useful in eliciting responses from patients with any urinary tract disorders. History-taking in elderly patients is time-consuming because they tend to digress and speak more slowly. Also, they may have difficulty recalling other medical conditions, previous medications, current medications, and previous operations. Often family members can be helpful in obtaining the history. They also aid in supervising patient adherence to instructions so as to gain the best advantage in both diagnosis and therapy (see Chapter 3).

Obviously the primary questions are directed at determining both the level of the patient's disability from urine loss and the precise details regarding quantity, frequency, timing, and circumstances of absence of voiding control. From the start, pads can be worn, changed at designated intervals, and weighed, thereby providing valuable information. Such information becomes especially useful when accompanied by a diary describing associated fluid intake, activities, and events.

By way of illustration, certain elements in the history that must be drawn from the patient are presented in Table 5-8. Although the verbal assessment process may seem tedious, such disclosures may help immeasurably in producing the highest tier of therapcutic success.

The ability to locomote and perform the activities of daily living are important considerations because some patients are incontinent simply due to their inability to reach a toilet in time. Vaginal bleeding frequently is present and is usually due to irritation and friction involving atrophic mucosal surfaces. However, neoplasm must be ruled out by appropriate tests, as indicated, before hormone replacement therapy, so vital to good results, is initiated. In the same vein, awareness of previous breast disease, especially cancer, now so common, and of recent mammography results is essential. As fundamental as any other information is a detailed description of any and all symptoms relating to pelvic floor and cardinal-uterosacral relaxation. Obviously questions regarding protrusion and pressure are foremost. A history of urinary tract infections, pulmonary problems, diabetes, other debilitating medical conditions, and all previous surgery, especially pelvic operations, including hospital records, should be obtained as indicated. Other considerations include the use of drugs, particularly psychoactive and cardiovascular medications that may exert profound effects on urethral and vesical function, causing either retention or involuntary elimination of urine. Assessment of menopausal status is important because disability from incontinence and prolapse most commonly does not surface until a true estrogen deficiency state is established. The importance of the attenuating effects of such physiologic deprivation is poignantly highlighted by the discovery in recent years of estrogen receptors throughout the lower urinary system, especially the urethra and trigone.

Never to be neglected, the attitudinal and mental status, both cognitive and effective, must be astutely observed and assessed. Psychiatric disorders hamper diagnosis and treatment of incontinence, not to mention the adverse effects some of the psychotropic drugs may have on urinary tract function.

The urolog or voiding diary is a 24-hour journal of spontaneous micturition. It is an extremely cost-effective method of obtaining the history of voiding habits and functional bladder capacity. A simplified diary, preprinted in columns for the patient to complete at home before her first visit, is illustrated in Table 5-9. In it, the patient must indicate the time of each spontaneous micturition and the amount voided. There are also columns for the patient to record urgency experiences and involuntary urine leakages at various times during the day. Importantly, another column must display fluid intake during the same 24 hours. The patient is usually given a list of instructions, with explanations, to help her and to encourage her to complete this form accurately. Thus, the physician is provided with a reliable global view of drinking and voiding habits, including urinary idiosyncrasies. Such a record magnifies in value if it is continued for 3 to 4 days. It is a pragmatic approach to the evaluation of urethral and vesical function through delineation of storage and excretory capabilities.

Physical Examination

The urogynecologic physical examination is more function specific than the usual gynecologic examination. When performed, simple clinical tests can be carried out as indicated simultaneously (Table 5-10).

A neurologic evaluation must be included to assess the sensory, motor, and proprioceptive function of nerve roots L5 to S4. Reflexes such as the anal and

TABLE 5-9 Voiding Diary

Time	Amount Voided	Activity	Leak Volume	Urge Present	Amount/Type of Intake

clitoral reflexes should be elicited. Assessment of sensation to sharp and dull stimuli and motor strength of the lower extremities are important in this evaluation to rule out neurologic causes for urinary tract symptoms. Comparing any areas of abnormal sensation with a dermatome chart can point to possible neurologic deficits (Figure 5-4). Motor strength is tested by inverting and everting the foot and extending and flexing the hip, knee, ankle, and toe joints (Figure 5-5). The remainder of the physical examination is similar to the gynecologic physical examination with emphasis on detection of weaknesses and defects throughout the entire pelvic musculofascial network.

A so-called provocative vaginal examination, in the assessment of precise degrees of pelvic relaxation, is initiated by the insertion of the posterior blade of the

TABLE 5-10 Evaluation—Phase II:
Physical Examination

General
Neurologic
Vaginal (provocative)
    Lithotomy
    Standing
Rectal
Pelvic muscular tonicity

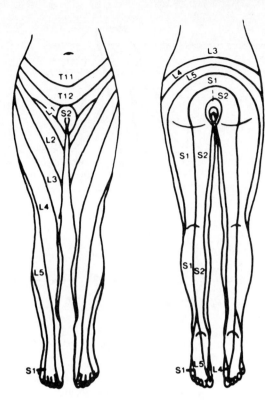

Figure 5-4 Front and rear views of dermatome segments corresponding to the denoted spinal nerves.

bivalve speculum independently into the posterior vaginal area, exerting pressure on the rectum. Then, while the patient bears down, the anterior vaginal wall is observed. If they are present, a hypermotile urethra, a cystocele, an anterior vault prolapse, or a cervical descensus can then be perceived. Similarly, the speculum can be rotated 180 degrees to observe the posterior wall. Again, during Valsalva, any posterior vault weakness, enterocele, or rectocele may be visually delineated. After the speculum is removed, two fingers are inserted into the vagina and the patient is again asked to strain maximally following a cough. The tactile stimulation of the examining fingers pointed anteriorly, posteriorly, laterally, and superiorly will determine the presence and degree of anterior, posterior, lateral, or superior vaginal wall defects in patients as they strain. The presence and degree of descent of the cervix or vagina may also be apprised during this maneuver. It is important to emphasize to the patient that, during bearing down, she should undertake a maximal effort and not be embarrassed by any involuntary loss of urine or rectal gas. Abnormal anatomic findings of pelvic floor relaxation often coexist with lower urinary tract symptoms. However, they may be present in the absence of incontinence. The digital examination must be repeated with the patient standing, particularly because defects and prolapses can be most accurately delineated only in this posture. Practically speaking, the older the patient, the more apt you are to

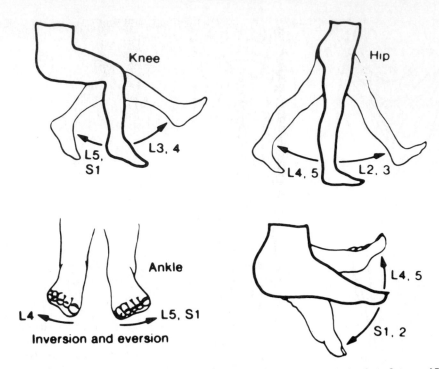

Figure 5-5 Motor tests of the lower extremities. (Reproduced with permission from Ostergard DR, Bent AE, eds. *Urogynecology and Urodynamics*. 3rd ed. Baltimore: Williams & Wilkins; 1991:103.)

learn what is wrong when she is standing rather than in the lithotomy position. Finally, as the digital examination is being completed, pelvic floor, vaginal, and rectal striated muscle tone should be checked and noted via the usual isotonic squeezing exercise.

Simple Clinical Tests

The Q-tip or swab urethral test is easily performed at the time of the examination (Table 5-11). A cotton swab lubricated with anesthetic jelly is gently placed

TABLE 5-11 Evaluation—Phase II: Simple Clinical Tests

Q-tip (cotton swab) test
Cough stress test
Postvoid residual urine
Urethral calibration

through the urethra so that the cotton tip is at the bladder neck.[15] This anatomic position can be found by gently placing the cotton applicator through the urethra into the bladder until the resistance disappears and then pulling back until resistance is felt again. Any sensation of markedly reduced resistance should be noted because it may predict an incompetent or poorly functioning urethra. The patient should be in the supine lithotomy position. The angle the Q-tip makes with respect to the long axis of the body is measured with an orthopedic goniometer with a leveling bubble affixed to it. If the wooden end of the cotton swab or applicator is parallel to the long axis of the body, it is considered to be at 0 degrees. The patient is asked to strain maximally and then cough; if there is significant rotational descent of the bladder neck, the wooden end of the cotton swab will point upward. The change in the angle from 0 degrees (arbitrarily chosen to be parallel to the long axis of the body) upward will be measured in positive degrees. Anything greater than a 30-degree deflection from the horizontal is considered abnormal, constituting evidence of rotational descent of the bladder neck (Figure 5-6). Patients who have a fixed urethra may have no descent at all, and patients who have had previous retropubic surgery may even have negative resting and straining angles. This test is essential for helping to determine whether or not patients are usual surgical candidates, because patients who have a fixed urethra may often not be candidates for conventional incontinence surgery, particularly if they have abnormal urethral pressure on urodynamic testing. One must be sure that the patient understands fully how to produce the Valsalva maneuver (bear down or strain). Although this command may seem rather simple to clinicians, sometimes the patient does not understand what we mean when we say bear down and a word of explanation is required.

The patient performs the cough stress test with a full bladder, in the standing position, often with one foot placed on a low stool, while she is asked to cough. Patients with genuine stress incontinence usually lose urine in spurts synchronous with each cough. Patients with cough-induced instability will have some short delay in the loss of urine after the cough. They will also have urgency, whereas those with stress incontinence in general do not. The cough stress test alone, however, is not sufficient to diagnose either genuine stress incontinence or vesical instability. Combining the cough stress test with single-channel cystometry can carry 95% positive predictive value in genuine stress incontinence in younger patients, but it is probably not as accurate in the elderly who are more likely to have low pressure urethral dysfunction causing incontinence.[16]

Determining the residual urine is often overlooked and, if not performed, needless error may result when trying to pin down a diagnosis in women with lower urinary tract dysfunction. Patients with significant residual urine can appear superficially to have either genuine stress incontinence or vesical instability, when in reality they have overflow incontinence. *No patient should be brought to the operating room or given a treatment for vesical instability without adequate determination of residual urine.* Significant residual urine may also predispose

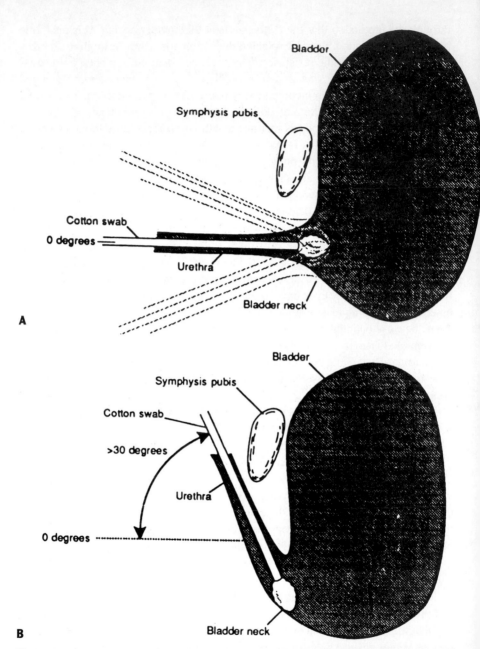

Figure 5-6 A, Resting Q-tip test—genuine stress incontinence. B, Straining Q-tip test—genuine stress incontinence. (Reproduced with permission from Scotti RJ. Urethral syndrome and urethral infections. *Infect Surge.* 1989;8:102-112.)

TABLE 5-12 Evaluation—Phase III: Simple Urodynamic and Endoscopic Studies

Uroflowmetry
Cystometry
Cystourethroscopy
Urethral profilometry (single channel)

patients for recurrent urinary tract infections. The postvoid residual is simple to determine and should never be overlooked! It is easily performed after spontaneous uroflowmetry or spontaneous voiding. It is mandatory, particularly in elderly patients, who often have incomplete voiding.

When urethral obstruction is suspected, urethral calibration may be performed with urethral dilators, measuring in French units. It should be performed only to rule out urethral stenosis. It is of little value in patients without urgency or without impaired flow. It can be performed at any time during the work-up, but should not be performed just prior to cystourethroscopy or it may traumatize the urethra and introduce artifact into urethroscopic visualization.

EVALUATION—PHASE III: SIMPLE URODYNAMIC AND ENDOSCOPIC TESTS

These procedures (Table 5-12) are simple to perform and can usually be accomplished by a generalist with minimal urodynamic equipment.

Uroflowmetry

Uroflowmetry is simply the measure of the urinary flow rate expressed in milliliters per second. Average uroflowmetry can be performed with a stopwatch and a urine collection pan. The calculation is simple:

$$\text{Flow} = \frac{\text{Amount Voided (mL)}}{\text{Time (s)}}$$

Ideal uroflow values are based on a 200-mL voided volume. The patient should void to completion within 20 seconds with a peak flow rate of 20 mL/s and an average flow rate of at least 10 mL/s. Many patients do not follow these ideal parameters; however, if the patient can void to completion comfortably without residual urine, undue straining, or splinting of the vagina or perineum, she can be considered to have essentially normal voiding function. Uroflow is really a screening tool for assessing urethral relaxation and bladder contraction, but it measures these indirectly as a function of flow.

If the patient has impaired flow, the voiding mechanism or voiding pressure, which measures urethral pressure, vesical pressure, and flow (phase IV), must be assessed urodynamically; urethral calibration must also be performed to rule out urethral stenosis. The value of uroflow as a study is somewhat limited unless it corroborates urethral stenosis as a cause for urinary urgency, retention, or urethral syndrome. It is an excellent screening tool particularly in patients with high residuals. In general, if the patient can void to completion without high residuals, uroflowmetry adds little but may prove important as a base when following these patients later.

Uroflowmetry has value subsequent to incontinence surgery, when indicated, to rule out obstruction and to follow patients postoperatively. It is also useful in patients with advancing urogenital prolapse to assess changes in flow resulting from obstruction. Uroflowmetry can also be used to follow patients who have had previous urodynamically diagnosed voiding disorders in which obstructed flow is a component. Occasionally, it may play a diagnostic role in patients with impaired vesical contractility subsequent to radical hysterectomy or abdominal-perineal resections. Uroflowmetry cannot, however, by itself, discern between obstructive flow and poor bladder contractility; to make this determination, a voiding pressure study must be performed (phase IV).

Spontaneous uroflowmetry can be conveniently performed on the first visit, even before obtaining results of culture and sensitivity, because it is a noninvasive test. If it is abnormal, it should be repeated. If the patient voids at least 200 mL and the flow is normal, she should be expected to void to completion without residual urine. The determination of residual urine by catheter or ultrasound can be performed immediately after spontaneous uroflowmetry.

Despite the aforementioned shortcomings, uroflowmetry is a simple test yielding much valuable information and should be carried out in all patients with lower urinary tract symptoms. Several characteristic flow patterns are illustrated graphically in Figures 5-3 and 5-7.

Cystometry

Cystometry is probably the most useful tool in the work-up of the incontinent patient. Without it, one cannot diagnose genuine stress incontinence or vesical instability because the definition of the former excludes and of the latter includes spontaneous or uninhibited detrusor contractions. This study can be performed with modern urodynamic equipment, using electronic pressure transducers, or with simplified equipment using a manometer attached to an intravenous pole, a Foley catheter, and an intravenous solution of sterile saline or water at 38°C, which is infused into the bladder via an ordinary single-channel catheter (Figure 5-8). Glucose-containing solutions should not be used because they may promote urinary tract infections when instilled into the bladder.

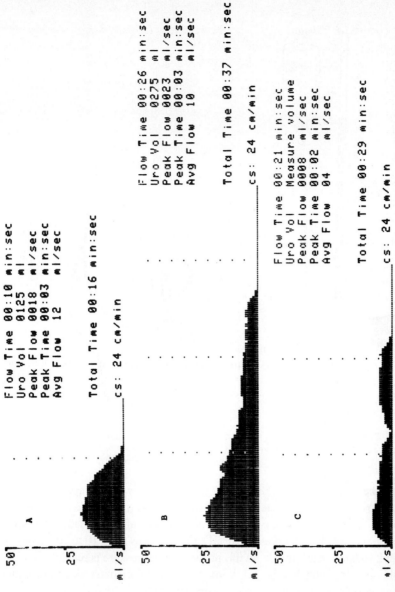

Figure 5-7 Sample uroflowmetry studies. A, Normal flow rate, normal flow time. B, Normal flow rate, abnormal flow time. C, Prolonged intermittent obstructed flow.

A

```
Flow Time 00:10 min:sec
Uro Vol    0125 ml
Peak Flow  0018 ml/sec
Peak Time 00:03 min:sec
Avg Flow    12 ml/sec

Total Time 00:16 min:sec

cs: 24 cm/min
```

B

```
Flow Time 00:26 min:sec
Uro Vol    0275 ml
Peak Flow  0023 ml/sec
Peak Time 00:03 min:sec
Avg Flow    10 ml/sec

Total Time 00:37 min:sec

cs: 24 cm/min
```

C

```
Flow Time 00:21 min:sec
Uro Vol   Measure volume
Peak Flow  0008 ml/sec
Peak Time 00:02 min:sec
Avg Flow    04 ml/sec

Total Time 00:29 min:sec

cs: 24 cm/min
```

117

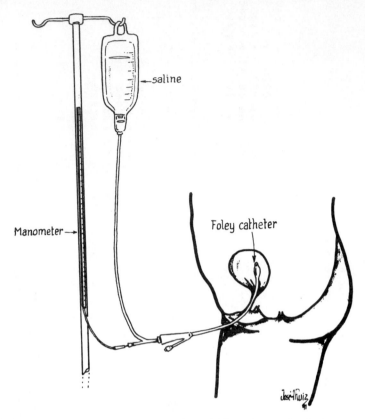

saline

Manometer→

Foley catheter

Figure 5-8 Simple cytometry using readily available equipment. A spinal manometer, Foley catheter, and adapters are all that are needed.

With the patient standing, her bladder is filled at a flow rate of approximately 80 to 100 mL/min. The manometer or transducer is set to atmospheric pressure which is given the arbitrary pressure of 0 cm of water pressure after the bladder is emptied. The normal empty bladder pressure in all patients varies from 10 to 20 cm of water pressure, so one can arbitrarily set this pressure. The pressure is readjusted to 10 to 20 mL once infusion has begun, particularly if the catheter does not contain separate ports for pressure and flow. Any spontaneous bladder contractions in excess of 15 mL of water pressure from the baseline, almost always accompanied by urgency, is prima facie evidence that the patient has vesical instability (Figure 5-9A). If the patient loses urine synchronous with cough during the test, in the absence of uninhibited vesical contractions, she has by definition, genuine stress incontinence.

As the bladder is filled, the first sensation of bladder filling, the sensation of bladder fullness, and the maximum bladder capacity are all recorded at the particular volume of infused liquid. Using water or saline as the infusing medium, most

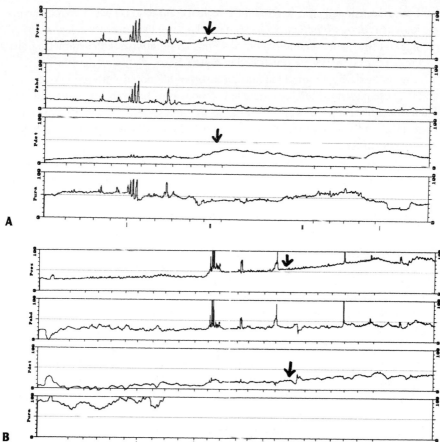

Figure 5-9 A, Vesical instability. Arrow indicates the beginning of a large detrusor contraction. B, Loss of bladder compliance. Note the steady upward increase beginning at the arrows.

premenopausal patients will experience the first sensation of fluid in their bladders between 100 and 150 mL; they will announce fullness between 150 and 250 mL and reach maximum bladder capacity between 250 and 600 mL. These values are idealized and are age dependent. They also depend on the size of the bladder as well as the physical characteristics of the patient. Postmenopausal patients may reach maximum capacity at 250 mL and may also have decreased compliance (Figure 5-9B). If CO_2 is used as the infusing medium, the values are somewhat lower owing to probable irritation of the bladder wall with CO_2 or its dissociation into HCO_3.

During the procedure, the patient is asked at periodic intervals (usually with every 100-mL increment) to cough and to bounce on her heels. The cough maneuver may elicit cough-induced vesical instability. This is often a delayed phenomenon, and the tracing or the manometer should be observed carefully over a 15-second interval. After this maneuver is completed, the patient is asked to bounce on her heels. Occasionally this will induce a vesical contraction. These two maneuvers are known as *detrusor activating procedures* because they may stimulate a vesical contraction in a symptomatic patient who has an otherwise flat cystometrogram. Examples of cystometry are illustrated in Figure 5-9.

A nonreflexic hypotonic bladder can also be diagnosed with the cystometrogram. These patients often have delayed responses of first sensation and fullness. Their maximum bladder capacity can be as high as 800 mL to several thousand milliliters without a strong urge to void. Many diabetic patients have this cystometric finding.

In summary, the cystometrogram is probably the single most valuable study in the evaluation in incontinence. Its diagnostic importance cannot be overemphasized. The cystometrogram must be performed in all patients complaining of urgency, urge incontinence, or stress incontinence.

Cystourethroscopy

The term *dynamic urethroscopy,* coined by Robertson, underscores the functional import of this study. According to various investigators, during filling or when the patient is asked to strain or hold her urine, the normal bladder neck closes during urethroscopic observation.[17-19] The technique is usually performed in the supine position with a 0-degree female urethroscope.

The functional urethroscopic features observed are closure of the bladder neck in continent women and, conversely, failure of closure of the bladder neck in incontinent women during filling or after a command to "hold the urine" or "squeeze the rectum" is given by the examiner. The bladder neck may also not close in incontinent women during coughing or straining. The technique of urethroscopy may be performed using CO_2 or water as the insufflating or infusing medium. Urethroscopy, however, can give functional information about stress incontinence with only 75% positive predictive accuracy.[20] It is not nearly as reliable as multichannel urodynamics in functional disorders such as stress incontinence and vesical instability.[20]

Urethroscopy is much more valuable for anatomic conditions. Marked pallor of urethra suggests hypoestrogenism. With the growing number of postmenopausal women in the population, urethral symptomatology related to hypoestrogenism has vastly increased, and urethroscopy is a useful tool for assessing the hormonal status of the urethra. Urethroscopy can also delineate other anatomic conditions, such as chronic urethritis, acute urethritis, urethral diverticula (Figure 5-10), polyps, fronds, and urethral spasm, although functional studies such as urethral pressure profiles are more suitable for the diagnosis of urethral spasm. Cystourethroscopy is not indicated for all patients with lower urinary tract symptoms but should be done specifically on those who complain of urgency or who are suspect for urethral diverticulum or urethral infection. Also, symptoms of the urethral syndrome, such as urgency, frequency, suprapubic pain, and urethral pain, demand urethroscopic investigation.

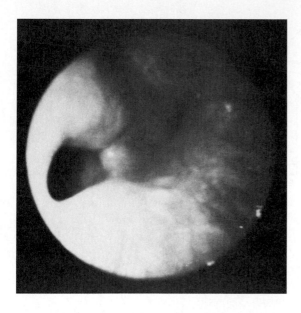

Figure 5-10 Urethral diverticulum. Note large orifice at 8 o'clock. (Courtesy of Jack R. Robertson, MD, Las Vegas.)

Single-Channel Urethral Pressure Profile

Numerous investigators have described the low pressure urethra and the high failure rate of conventional retropubic surgery in patients with a low pressure urethra.[21–24]

The *low pressure urethra* is defined as a resting urethral pressure less than 20 mL of water. It is present in patients with a dysfunctional urethra, i.e., when the urethra itself is weak and cannot exert sufficient pressure to contain fluid in the bladder. Patients at risk for a low pressure urethra are women over age 60, women who have had previous incontinence procedures resulting in neuropathy or scarring (the so-called drain pipe urethra), and women with other neurologic deficits. These patients often have no descent of the bladder neck or proximal urethra outside the abdominal pressure zone during straining or coughing as a mechanism for their incontinence. They are likely to have poor urethral tone as a cause for their incontinence. This is also called type III stress incontinence.

Because of the increasing incidence of this condition, especially in the aging population, single-channel urethral pressure profiles should be performed before undertaking periurethral or incontinence surgery on all patients over 65 years of age, patients who have had previous failed incontinence surgery, women with neurologic disease, and probably those with mixed stress and urge incontinence. This can be done most simply with a single-channel urodynamics monitor. The urethral closure pressure can be determined by pulling a microtransducer or a water pressure transducer through the urethra. One will record the bladder pressure as well as the peak urethral pressure (Figure 5-11A). The difference between these

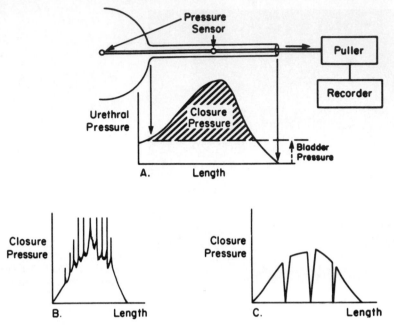

Figure 5-11 A, The double microtip electronic catheter is pulled through the urethra. The microtransducer (pressure sensor) at the tip of the catheter continuously monitors bladder pressure, while the second transducer monitors urethral pressure along its entire length. The tracing generated depicts a normal status (resting) urethral pressure profile. B, A normal stress (cough) urethral pressure profile. Note that the urethral pressure is always higher than bladder pressure in a continent patient. C, An abnormal stress urethral pressure profile. Note that the urethral pressure is equal to bladder pressure with cough in an incontinent patient.

will be the urethral closure pressure (Figure 5-11B). A closure pressure less than 20 mL of water constitutes a low pressure urethra (Figure 5-11C). Currently Horbach and colleagues[22] and McGuire and coworkers[25,26] recommend a sling procedure on patients with a low pressure urethra. Other incontinence procedures have not been adequately evaluated at this time. However, Meschia and colleagues have recently reported successful Burch procedures for the low pressure urethra.[27] These operations and the objective criteria for their choice will be discussed in the next chapter.

EVALUATION—PHASE IV: MULTICHANNEL URODYNAMICS, SPECIAL IMAGING, AND ELECTRODIAGNOSTICS

Multichannel Urethrocystometry

Fewer than 10% of patients actually require complete multichannel urodynamic assessment (Table 5-13). Patients who reach this phase should be those with

TABLE 5-13 Evaluation—Phase IV:
Complex Technical Studies

Multichannel urodynamics
   Urethrocystometry
   Pressure voiding study
   Electromyography

Prolapse reduction test

Imaging analyses
   Double-balloon urethrography
   Resting and straining cystography
   Voiding cystourethrography
   Video cystourethrography

Neuromyographic testing
   Pudendal nerve latency
   Perineal nerve latency
   Nerve fiber density

unresolved mixed symptoms of urgency and stress incontinence and those anticipating repair of a very large cystocele, enterocele, or vaginal vault prolapse. Also to
be included are situations of continued doubtful diagnosis, previous failed incontinence surgery, and suspicion of neuropathy.

Multichannel studies are recorded on instruments available from various manufacturers or on any polygraph adapted for this specific purpose. Multichannel
urodynamic monitors measure urethral, bladder, and abdominal pressures and
calculate the urethral closure pressure and the true detrusor pressure.

The *urethral closure pressure* is defined as the pressure in the urethra in excess
of bladder pressure and is obtained urodynamically by subtracting bladder pressure
from urethral pressure ($P_{ur} - P_{ves} = P_{uc}$). It is precisely this pressure in the urethra
that keeps the patient from leaking urine. The higher the urethral closure pressure
during cough, the more likely is the patient to remain continent. It is a significant
determinant of continence. Figure 5-12 illustrates the reverse during cough in a
woman with genuine stress incontinence. The urethral closure pressure drops
distinctly below bladder pressure and urine spurts.

The true detrusor pressure isolates the bladder pressure from abdominal pressure. A transducer placed in the bladder will measure vesical (detrusor) pressure.
Abdominal pressure is measured by a separate transducer placed in the vagina or
rectum. Subtracting the abdominal pressure from the intravesical pressure yields
the *true detrusor pressure* ($P_{ves} - P_{abd} = P_{true\ det}$). The urodynamic monitor will
perform the subtraction and record the true detrusor pressure, thereby eliminating
artifact that could occur in the unsubtracted bladder lead if the patient inadvertently
strains.

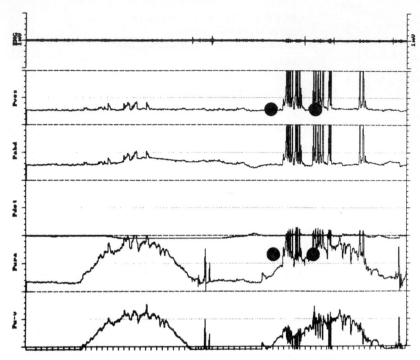

Figure 5-12 A cough profile in an incontinent patient. The resting profile shows normal pressure. The cough profile, indicated by multiple cough spikes, demonstrates that urethral pressure becomes equal to or drops below bladder pressure during cough, accompanied by urine loss.

Simultaneous flow and electromyography can also be measured. Multichannel urethral pressure profiles, cystometry, and voiding pressure studies can thus be performed (Figure 5-13).

Multichannel urethrocystometry can also be performed to determine if other variables, such as urethral instability or voluntary increases in intra-abdominal or vesical pressure, contribute to symptoms of incontinence. It gives similar results to those of single-channel cystometry for bladder parameters, but because it continuously monitors urethral pressure, it enables the clinician to diagnose urethral instability, urethral spasm, and uninhibited urethral relaxation (Figure 5-14). It also enables measurement of true detrusor pressure and synchronous or nonsynchronous events in the bladder and urethra. One may also measure bladder compliance with multichannel as well as single-channel cystometry.

Multichannel Resting (Static) Urethral Pressure Profiles

When catheters placed in the bladder are pulled through the urethra, resting (static) urethral pressure profiles are generated. Both urethral length and pressure can be

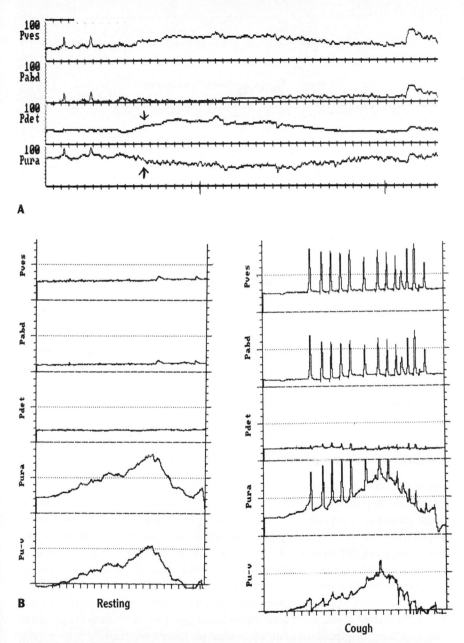

Figure 5-13 A, Multichannel urethrocystometrogram shows vesical instability with concomitant urethral relaxation (arrows). B, Multichannel urethral pressure profile, both static (resting) and stress (cough). Both are normal. C, Multichannel voiding pressure study. When the patient voids, the urethra relaxes followed in 3 to 5 seconds by a bladder contraction with concomitant flow. Note that this patient had intermittent flow after the initial bladder contraction caused by repeated Valsalva. At the conclusion of flow, the resting urethral pressure recovers to the same (or in this case, higher) pressure as the original resting pressure.

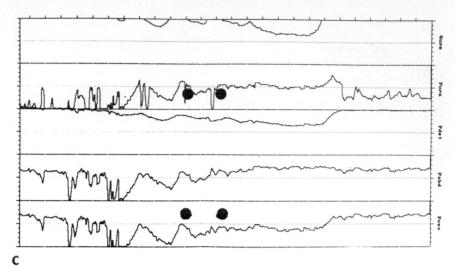

C

Figure 5-13 *Continued*

determined although urethral pressure is the only real significant determinant of urethral function. The bladder and abdominal pressures are continuously monitored while urethral pressure and length are measured. The patient is asked not to cough or strain.

Multichannel Urethral Cough Profile (Stress Profile)

The cough profile is a urethral pressure profile performed during coughing. It is particularly important to distinguish between the resting or static profile and the cough profile (see Figures 5-12 and 5-13B). Most patients with genuine stress incontinence will have normal urethral resting profiles and low or absent urethral closure pressure during a cough. This is logical because these patients are only incontinent during a cough or other increase in intra-abdominal pressure. When the static profile shows normal urethral pressure and the cough profile is positive (the pressure becomes equal to bladder pressure), the urodynamic test indicates that during the instant of cough (or other stress that triggers incontinence) the proximal urethra is being displaced out of the abdominal pressure zone, thereby momentarily creating a loss of pressure in the urethra relative to the intra-abdominal bladder. Thus, a momentary pressure gradient develops with involuntary flow from bladder through urethra at the moment of cough. Patients with a positive cough profile and a history of the symptom of stress incontinence are urodynamically diagnosed as having genuine stress incontinence.

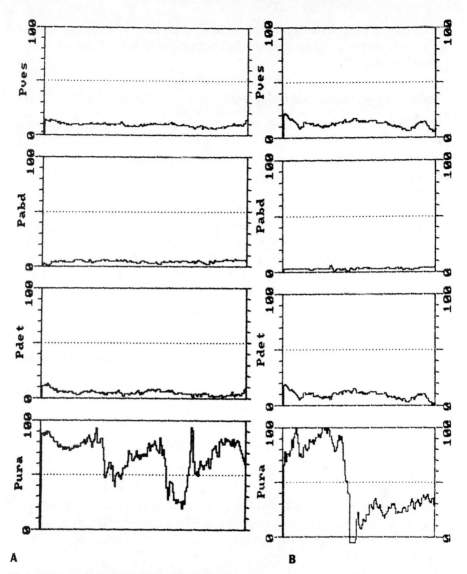

A   **B**

Figure 5-14 A, Urethral instability. Note the fluctuating urethral pressure. This is often accompanied by urgency or urge incontinence. B, Uninhibited urethral relaxation. Note the drop in urethral pressure, which is usually accompanied by incontinence.

Voiding Pressure Studies

The voiding pressure study is a functional blueprint of events that occur during micturition. The patient is asked to void with catheters in place. In a normal subject, urethral relaxation and quieting of the electromyogram will be the first physiologic events recorded. These will be followed in 3 to 5 seconds by a vesical contraction.

Abdominal pressure usually remains unchanged. Patients with voiding disorders (e.g., neuropathy, previous radical hysterectomy) may have abnormal voiding pressure studies.[28]

The Pessary (Prolapse Reduction) Test

This test is used for surgical candidates with large cystoceles, large enteroceles, or vaginal vault prolapse, in whom a kinking effect on the urethra by the large urogenital prolapse prevents urine loss during cough or straining.[29,30] Many of these patients may develop stress incontinence postoperatively after surgical correction of the vaginal relaxation because the urethral obstruction may be relieved by reducing the large cystocele or prolapse if the hypermobile urethra, even though asymptomatic preoperatively, is not simultaneously repositioned. Before surgery, multichannel urodynamic cough profiles should be performed with the cystocele, rectocele, or prolapse reduced by a pessary, a Sims speculum, or a vaginal finger pointed to S3 to S4 (that does not occlude the urethra), and then repeated after the patient strains and the prolapse redescends. Patients whose urogenital prolapse causes a kinking effect of the urethra while the prolapse is extended will have high urethral pressures and continence. These same women may have low pressure, frank leakage, or reduced margins to leakage when the prolapse is reduced[31] (Figures 5-15 and 5-16). Cases showing a marked diminution in urethral pressure with the prolapse reduced are candidates for concomitant urethropexy as part of the total repair of the urogenital prolapse. Many authors have warned about the spontaneous development of stress incontinence in patients who have vaginal relaxation repaired without prior urodynamic assessment and without some suspension of the bladder neck at the time of vaginal repair if indicated.[29–32]

Special Imaging Studies

The voiding cystourethrogram and the double-balloon positive pressure urethrography offer methods for diagnosing urethral diverticula. They are far more accu-

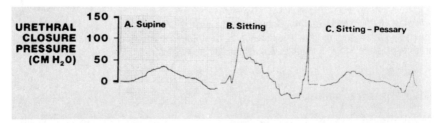

Figure 5-15 Urethral pressure profile in urogenital prolapse. The resting urethral pressure is high when the prolapse is extended in the sitting position (B). Resting profile with prolapse is reduced either by placing the patient in a supine position or by inserting a pessary, thereby unkinking the urethra and causing a lowered pressure (A, C).

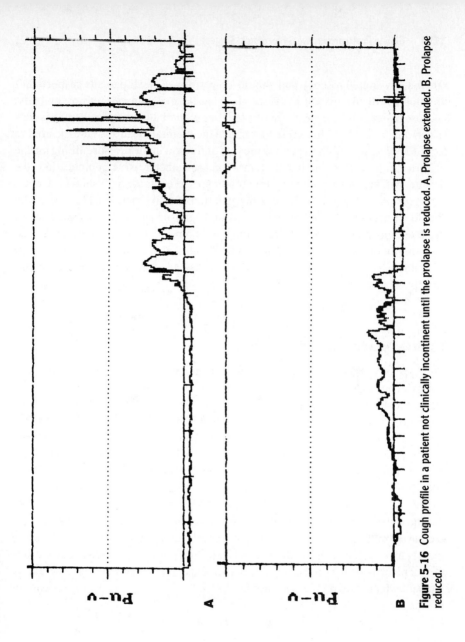

Figure 5-16 Cough profile in a patient not clinically incontinent until the prolapse is reduced. A, Prolapse extended. B, Prolapse reduced.

rate than cystourethroscopy and should be performed in all patients suspected of urethral diverticula, even if a diverticulum has been diagnosed urethroscopically, because diverticula can often be multiple. The double-balloon catheter study is easy to perform, as balloons in the bladder and at the urethral meatus isolate the urethra from the bladder and the external meatus and allow high pressure filling of the urethra.[33] Injection of dye into a channel in the catheter, which empties into the urethra, will then fill any diverticulum under pressure. Figure 5-17 shows a Tratner catheter study performed with the demonstration of a diverticulum. Urethrography should be performed in all patients with undiagnosed suburethral masses and in those complaining of postvoid dribbling in whom urethroscopy does not reveal urethral diverticular orifices. These studies should also be performed in patients with clinically or urethroscopically diagnosed diverticula to rule out the presence of multiple diverticula.

Video Cystourethrography

This type of sophisticated testing can record the multichannel urodynamic tracing alongside an x-ray of the bladder and urethra on the same video screen. It is an attempt to display simultaneously both anatomic and functional data. Although this technique is popular in Europe and the United Kingdom, it has not reached widespread usage in the United States and Canada because it requires concomitant radiologic technology creating obvious space and personnel complexities. With more widespread usage of ultrasound techniques and the availability of digital recording of ultrasound images, ultrasound techniques may replace x-ray in the future.

The value of imaging the bladder and urethra while performing urodynamics has certain advantages. It may give useful information about anatomic abnormalities of the bladder such as diverticula, fistulae, and funneling. It also may indicate improper placement of transducers or displacement of transducers during urodynamic studies (which would otherwise not be noticed), giving erroneous or misleading results.

Electrodiagnostic Testing

Pelvic floor electrophysiologic testing has been added to the diagnostic armamentarium of the urogynecologist. It has been suggested by Snooks and colleagues that normal vaginal delivery may lead to pudendal or perineal nerve damage that could become permanent.[34] Neurophysiolgic weakness of the pelvic floor will then develop and may be a factor in the genesis of incontinence. The neurogenic hypothesis of stress incontinence[34] presumes that chronic partial denervation of the pelvic musculature occurs progressively following injury initiated during child-

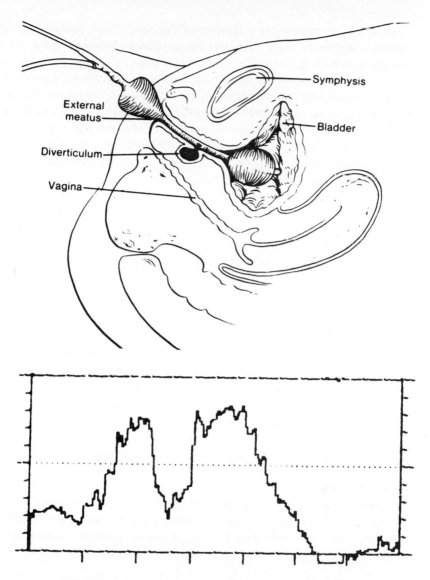

Figure 5-17 A, The double-balloon Tratner catheter. The channel opens into the urethra. Radiopaque fluid is injected into this channel to opacify urethral diverticula, allowing them to be readily seen by x-ray. B, Urodynamic tracing of a patient with a diverticulum. Note the reduction in urethral pressure at the area of the diverticulum.

birth, especially if sustained by repeated stretch-induced injury during straining from other subsequent activities, especially those that increase intra-abdominal pressure. Third or fourth degree lacerations at the time of delivery have also been shown to lead to decreased rectal sphincter tone and strength as well as decreased puborectalis function despite repair at the time of injury.[36–38]

To assess neurophysiologic function of the pelvic floor, pelvic electromyography is performed using either needle or surface electrodes connected to a polygraph. Recording electrostimulation techniques[39] offer objective information of neuromuscular function by stimulating the pudendal nerve on either side of the pelvis and measuring the time (latency) from stimulation to response. This test is performed by using an electrode attached to a glove, thereby permitting the examiner's finger to correctly place the electrode transrectally or transvaginally on the pudendal nerve. Information obtained by these techniques includes motor and sensory latency and evoked potentials of both pudendal and perineal nerves. This information is especially useful in patients with low pressure urethra without anatomic defects because neuropathy may be the cause for incontinence in this group of patients. Patients with poor rectal tone, poor levator tone, other neurologic abnormalities, or a history suggestive of neurologic injury are candidates for electrophysiologic testing. Perineal nerve testing can also be performed using an electrode attached to a special bladder catheter.

SUMMARY

The multiplicity of diagnostic procedures available for the assessment of patients with lower urinary tract symptoms illustrates that no one or two tests can provide definitive information. In general, clinicians should proceed with simple to more complex tests only if an accurate diagnosis cannot be made by more simple tests.

The most cost-effective and time-efficient tests that yield the most focused information and indicate direction for further testing are the cough stress test, single-channel cystometry, Q-tip test, and postvoid residual. After ruling out infection and a thorough history and physical examination, these simple studies are invaluable and should never be omitted.

All tests, however, should be considered as relatively soft data to be placed into the clinician's biocomputer for careful consideration. It is the astute clinician who can reasonably synthesize these data and arrive at an accurate diagnosis and a rational treatment plan based on this information.

Acknowledgment
The author would like to acknowledge the assistance of Raul Mendelovici, M.D., in the preparation of this manuscript.

REFERENCES

1. Hilton P, Millard PH. The elderly. In: Stanton SL, ed. *Clinical Gynecologic Urology.* St. Louis: CV Mosby; 1984:354.

2. Young JZ. *An Introduction to the Study of Man.* Oxford: Oxford Clarendon Press; 1971:331.

3. Studd J, Chakravarti S, Oram D. The climacteric. *Clin Obstet Gynecol.* 1977;4:3–29.

4. Urinary Incontinence Consensus Conference. *JAMA.* 1989;261:2685–2690.

5. Mohide EA. The prevalence and scope of urinary incontinence. *Clin Geriatr Med.* 1986;2:639–657.

6. Milne JS. Urinary symptoms in older people. *Mod Geriatr.* 1972;2:198–212.

7. Milne JS. Prevalence of incontinence. In: Willington FL, ed. *Incontinence in the Elderly.* London: Academic Press; 1976:9–21.

8. Adams GF, McIlwraith PM. *Geriatric Nursing.* Oxford: Oxford Press; 1963:34.

9. Beck RP, Armsch B, King C. Results in treating 210 patients with detrusor overactivity incontinence of urine. *Am J Obstet Gynecol.* 1976;125:593.

10. Brocklehurst JC, Dillane JB. Studies of the female bladder in old age. II: cystometrograms in non-incontinent women. *Geront Clin Basel.* 1966;8:285–305.

11. Resnick NM, Yalla SV, Laureno E. The pathophysiology of urinary incontinence among institutionalized elderly persons. *N Engl J Med.* 1989;320:1–7.

12. Lewis WH Jr, Alving AS. Changes with age in the renal function of adult men. *Am J Physiol.* 1938;123;500–515.

13. Bates P, Bradley WE, Glen E, et al. First report on the standardization of terminology of lower urinary tract function. Urinary incontinence. Procedures related to the evaluation of urine storage-cystometry, urethral closure pressure profile, units of measurement. *Br J Urol.* 1976;48:39–42; *Eur Urol.* 1976;2:274–276; *Scand J Urol Nephrol.* 1976;11:193–196; *Urol Int.* 1976;32:81–87.

14. Rife CC, Farrow GM, Utz DC. Urine cytology of transitional cell neoplasms. *Urol Clin North Amer.* 1979;6:599–612.

15. Scotti RJ, Ostergard DR. Investigating symptoms of lower urinary tract disease. *Contemp Obstet Gynecol.* 1986;27:79–97.

16. Scotti RJ, Myers DL. Predictive accuracy of the cough stress test and single channel cystometry compared to multichannel urodynamics. Presented at the American College of Obstetricians and Gynecologists 39th Annual Clinical Meeting, New Orleans, May, 1991.

17. Scotti RJ, Meyers DL. A comparison of the cough stress test and single-channel cystometry with multichannel urodynamic evaluation in genuine stress incontinence. *Obstet Gynecol.* 1993;81:430–433.

18. Kelly HA, Burnam CF. Diseases of the kidneys, ureters and bladder. First volume. New York: Appleton; 1992. *Gynecology.* 1983;61:144.

19. Ball TZ. *Gynecologic Surgery and Urology.* St. Louis: CV Mosby; 1957;145–152.

20. Robertson JR. Gynecologic urethroscopy. *Am J Obstet Gynecol.* 1972;115:986.

21 Scotti RJ, Ostergard DR, Guillaume AA, Kohatsu KE. Predictive value of urethroscopy as compared to urodynamics in the diagnosis of genuine stress incontinence. *J Reprod Med.* 1990;35:772–776.

22. McGuire EJ. Urodynamic findings in patients after failure of stress incontinence operations. *Prog Clin Biol Res.* 1981;78:351–357.

23. Horbach NS, Blanco JS, Ostergard DR, Bent AE, Cornella JL. A suburethral sling procedure with polytetrafluoroethylene for the treatment of genuine stress incontinence in patients with low urethral closure pressure. *Obstet Gynecol.* 1988;71:648–652.

24. Sand PK, Bowen LW, Panganipan R, Ostergard DR. The low pressure urethra as a factor in failed retropubic urethropexy. *Obstet Gynecol.* 1987;69:399–404.

25. Bowen LW, Sand PK, Ostergard DR, Franti CR. Unsuccessful Burch retropubic urethropexy: a case controlled urodynamic study. *Am J Obstet Gynecol.* 1989;160:452–458.

26. McGuire EJ, Lytton B. Pubovaginal sling procedure for stress incontinence. *J Urol.* 1978;119–82.

27. McGuire EJ, Bennett CJ, Konnak JA, Sonda LP, Savastano JA. Experience with pubovaginal slings for urinary incontinence at the University of Michigan. *J Urol.* 1987;138:525–529.

28. Meschia M, Barbacini P, Carena M, Marri R, Mele A. Unsuccessful Burch colposuspension: analysis of risk factors. *Int Urogyn J.* 1991;2:19–21.

29. Scotti RJ, Bergman AA, Bhatia N, Ostergard DR. Urodynamic changes in urethrovesical function subsequent to radical hysterectomy. *Obstet Gynecol.* 1986;68:111–120.

30. Bhatia NN, Bergman A. The pessary test in women with urinary incontinence. *Obstet Gynecol.* 1985;65:220.

31. Richardson DA, Bent AE, Ostergard DR. The effect of uterovaginal prolapse on urethrovesical pressure dynamics. *Am J Obstet Gynecol.* 1983;146:901.

32. Bump RC, Fantl JA, Hurt WG. The mechanism of urinary continence in women with severe uterovaginal prolapse: results of barrier studies. *Obstet Gynecol.* 1988;72:291–295.

33. Scotti RJ. Repair of genitourinary prolapse in women. *Curr Opin Obstet Gynecol.* 1991;3:404–412.

34. Davis HJ, Cain LG. Positive pressure urethrography: a new diagnostic method. *J Urol.* 1956;75:753.

35. Snooks SJ, Swash M, Mathers SE, Henry MM. Effect of vaginal delivery on the pelvic floor: a 5-year follow up. *Br J Surg.* 1990;77:1358–1360.

36. Swash M. The neurogenic hypothesis of stress incontinence. *Ciba Found Symp.* 1990;151:156–175.

37. Laurberg S, Swash M, Henry MM. Delayed external sphincter repair for obstetric tear. *Br J Surg.* 1988;75:786–788.

38. Go PMNYH, Dunselman FAJ. Anatomic and functional results of surgical repair after total perineal rupture at delivery. *Surg Gynecol Obstet.* 1988;166:121–124.

39. Haadem K, Dahlstrom JA, Ling L, Ohrlander S. Anal sphincter function after delivery rupture. *Obstet Gynecol.* 1987;70:53–56.

40. Pescatori M, Ravo B. Diagnostic anorectal functional studies—manometry, sphincter electromyography and defecography. *Surg Clin North Am.* 1988;68:1231–1247.

The Treatment of Genuine Stress Incontinence

Richard J. Scotti

The diagnosis of genuine stress incontinence, generally made urodynamically, has been described in detail in the previous chapter. After evaluation is completed and a diagnosis made, a variety of treatment options may be considered. These choices depend on many variables, some of which are not easily ascertained. The most important caveat in decision-making for treatment is that it must always involve the patient and her preferences. In other words, having been fully informed, coupled with objective guidance by the physician, the patient should always be encouraged to actively participate in the selection of therapy.

DECISION-MAKING

The most important variables in arriving at a decision for nonsurgical or surgical treatment are enumerated in Table 6-1. They are discussed below.

MEDICAL CONDITION AND AGE   Probably the most important factor in choosing a surgical or nonsurgical approach is status of health. Medical problems such as diabetes, chronic pulmonary disease, coronary artery attrition, previous cerebrovascular accident, generalized neuropathies, Alzheimer's disease, and systemic debilitation are all valid considerations as negative factors. Age is probably not as important a variable as the general medical condition of the patient. Hosking and colleagues have shown no difference in mortality or morbidity from

TABLE 6-1 Important Considerations in Surgical or Nonsurgical Decision-making

1. Medical condition and age
2. Severity of symptoms
3. Patient's choice: no surgery or surgery
4. Patient's suitability for surgery
5. Presence of other pelvic conditions necessitating simultaneous treatment
6. Strength of the pelvic floor
7. Presence or absence of low-pressure urethra
8. Presence or absence of urethral mobility
9. Presence or absence of detrusor instability or voiding difficulty
10. Presence or absence of pelvic floor neuropathy
11. History of previous surgery
12. Presence or absence of urethrovesical funneling

surgical procedures in patients between ages 65 and 90 from those in the same population not undergoing surgery, if they have no medical contraindication to surgery.[1] Gillon and Stanton have reported comparable surgical cure rates in elderly and younger age groups undergoing incontinence surgery.[2]

SEVERITY OF SYMPTOMS Unfortunately, most studies in the literature do not grade the severity of the symptoms when considering the success rate for cure of genuine stress incontinence. Confounding this lack of information are the patient differences in how symptoms affect life-style. An active athletic 40-year-old person may be affected differently from a mostly sedentary 70-year-old woman, and the converse may also be true. Personality differences also affect how individuals may variously react to mild degrees to severe degrees of incontinence. A more objective clinical assessment such as pad weights[3] may be useful in deciding degree of loss. A standing cough stress test[4] with a known amount in the bladder (by first emptying then filling) may also be useful, provided the patient is encouraged to cough with maximal effort. Certainly if a patient leaks urine with a cough in the supine position with a relatively empty bladder, she has fairly severe stress incontinence. Despite the utility of pad tests and clinical observation, the best judge of severity of symptoms is the patient herself.

PATIENT'S CHOICE: NO SURGERY OR SURGERY Certainly no responsible physician, patient advocate, or legal advisor would recommend surgery if the patient clearly does not want it except in the case of certain lifesaving procedures or in minors or other individuals who are unable to give their own consent. The question has broader ramifications when one considers the desirability for surgery in the patient with genuine stress incontinence. Because the most important issue is the quality of life in respect to incontinence, one must first ask questions regarding the impact of incontinence on the individual's life-style.

There is certainly vast individual variability in response to this question. As physicians, we are obliged to inform our patients about all the various options and chances for cure for each option, and allow the patient to pick the option most suitable for her. Borcier[5] has reported that 60% or more of patients when given a choice between a surgical and nonsurgical approach will opt for a nonsurgical approach. It is again the role of the responsible physician to offer the patient various conservative approaches, when appropriate, until either failure or success of conservative modalities is clear, thus arriving at the next phase of decision-making. At that point the patient may opt for a surgical approach if conservatism has failed. It is also reasonable to let the patient know when nonsurgical approaches really will not work or will not be satisfactory.

CONNECTIVE TISSUE STATUS Inherent collagen inadequacies[6] are unquestionably major factors in both the cause of genuine stress incontinence and the level of success of surgery to correct this condition. A wide variety of stresses and strains as life progresses compromise the quality of connective tissue of the body in general and that of the pelvis, at the bottom of the torso, in particular. Often optimal operative efforts are unsuccessful when performed in the presence of significant shortcomings in this category. The full gamut of congenital collagen deficiency syndrome and connective tissue atrophy, with special reference to the urinary system, is thoroughly discussed in Chapter 1.

PRESENCE OF OTHER PELVIC CONDITIONS NECESSITATING SIMULTANEOUS TREATMENT Many patients require surgery because of intractable vaginal bleeding, the presence of cervical or endometrial carcinoma, the presence of genitourinary prolapse, and so forth. These patients may have concomitant stress incontinence. Because they are candidates for surgical correction of their other conditions, the choice and route of surgery for stress incontinence may depend somewhat on the choice and route of surgery for the associated primary conditions. For example, a patient with intractable vaginal bleeding may elect to have a vaginal hysterectomy. The choice of a vaginal procedure for stress incontinence may be an important consideration. If, however, an abdominal route for stress incontinence may yield the highest cure rate, an abdominal hysterectomy should probably be considered. Similarly, a patient with vaginal vault prolapse or a large cystocele may be best served by a vaginal repair and wish to have both correction of genuine stress incontinence and pelvic relaxation performed vaginally at the same time.

The most important determinant that dictates the choice of surgical procedure for genuine stress incontinence is probably the objective success rate of the surgeon performing the procedure, with the same set of preoperative variables, alone or in combination with other pelvic surgical procedures. In our experience, we might perform a vaginal repair of symptomatic prolapse and an abdominal repair for incontinence to effect the best individual cure rates for each of these conditions. The vaginal route may be the best choice for genitourinary prolapse, whereas an abdominal retropubic urethropexy and colposuspension may be the most logical choice for incontinence. The best operation for each condition should be chosen and not necessarily the simplest, quickest, or most convenient for the surgeon. The failure rates of these simpler more convenient procedures must be factored into the equation for the surgical decision because reoperation in the future is likely to be much more complex, costly, and inconvenient.

STRENGTH OF THE PELVIC FLOOR For this evaluation, both electrical and pressure transducers have been used. The disadvantage of a pressure transducer such as a perineometer is that the device, when placed in the vagina, will measure not only pelvic floor contractions but also those of the abdominal wall. The simplest clinical method for assessing pelvic floor strength, as mentioned in the previous chapter, is physical assessment performed digitally by the examiner in both the vagina and rectum. By asking the patient to squeeze the rectum and vagina around the examining fingers, one can assess the relative strength of both the levator muscles and the external anal sphincter. We will usually ask the patient to stimulate rectal tightening as she would to prevent the loss of stool rectally in situations where a restroom is not immediately available. While digitally feeling the quality of first the levator and then the external anal sphincter tone, the examiner can assess both the resting and contracting muscle tone. Testing pelvic floor strength will indicate whether or not the patient may benefit from pelvic floor reeducation. If it is good, Kegel's or other exercises may not improve incontinence or increase muscle tone in patients with pelvic relaxation. For example, if the patient has severe stress incontinence with moderate to severe genitourinary prolapse, the determination of pelvic floor strength is somewhat academic because this patient needs surgery anyway. Certainly patients with mild incontinence producing minimal urine loss on cough or strain may derive great benefit both in terms of improvement or cure by conservative management such as pelvic floor stimulation or reeducation. Assessing the strength of the pelvic floor will therefore enable the clinician to make a decision regarding the effectiveness of pelvic floor exercise or electrical stimulation therapy.

PRESENCE OR ABSENCE OF LOW PRESSURE URETHRA McGuire[7] was the first author in the era of modern urodynamics to ask and answer the question "Why do patients fail incontinence surgery?" In his retrospective review of 114 patients, he concluded that "failure of multiple operations was associated with 75% incidence of type III sphincter dysfunction or a low resting urethral pressure (less than 20 cm H_2O) with or without hypermobility ... The majority [of patients in his study] had a well supported urethra in normal anatomic location ... which failed to exert sufficient closure pressure."[7] He was the first to

TABLE 6-2 Groups at Risk for Dysfunctional (Low-Pressure) Urethra

1. Over age 65
2. Previous incontinence surgery
3. Neuropathy of pelvic floor
4. Continuous or insensible urinary loss
5. Mixed urge and stress incontinence
6. Urinary loss with a well-supported bladder neck (negative Q-tip test)

analyze urodynamically and radiologically characteristics of patients who had failed previous surgery. He reported the type of previous procedure performed in the study group, but since his study is retrospective, there is no assessment of the multiple surgical procedures done on the patients who had successful surgery, or adequate reporting of the preoperative evaluation. The finding of a low-pressure or dysfunctional urethra has been surveyed by many authors.[8–10] A low-pressure urethra is generally thought to be a result of aging itself, neuropathy, previous denervating or devascularizing surgery, and scarring subsequent to infection or previous surgery.

Other authors have tried to answer the questions unanswered by McGuire's study. Sand and colleagues[8] found that 54% of patients with low-pressure urethra failed a modified Burch procedure in comparison to an 18% failure rate in patients with normal urethral pressure. In a later study, Bowen and co-workers[9] found a low-pressure urethra to be an independent variable for failed Burch urethropexy. It is therefore essential to evaluate adequately patients at risk for a low-pressure urethra. Risk groups include women over 65, those with previous incontinence surgery, patients suspect for pelvic floor neuropathy, women with continuous or insensible urinary loss, cases of mixed urge and stress incontinence, and those with urine loss despite a well-supported bladder neck (Table 6-2).

PRESENCE OR ABSENCE OF URETHRAL MOBILITY   It is essential to assess the preoperative presence or absence of mobility of the bladder neck especially in those with previously failed surgery. It is obvious that patients who had no mobility of the bladder neck, based on a cotton swab (Q-tip) urethral axis test or x-ray evaluation, would be poor candidates for conventional surgical approaches, which elevate the urethra into an intra-abdominal position. Because these patients already have good elevation, it is conceivable and understandable that little would be gained from surgery. These patients particularly should undergo mandatory urodynamic evaluation, including urethral pressure profilometry. Many may have a low-pressure dysfunctional urethra rather than descent of the vesical neck as the etiology for their stress incontinence (McGuire's type III stress incontinence[7]). Serious consideration should be given in this group of patients before any commitment to surgery because they are at high risk for failure. Summit and colleagues[10] have found an 80% failure rate in patients undergoing a sling procedure who have a low-pressure urethra and a negative Q-tip test (poor mobility of the bladder neck) as compared to a 93% success rate of the sling procedure with a positive Q-tip test (hypermobility of the bladder neck). Bergman and coworkers[11] report high failure rates in patients with little mobility of the bladder neck irrespective of urethral pressure. To minimize surgical failures, the practitioner would do well to follow this axiom: "Do not perform conventional incontinence procedures in patients with minimal or no mobility of the bladder neck." *These cases demand expert urodynamic assessment.*

PRESENCE OR ABSENCE OF DETRUSOR INSTABILITY OR VOIDING DIFFICULTY   It is well known that patients with uninhibited detrusor instability can be worsened by surgical treatment for genuine stress incontinence. Zealous overcorrection of the urethrovesical junction may also cause or worsen detrusor instability. This has been borne out by several authors[12,13] who have found that correction of the pressure transmission ratio above 100% is associated with significant stricture in the urethra with concomitant failure to cure detrusor instability and may cause de novo development of detrusor instability. The mostly likely reason for the genesis of postoperative detrusor instability or worsening detrusor instability after surgery is partial obstruction to urinary flow. Increased postvoid residual urine volumes have been reported in many of these women. It is well known that outlet obstruction is an important clinical[12–14] and experimental[15] cause of detrusor instability.

Voiding dysfunction, including poor bladder contractility with high postvoid residual urine, is also an important factor in the choice of treatment for genuine stress incontinence. Certainly patients who are unable to empty their bladders well are at further risk for obstructive voiding, higher postoperative postvoid residual urine volumes, and the development of detrusor instability, particularly if they undergo an obstructive procedure such as suburethral sling. They should be forewarned of this possibility and evaluated for the ability to perform intermittent self-catheterization before any surgical attempt at cure for genuine stress incontinence. They must be particularly evaluated urodynamically before any proposed surgery. The patient must also face the question, "If surgery cures my incontinence, can I learn to live with catheterizing myself to empty my bladder after voiding?" To demonstrate the ease of self-catheterization, I have my patient close her eyes and place one finger in her ear. If she performs that exercise correctly, she can usually be convinced that only she can catheterize her own urethra blindfolded! Enlisting spousal or other caretaker support with physical assistance can also minimize the fear of self-catheterization. Even if the chance of postoperative urinary retention is small, for the sake of informed consent, the patient should be forewarned of retention as a possible consequence, and be told to expect "self-cath" if prolonged catheterization is anticipated.

PRESENCE OR ABSENCE OF PELVIC FLOOR NEUROPATHY   In recent years, much attention has focused on nerve damage to the pelvic floor (see Chapter 1). For decades as gynecologists we have come to believe that pelvic relaxation is a result of a weakness in the pelvic fascia. Snooks and coworkers[16,17] and others[18,19] have causally linked urinary incontinence to neuropathy of the muscles of the pelvic floor. The logic of this hypothesis is obvious. Because the levator group of muscles receive innervation from the pudendal nerve, these authors postulate that denervation of the levator could cause pelvic relaxation with attendant urinary and anal incontinence. Smith and colleagues[18] and Gilpin and coworkers[19] demonstrated increased motor latency (nerve transmission time) with decreased stainable nerve in pelvic tissue of patients who had undergone long labors. They compared these to a control group of women who had never been in labor. They found that women who have had labor demonstrate varying degrees of impaired nerve transmission to the pelvic floor with diminution in the amount of stainable nerve tissue, presumably brought about by stretching and damage to the pudendal and perineal nerves during fetal passage. The diagnosis of pelvic floor neuropathy can explain a urethra with low resting pressure. For a definitive diagnosis, however, nerve conduction studies must be performed. Although no data are available to ascertain the correct management of patients with pudendal or pelvic nerve neuropathy, it is generally assumed that a patient with significant descent of the bladder neck with a low-pressure urethra can be cured by partially obstructive surgery, such as a suburethral sling[8–10] or a Ball-Burch procedure[20] and patients with no mobility and low-pressure urethra require urethral bulking agents or an artificial sphincter. These modalities will be discussed later in this chapter.

HISTORY OF PREVIOUS SURGERY   The history of previous surgery and the type of surgery that has failed are other important considerations. The patient with failed surgery is at high risk for subsequent failure and may have a dysfunctional low-pressure urethra in the presence or absence of urethrovesical descent. She must be meticulously evaluated before any surgical decision is made. Evaluation of such a patient is outlined in the previous chapter. Certainly any woman who has continuous leakage without urethrovesical descent or with high-volume postvoid residual urine needs a careful and thorough urodynamic evaluation including multichannel urethrocystometry and urethral pressure profilometry. We have proposed a schema for triaging patients with a history of previous failed surgery.[21] The important patient variables are the presence or absence of descent of the vesical neck, the presence or absence of postvoid residual urine, and the presence or absence of a low-pressure urethra or periurethral scarring. Tissue quality and surgical and medical conditions are also important. If there is descent of the bladder neck (hypermobility) with a normal urethral pressure, the patient may be a candidate for almost any of the surgical procedures listed below provided the operator has experienced success with the proposed surgical procedure. As we have previously mentioned, if the patient has descent of the bladder neck with a low-pressure urethra, she is probably a candidate for a suburethral sling[8-10] or a Ball-Burch[20] procedure. If the patient has no descent with a low-pressure urethra, she is a candidate for a periurethral bulking agent or an artificial sphincter, as described below.

PRESENCE OR ABSENCE OF URETHROVESICAL FUNNELING   There has been much theorizing over the condition of urethral funneling without much objective data. It is generally believed that funneling represents inherent urethral muscular weakness at the bladder neck and may be responsible for concomitant vesical instability on the experimental basis that fluid entering the urethra in animals causes a vesical contraction.[22] Correction of funneling during incontinence procedures may explain the 30% to 60% cure of concomitant vesical instability in these patients.[23] The Ball operation, a plication of the urethrovesical junction transabdominally, may reduce funneling as well as increase intrinsic urethral pressure, as reported by Bergman and colleagues.[20] In our preliminary study of 11 patients presenting with urgency, genuine stress incontinence, and radiographic demonstration of funneling, we have found 10 of 11 patients cured of urgency after a Ball-Burch procedure.[24]

CONSERVATIVE MANAGEMENT

Before any surgical decision is reached, the clinician should discuss the advisability and likelihood of success of conservative treatment, as alluded to at the outset. The risk-benefit analysis of conservative treatment as compared to surgical treatment should be reviewed with respect to severity of symptoms, need for anatomic surgical correction, and likelihood of success of conservative management. Conservative nonsurgical approaches consist principally of intravaginal (or intraurethral) estrogen, pelvic floor electrical stimulation, pelvic floor reeducation (exercise), and vaginal pessaries.

ESTROGEN   Because most postmenopausal women present with hypoestrogenism in the urethra and vagina, in the presence of genuine stress incontinence, estrogen is the most logical first choice of therapy in the perimenopausal or postmenopausal patient (see Chapter 1).

Some postmenopausal patients will already be on an oral maintenance dose of hormone replacement including estrogen. It is not uncommon, however, for these patients to have symptomatic disease in the lower urinary tract, including incontinence, despite adequate oral maintenance. Addition of intravaginal estrogen may more effectively treat the target organs, specifically, the urethra, trigone, and vagina. The most likely route, therefore, to increase the tone of the urethra and vagina as well as the levator muscles is intravaginal. Hilton and Stanton[25] and Rud[26] have found increases in intrinsic urethral tone after the administration of estrogen. Although these effects are not documented in other studies, many patients get some symptomatic relief from intravaginal estrogen.[27,28] It certainly is a logical, simple, relatively safe first step in approaching treatment in the patient with genuine stress incontinence. Intravaginal estrogen also prepares tissues in the vagina and urethra for eventual surgery by strengthening them and increasing the blood supply to these estrogen-sensitive organs. Serum estradiol levels may also be obtained, but clinical symptoms can usually be followed as a gauge to response.

PELVIC FLOOR ELECTRICAL STIMULATION   This procedure has been advocated by many[29,30] for treatment of genuine stress incontinence. It is usually in the form of functional electrical stimulation, using one of several devices currently commercially available. The purpose of electrical stimulation is strengthening the muscles of the pelvic floor and the periurethral skeletal muscles. It may also suppress abnormal detrusor contractions in patients with concomitant stress and urge incontinence. Frequencies for stress incontinence and urge incontinence are different, necessitating the use of two frequencies in the same patient. Most currently available devices are capable of delivering two frequencies to the pelvic floor. The electrode plug is placed intravaginally, or intrarectally if the vagina is stenotic, and adjustments appropriately made until reflex contractions of the pubococcygeus (anal "wink") can be registered by the examiner. The voltage is noted and the patient instructed to begin using stimulating voltage at that level or at the highest tolerable level. She is given a schedule, which consists of 15- to 30-minute treatments twice daily over a period of 8 to 12 weeks or longer depending on her response. The indication for usage of these devices for stress incontinence depends principally on the presence or absence of levator tone. In a patient who has good levator tone on physical examination (often one who has previously performed Kegel's exercises), the device may be of limited use. Patients with moderate to severe incontinence with marked degrees of urethrovesical descent will probably not respond to electrical stimulation. In general, electrical stimulation is associated with 30% to 60% improvement in the symptom of stress incontinence and is most effective in patients with mild stress incontinence with poor pelvic muscle voluntary contraction, that is, poor tone. Patients with major pelvic relaxation, such as those with large cystoceles, rectoceles, enteroceles, or vault prolapse, are not good candidates for electrical stimulation as the primary mode of therapy. This form of treatment may also help patients to identify the muscles of the pelvic floor and to enhance contraction by voluntary effort.

PELVIC FLOOR REEDUCATION   Generally, pelvic floor reeducation refers to the use of Kegel's exercise or its functional correlate, exercise with vaginal cones.

Arnold Kegel[31] was the first to describe the use of pelvic floor exercise in incontinent women. The exercise calls for daily repetitive contraction of the pelvic floor to strengthen levator tone. Compliance, however, may be a major impediment to the effectiveness of Kegel's exercises. Plevnik developed sequentially weighted vaginal cones; he and his coworkers found that patients were more likely to comply with the use of cones[32] than Kegel's exercises, reporting a 70% improvement in symptoms of patients with genuine stress incontinence. The cones are placed intravaginally while the patient is asked to contract the pelvic floor for 15 minutes twice a day. Once the patient has mastered the lowest weighted cone (10 or 20 g), she moves up to the next highest weight and successively increases in 20-g increments up to 80 to 100 g. The patient who cannot hold a cone in place will revert to the lower weighted cone until she is successfully able to maintain the cone in a high intravaginal position by contracting the pelvic musculature. As the patient develops more and more control over her pelvic floor, she may become capable of holding the highest weighted cone in place successfully. Patients who already have good levator tone with a good increase in it with voluntary contractions may sustain limited benefit from vaginal cones. Similarly, as for electrical stimulation, patients with moderate to severe incontinence or with severe degrees of pelvic relaxation are primarily surgical candidates and not candidates for conservative regimens such as Kegel's exercise or vaginal cones.

The assignment of pelvic floor exercises does give the patient a positive incentive to do something for herself, improves her self-perception, and enhances her sense of well-being, by reinforcing the idea that she, by herself, can derive some benefit through pelvic exercise. Supporting the patient's own ability to achieve a cure also tends to minimize her feelings of helplessness.

VAGINAL PESSARY   Pessaries have been commonly used in patients with pelvic relaxation. They may also increase urethral closure pressure and urethral functional length[33] in patients with mild to moderate cystoceles. Bhatia and colleagues report good results in 60% to 75% of such selected patients.[33] The mechanism of continence appears to be either increased urethral pressure, probably by obstruction of the urethra, or elevation of the proximal urethra into the abdominal pressure zone. These patients are at risk for urinary retention and should be thoroughly instructed in removing or deflating the pessary at regular intervals, probably daily, and cautioned and checked for the presence of retained urine and urinary tract infection. Some reports[34,35] have suggested an increase in the incidence of vaginal cancer in patients wearing pessaries, particularly if neglected. Neglected pessaries have also been known rarely to erode into the bladder or rectum.[36]

We have had much success with inflatable pessaries because they decompress for easy insertion and can be inflated to variable sizes. These may be self-managed. Pessaries require a certain degree of manual dexterity and a positive comfortable attitude in their usage and care. Encouragement and considerable instruction in their use are essential. The newest pessary developed by Biswas and colleagues is a silicone device with two extension arms to support the bladder neck; it is still undergoing clinical trials, but initial results are promising.[37]

Patients with a markedly relaxed vaginal outlet may not be able to retain pessaries. Occasionally patients who are not candidates for extensive surgery can have a simple perineoplasty under local anesthesia to build a posterior "shelf," thereby optimizing pessary retention. Most patients who have difficulty using or retaining pessaries, however, are more satisfied with definitive corrective surgery.

OTHER CONSERVATIVE REGIMENS   Various other nonsurgical regimens have been reported in the literature including biofeedback, interferential therapy, α-stimulatory drugs, weight reduction, and others. All have had varying success rates of 10% to 90% in genuine stress incontinence depending on the centers that use them.[30]

Careful selection of patients is necessary when using conservative therapy. It has also been shown that a professional trained in the use of these methods, with whom the patient develops confidence and trust, will ensure compliance and a more nearly successful outcome.

SURGICAL TREATMENT FOR GENUINE STRESS INCONTINENCE

Patients who fail conservative regimens are usually surgical candidates. Patients who have good measurable pelvic floor strength, with severe degrees of prolapse or descent, or with severe stress incontinence, are also usually primary surgical candidates. There are also patients with troubling incontinence who have little patience for a 3-month trial of conservative treatment who elect surgery primarily. In this section, we discuss the choice of surgical procedures and describe various operations with their reported success rates.

The selection of patients for surgery is influenced by the variables mentioned in Table 6-1. There also exists considerable difficulty in assessing the efficacy of surgical procedures from any review of the literature for the many reasons enumerated in Table 6-3 and discussed below.

There are many differences in reporting the severity of symptoms and no uniform method for doing so currently exists. This makes it difficult to characterize accurately the presurgical conditions and consequently to assess the success or failure of the various surgical procedures of different surgeons. Patient characteristics such as age, parity, and previous surgery are not always stated in the literature, introducing further difficulty in evaluating multiple

TABLE 6-3 Difficulties in Evaluating Success of Incontinence Surgery

1. Differences in reporting of severity of symptoms
2. Patient variables (age, parity, previous surgery)
3. Nonrandomized retrospective studies
4. Varying degrees of preoperative evaluation
5. Individual surgeon variations and multiple surgical techniques
6. Varying length of follow-up
7. Inconsistent reporting of previous incontinence procedures
8. Performance of other procedures during incontinence surgery

variables in the different patient series reported. Selection bias is compounded by numerous nonrandomized retrospective studies which are subject to the known inherent weaknesses of these types of studies. There are also varying degrees of preoperative evaluation reported, ranging from none to simple to multichannel urodynamics.

Perhaps two of the most important variables for predicting success or failure of incontinence surgery are the wide differences among surgeons in performing a given procedure and the many surgical techniques reported. A single operation, although called by the same name in multiple scientific reports, may be as individual as the surgeon performing it. The follow-up interval may also vary from study to study, or the authors may not indicate the type and number of previous surgical procedures. The usual and often necessary practice of simultaneously performing other restorative procedures in concert with corrective incontinence surgery may also introduce confounding variables. These and other inconsistencies hamper the accurate reporting and recording of surgical success in genuine stress incontinence.

OBJECTIVE CRITERIA IN THE CHOICE OF SURGICAL PROCEDURE

Notwithstanding the numerous difficulties in assessing various surgical techniques, we have attempted to develop a set of objective criteria for choosing surgical procedures in patients with genuine stress incontinence. Probably the most important determinants in selecting a procedure are severity of the symptoms, presence or absence of mobility of the bladder neck, presence or absence of a low-pressure urethra, individual patient preferences, and patient suitability for a particular surgical procedure. For example, women with poor bladder emptying or those who require an obstructive procedure such as suburethral sling should also be forewarned that it may be necessary for them to perform intermittent clean self-catheterization postoperatively if they select a surgical procedure. On the other hand, they would be inappropriate candidates for an obstructive surgical procedure if they state beforehand unwillingness to accept the possibility of self-catherization postoperatively. Most of all, no patient should preoperatively be given any absolute guarantees, and the possibility of failure, despite the best surgical effort, must be understood by the patient and her family.

THE CHOICE OF SURGICAL PROCEDURE

In clinical practice, many surgeons for a variety of reasons, not always plausible, prefer to perform the simplest rather than the most effective operation. The use of anterior colporrhaphy as a sole operation for stress incontinence is currently unacceptable. Patients have also been influenced by the media where "no incision" operations have been touted by surgeons without any statement of objective results or preoperative evaluation. Once again, in general one should choose the best operation, not the simplest. This advice assumes that in the particular surgeon's hands, the best operation has the highest success rate and the simplest operation has the lowest success rate, but this is not always the case.

We will evaluate both the "simple" and the "best" operations in the light of our experience and the reported literature, keeping in mind that the single most important variable in the success or failure of the operation is the individual surgeon's objective cure rate for the particular operation with the same set of preoperative conditions. Because this information is not always available or forthcoming with most surgeons, one must critically view the success or failure rates reported in the literature. Individual surgeons must also honestly and critically evaluate their own techniques, over time, to assess objectively their own failure rates. Richardson has carried out a thoughtful analysis of the evaluation of different procedures and reiterates that the most difficult variable to assess is the skill of the operating surgeon.[18]

Anterior Colporrhaphy and Kennedy-Kelly Plication

The archaic dictum to operate from below first, and if this fails, to operate from above has influenced decades of surgeons in the treatment of genuine stress incontinence. This advice is antiquated and has no place in contemporary management of genuine stress incontinence. Numerous studies[39-43] have substantiated the high failure rates of anterior colporrhaphy and Kelly plication in the treatment of genuine stress incontinence.

Kelly and Dunn first described this procedure in 1914.[44] The purpose of the operation in Kelly's view was repair of the injured "sphincter muscle" at the level of the urethrovesical junction. He used two silk mattress sutures placed on both sides of the urethra to reunite the "sphincter" in the midline. Kennedy[45] extended sutures along the entire length of the urethra to plicate the "torn sphincter" along the entire length of the urethra. To perform the procedure, extensive dissection is necessary to free the urethra from the vaginal mucosa. Marked variability in success rates of the Kelly-Kennedy operation, ranging from 34% to 91%, exists in the literature.[38] Failure may be a consequence of our imprecise understanding of the pathophysiology of incontinence and urethrovesical anatomy. Moreover, this extensive dissection may cause nerve and muscle damage as proposed by Tanagho.[46] Since it has been discovered that there truly is no internal urethral sphincter as postulated by Kelly, or torn urethral sphincter as conceived by Kennedy, the surgery may be merely obstructive. However, it may elevate to some degree the proximal urethra into the abdominal pressure zone, which is the current theory of the cure of stress incontinence and why some, but not enough, of the Kelly operations worked.

Beck and McCormick[47] and Nichols[48] have reported acceptably high success rates with their individual variations of anterior colporrhaphy. Most surgeons, however, do not perform anterior colporrhaphy in the same manner. Beck[47] attaches the periurethral fascia or pubourethral ligaments (or both) to the pubic periosteum. This variation is mechanically somewhat similar to the abdominally performed Marshall-Marchetti-Krantz operation, described below. Considering the good results of the latter procedure, this may explain Beck's reported high success rate. Nichols[48] overlaps small segments of these tissues from both sides in a "vest over trouser" fashion (see Grody's "double-breasted" flaps in Chapter 7). Kujansau and coworkers[49,50] found a higher success rate with anterior colporrhaphy (91%) compared to colposuspension (55%), and they state that surgical failures in anterior colporrhaphy revealed inadequate postoperative urethral elevation, implying superiority of their techniques. This study, however, is at variance with a considerable body of literature showing significantly higher success rates of retropubic approaches over vaginal approaches in the treatment of genuine stress incontinence, in the hands of good operators. Nonetheless anterior colporrhaphy, Kennedy-Kelly plications, or variations of these are still used for stress incontinence by skillful surgeons who claim satisfactory results. Anterior colporrhaphy still remains the simplest, most accepted, and most effective method for treating central anterior vaginal wall prolapse (distention cystocele) when unaccompanied by genuine stress incontinence.

Retropubic Urethropexy

In 1949, Marshall, Marchetti, and Krantz[51] reported a new operation for the treatment of stress incontinence. They obtained a 90% cure rate overall in

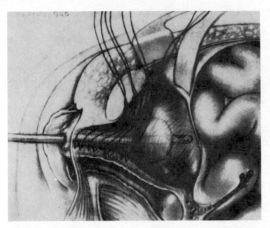

Figure 6-1 Marshall-Marchetti-Krantz procedure. Sagittal section shows location of four paraurethral sutures on left. (Reproduced with permission from Marshall, Marchetti, and Krantz.[51])

patients complaining of stress incontinence with a 76% cure rate in patients with previously failed incontinence surgery (Figures 6-1 and 6-2). This procedure was later modified by Burch[52] who found that attachment of the periurethral tissue to Cooper's (iliopectineal) ligament was simpler to perform on

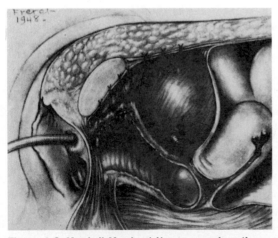

Figure 6-2 Marshall-Marchetti-Krantz procedure (from original paper). Same as Figure 6-1 except sutures tied—diagrammatic, as actually less space remains between origin and insertion of sutures. The sutures are bilaterally placed periurethrally and fixed through the pubic periosteum and cartilage. Most surgeons, including Krantz, no longer advocate placing sutures through the bladder as originally described and depicted in their photograph. (Reproduced with permission from Marshall, Marchetti, and Krantz.[51])

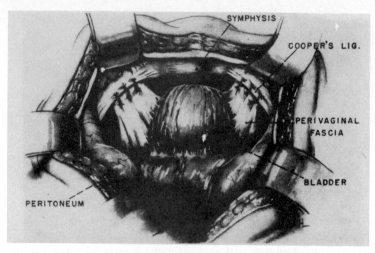

Figure 6-3 Burch modification. Lateral edges of vagina have been approximated to Cooper's ligament by using three interrupted sutures. (Reproduced with permission from Burch.[52])

certain patients and afforded higher retropubic placement (Figure 6-3). Various modifications have been proposed since Burch's original description, but the essential features remain the same. Most authorities have demonstrated that if permanent sutures are used, cure rates are as high as 95% for primary treatment of genuine stress incontinence in patients with a normal-pressure urethra (more than 20 cm H_2O) and urethrovesical mobility (more than 30-degree Q-tip test). Close apposition to Cooper's ligament is neither necessary nor desirable. The object is to create an endogenous sling of vaginal tissue to gently elevate the bladder neck into the abdominal pressure zone. Overcorrection may cause obstruction and vesical instability. Intraoperative indicators such as 0-degree Q-tip test or providing space for an index finger between the pubic bone and bladder may be useful in determining suture tension. Almost invariably a short suture bridge is left. In expert hands, there exists no significant difference in cure rates or morbidity between Marshall-Marchetti-Krantz or Burch procedures[38,53] with the exception of slightly increased incidence of obstructive voiding in patients undergoing Marshall-Marchetti-Krantz procedures in the first 3 postoperative months. A notable characteristic of retropubic cystourethropexy in general is the consistent cure rates from one surgeon to another. Mainprize and Drutz[54] found that the overall success rate of the Marshall-Marchetti-Krantz procedure was 86% (92% in primary procedures and 84% in repeat procedures). In our series, we have found a 93% success rate in primary Burch procedures with an 84% success rate in repeat Burch operations.[55]

Several variations of the Burch and Marshall-Marchetti-Krantz procedures have been reported in the literature; for instance, combining either operation with a Ball technique that plicates the urethra.[20] It may be advantageous to perform this variation in patients with severe funneling of the bladder neck or a low-pressure urethra or both.

Paravaginal Repair

Recently the paravaginal approach has received considerable attention. Both A. Cullen Richardson and Wayne Baden independently began describing paravaginal defects in the 1960s. These lesions are separations of the pubovesicocervical connective tissue bladder supports from their attachments to the arcus tendineus fasciae pelvis, which runs from the mid-symphysis to the ischial spine and overlies the medial aspect of the obturator internus muscle. At their distal locations, these defects are responsible for rotational descent of the urethrovesical junction, and thus are accompanied by overt or demonstrable stress incontinence. Defects of this nature may be unilateral or bilateral. In either case, they are also the cause of the paravaginal or distention type of cystocele, which often goes unrecognized simply because of ignorance that this type of impairment exists at all. Proponents of the paravaginal defects injury,[55-57] which can usually be demonstrated readily both clinically and during surgery, claim that the displacement cystocele resulting from it is probably more common than the distention cystocele, the central herniation under the bladder with which we are all familiar.

Repair of these defects has been reported as a reunion of the separated connective tissue of the area of both the urethrovesical junction and the bladder to the arcus tendineus ("white line") by a series of interrupted nonabsorbable sutures through a suprapubic approach via the space of Retzius. Initially each suture, after being anchored appropriately into the "white line" in the obturator internus fascia, as a safety measure, was also brought up to Cooper's ligament but this has been discontinued. Enthusiasts claim this method of repair as the most anatomic of approaches because, in bringing the urethrovesical junction back into the abdominal pressure influence and the lateral bladder supports to the "white line" in this manner, natural relationships are restored (Figures 6-4 and 6-5). Richardson and colleagues in 1981[55] and Shull and Baden in 1989,[56] based on substantial series and relatively long-term results, reported 95% and 97% very satisfactory results, respectively.

Modified Burch Colposuspension

Stanton[58] modified the Burch procedure by suspending not only the urethrovesical junction but also the entire length of vagina to Cooper's ligament to reduce coexisting cystocele. He does report, however, a high risk of enterocele,[59] which is understandable given the extreme anterior placement of the vagina. We

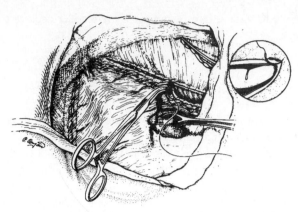

Figure 6-4 Starting the repair of the right paravaginal defects on the medial aspect of the right obturator internus muscle. (Reproduced with permission from Contemporary OB/GYN 1990;35[9]:100–109. Copyright 1990 Medical Economics Company Inc., Montvale, NJ.)

rarely use this procedure to suspend the mid-vagina, for which we prefer the paravaginal repair, or to suspend the apex, for which we prefer abdominal or vaginal colpopexy. We have found it useful in patients in whom colpopexy is difficult or impossible.

Combined Paravaginal and Burch Operations

Our current mode of performing incontinence surgery is to place retropubic sutures of the Burch type at the level of the urethrovesical junction into

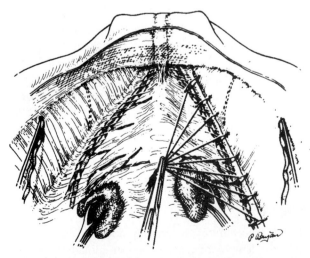

Figure 6-5 Completed paravaginal repair. (Reproduced with permission from Contemporary OB/GYN 1990;35[9]:100–109. Copyright 1990 Medical Economics Company Inc., Montvale, NJ.)

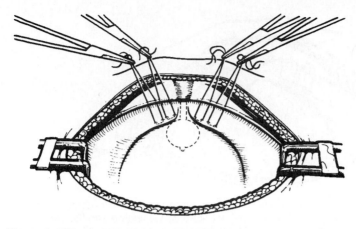

Figure 6-6 Modified Burch retropubic urethropexy. One or two figure-of-eight sutures are placed on each side of the urethrovesical junction and occasionally more distally. These are elevated and secured to Cooper's (ileopectineal) ligament. (Reproduced with permission from Hurt WG. *Urogynecologic Surgery.* Galthersburg, Md: Aspen; 1992:90.)

paravaginal tissue approximately 1 to 1.5 cm lateral to the urethrovesical junction on each side and then anchoring them into Cooper's ligament (Figure 6-6). Placing the stitches too close to the urethra may interfere with its nerve and blood supply. Placing them too far laterally may cause undue tension and tenting of the posterior vagina as the sutures are tied in their very anterior position. The amount of tension in the vagina may be tested by pulling up on the sutures in the direction of Cooper's ligament. If there is too much posterior vaginal wall tension, the stitches can be repositioned more medially but not closer than 1 cm from the urethra to avoid possible neurovascular compromise.[46] Posterior vaginal tenting, when present, does tend to diminish during the first 6 to 8 postoperative weeks as the compliant vagina tends to readjust.

The modified Burch procedure affords good retropubic positioning of the proximal urethra into the abdominal pressure zone without undue angulation of the urethra. We use nonabsorbable sutures of double-armed polyester (Dacron® or Ti-Cron®) or Gore-Tex®. A double bite is taken through the full thickness of the vagina followed by placement into Cooper's ligament. These stitches must be staggered so they can be tied across intervening fibers of Cooper's ligaments, that is, not in the same fiber plane (Figure 6-7). We also repair lateral wall defects if present as described by Richardson, Shull, and Baden, using the paravaginal abdominal approach. Our success rate for this combination operation compares favorably with those of other authors.[57]

The rationale for our choice of this combination of procedures has to do with the good results we have achieved using the Burch retropubic urethropexy in the treatment of incontinence and the high success recorded in the two major

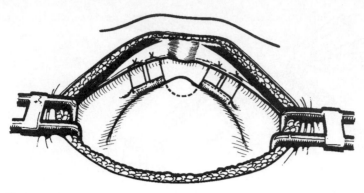

Figure 6-7 Modified Burch retropubic urethropexy. Colposuspension is performed by tying suspending sutures. They should elevate, but not obstruct, the urethrovesical junction. (Reproduced with permission from Hurt WG. *Urogynecological Surgery.* Gaithersburg, Md: Aspen; 1992:91.)

studies on paravaginal defects reported in the literature.[55,56] This combination more closely helps to approximate the normal axis of the vagina which should point more directly cephalad in the lower third and posteriorly in the upper two thirds (see Chapter 9).

There is a certain anatomic advantage gained by suture vectors pulled more anteriorly in the lower third of the vagina and more posteriorly in the upper two thirds of the vagina. Because of the occasional weakness in the obturator fascia, in our judgment, and the consistently strong quality of Cooper's ligament, we prefer not to use obturator fascia as a sole repair for genuine stress incontinence. Burch[52] initially fixed the paravaginal fascia to the "white line of the pelvis" as well, reporting an excellent anatomic result, but was fearful that not enough elevation would be provided. Thus, he used Cooper's ligament for what he thought would be a more pronounced lifting effect. Shull and Baden[56] initially recommended placing each paravaginal suture also through Cooper's ligament as well as the obturator fascia to offer a safety mechanism should any of the stitches in the tendinous arch not hold. As already mentioned, they have discontinued this practice.

Because of our experience and that reported by others, we continue to use Cooper's ligament for the fixation at the level of the bladder neck, and the obturator fascia or arcus tendineus ("white line") for fixing the mid-vagina and apex. We have also occasionally placed these mid-vaginal and apical sutures through the strong iliococcygeus fascia or the periosteum of the ischium itself under the surface of the iliococcygeus fascia and muscle. This strong tissue, when located, may be superior to the arcus tendineus. It can be found lateral to the ischial spines, underlying the obturator muscle. It is a safe zone for suture placement because it is posterior and medial to the obturator nerve and vessels and lateral to the major nerves and vessels exiting the pelvis through the greater sciatic foramen.

In our hands, this combination provides the best success for treating incontinence and the most anatomic placement of the mid and apical vagina. We generally leave a suture bridge, using permanent sutures only, at the bladder neck so as to pull it retropubically enough to achieve a zero to minus 5 Q-tip test during the operation. If we suspend the vagina more anteriorly by Stanton's technique, we tend to place the sutures more anteriorly in the lateral vagina, thus resulting in a long suture bridge between the vagina and iliopectineal ligament. In addition, we always perform a culdocleisis (Halbans and/or Moschkowitz) with permanent sutures to prevent the future development of enterocele. Since these patients are almost always climacteric, the risk of adhesion formation interfering with childbirth does not present a problem.

Distention Cystocele Repair

In our experience, large central pulsion type cystoceles must be rectified primarily transvaginally by a standard anterior colporrhaphy or by transabdominal cystocele repair for the highest success rate. We will correct central cystoceles transabdominally if the primary surgical incontinence procedure is performed transabdominally. This can be accomplished by carefully mobilizing the bladder off the vagina, removing a portion of the anterior vaginal wall, and closing the defect[60,61] (Figure 6-8A–D).

Laparoscopic Technique

Various laparoscopic approaches to retropubic urethropexy have been recently reported.[62] The basic procedure is similar to an open abdominal incision technique but uses a laparoscope in the retropubic space of Retzius. No reports of long-term success are currently available for this approach, although several investigators are currently attempting to carry out a randomized trial comparing the laparoscopic with the standard open abdominal approach.

Needle Endoscopic Suspension

In 1959, Pereyra described a simplified approach for the correction of stress incontinence in women by placing sutures through the pubourethral ligaments, attaching them by needle passage from above through the retropubic space to the anterior abdominal fascia.[63] This procedure was later modified by Stamey,[64] who used a narrow plastic buttress around the suture to prevent it from pulling

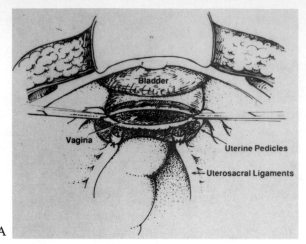

A

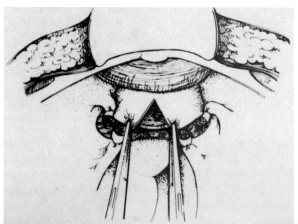

B

C

Figure 6-8 Abdominal cystocele repairs. A, Hysterectomy has been completed. The angles of the vagina are grasped with long Kochers. The uterosacral pedicles have been isolated for later plication. B, The bladder is mobilized off the anterior vaginal wall by sharp dissection. C, An equilateral triangle is then excised from the anterior vaginal wall. D, The vaginal walls are sutured in the midline. (Reproduced with permission from Drutz, Baker, and Lemieux.[60])

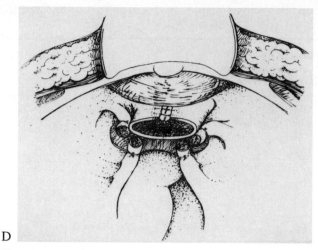

D

Figure 6-8 *Continued*

through the paravaginal connective tissue. Later Raz used a double-needle technique passing sutures in helix formation through the fibromuscular coat of the vagina paraurethrally.[65] Stamey, Muzsnai, and colleagues also placed sutures through a portion of the vagina.[66] Still later Gittes and Roughlin placed the sutures through the entire thickness of vaginal wall.[67]

Success rates for these techniques are reported variously from 40% to 95%[38,43,63–69] (Table 6-4). Suture fixation of these various techniques is illustrated in Figure 6-9. Although these methods enjoy widespread usage and good cure rates in some hands, they have not apparently enjoyed the consistent operator-to-operator long-term success rate of the various retropubic approaches. At the current time we do not recommend them for primary or secondary treatment of genuine stress incontinence because of the higher failure rates compared to abdominal retropubic techniques. Kelly and colleagues recently reported only a 51% cure rate from endoscopic Raz needle suspensions.[68] We have reserved endoscopic suspension for patients with potential incontinence, that is, patients with large cystoceles or genitourinary prolapse without overt incontinence who demonstrate lowered urethral pressure and frank leakage with positive urodynamic urethral cough profiles after prolapses have been reduced digitally or by a pessary or a speculum.[70–73] To assess the possibility of potential incontinence we prefer to reduce the prolapse digitally by placing one or two fingers into the vagina and directing the apex of the vagina to its normal axis, toward S-3.[74] Care is taken not to place any pressure in the anterior direction against the urethra because this maneuver may cause partial obstruction of the urethra, leading to misleading test results. This maneuver is performed with the patient sitting erect in the urodynamics chair, since most

TABLE 6-4 Objective and Subjective Comparative Rates of Various Endoscopic Needle Procedures

Author, Year and Reference*	Number of Patients	Follow-up Period	Type of Procedure	Cure Rate (%)	Objective (O)[†] or Subjective (S)[‡]
Bergman, 1989[43]	107	1 y	Pereyra	65	O
Weil, 1984[40]	86	6 mo	Pereyra	50	O
Muzsnai, 1982[66]	98	>6 mo	Muzsnai (Raz)	95	S
Karram 1992[94]	103	1 y	Pereyra	60	O
Hilton, 1989[95]	21	6 mo	Stamey	80	O
Mundy, 1983[96]	51	1 y	Stamey	40	O
Kelly, 1991[68]	145	3–5 y	Pereyra	51	S
Bhatia and Bergman, 1985[69]	64	1 y	Pereyra	85	O

*Reference number in this text.
[†] Objectively determined by postoperative urodynamic evaluation.
[‡] Subjectively determined by symptom analysis, telephone follow-up, and so on.

patients can void or strain easily in this position, as well as for reasons of standardized urodynamic conformity. Patients with potential or latent incontinence are good candidates for needle endoscopic procedures.

Suburethral Sling Operations

Suburethral sling operations have been in clinical usage for almost a century.[75,76] Originally they were used to treat all types of incontinence, but because of their high complication rate, including obstruction, detrusor instability, urethral compression, both urethral and vaginal erosion, and high postvoid residuals, their usage is usually reserved for patients with previous failed surgery or patients with a dysfunctional low-pressure urethra.[77–79] An autologous or heterologous graft is placed suburethrally at the urethrovesical junction and firmly tied from either side to the anterior rectus fascia. Alternatively slings have been tied to Cooper's ligament. The most commonly used autologous materials have been either rectus fascia or tensor fascia lata. Various synthetic materials, such as Mersilene® and Gore-Tex®, have been used.[77,78] Significant infection rates requiring replacement have been found with Gore-Tex®.[78] Summitt and co-workers have reported a high success rate with the sling operation in patients with low-pressure urethra who have good mobility of the bladder neck as compared to those patients with no such mobility.[10]

At the current time, we also use suburethral slings in patients who have a low-pressure urethra with good mobility of the bladder neck. Many of these women might have had previous failed incontinence surgery, but we still use

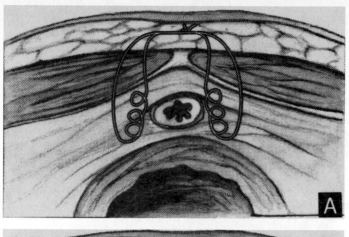

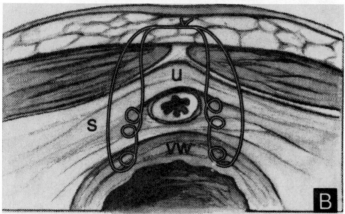

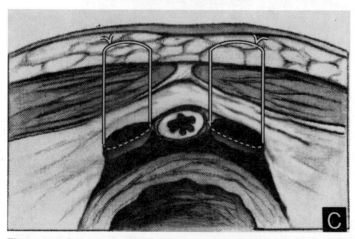

Figure 6-9 Cross-section view of various anchoring sutures used in commonly performed needle procedures. A, Modified Pereyra procedure—helical stitch through pubourethral ligament and detached endopelvic fascia. B, Raz procedure—helical stitch through detached endopelvic fascia and anchored in vaginal wall. VW = vaginal wall; U = urethra; S = symphysis. C, Stamey procedure—buttresses placed in pubocervical fascia on each side of bladder neck. D, Gittes procedure—stitches through full thickness of vaginal wall. E, Muzsnai procedure—two stitches on each side through vaginal wall (excluding epithelium). (Reproduced with permission from Karram MM. In: Hurt WG, ed. *Urogynecological Surgery.* Gaithersburg, Md: Aspen; 1992:63.)

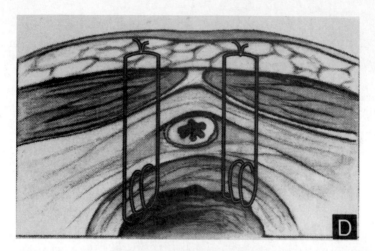

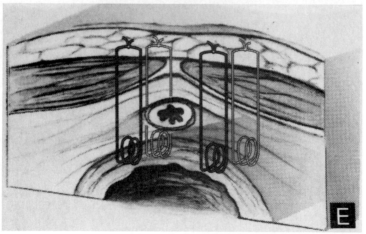

Figure 6-9 *Continued*

the same criteria regardless. We attach the sling through the rectus muscle and fascia to take advantage of rectus contraction during cough, which further tightens the sling. It should be emphasized that a sling to be most effective should obstruct the urethra somewhat during cough or strain, But tying it too tightly may cause obstructive voiding or severe urgency, not to mention erosion. Therefore, placing the sling loosely without tension is probably the best method. The intraoperative indicators most commonly used to judge the degree of sling tension include the following: (1) placing a Q-tip in the urethra and tightening the sling until a Q-tip angle of 0 degrees is reached; (2) using a Q-tip or   a small meatal dilator to assess urethral resistance while tightening the sling; (3) inserting a 0-degree urethroscope and observing tightening of the sling until closure of the urethrovesical junction is seen through the scope; (4) tightening the sling to minimum tension, so that it just elevates the urethra, as felt vaginally. Unfortunately the range of efficacy is small in respect to sling tension such that tying the sling either too tightly or too loosely makes it either ineffective or causes constriction, respectively.

Various other methods have been used to assess how obstructively the sling should be tied to avoid failure, including urodynamic determinations. This can be notoriously inaccurate during general anesthesia, which produces varying degrees of neuromuscular blockade, thereby precluding accurate assessment of urethral pressure during sling placement. Removal of the sling for obstruction or infection can be as high as 30%. After removal or revision of an overly tight sling, incontinence can return in 10% to 15% of patients. The complications of slings must be weighed carefully before contemplating their use, especially if patients have a normal-pressure urethra with hypermobility. These cases may benefit from the less complicated Burch procedure. We continue to maintain that the only indication for sling placement is low-pressure urethra with a mobile (more than 30 degrees Q-tip test preoperatively) urethra. Table 6-5 summarizes indications, complications, and success rates for al the incontinence procedures.

Other Slinglike Approaches

Zacharin[80] described a type of suburethral sling attaching rectus fascia to pubourethral ligaments. In our opinion these ligaments are often attenuated and difficult to find, and this procedure seems more difficult to perform than other methods of sling placement since it involves considerable abdominal and perineal dissection.

Raz[81] describes a four-corner vaginal wall sling operation that essentially leaves an undissected strip of vaginal mucosa over the proximal urethra and bladder neck. He attaches each of the four corners of the patch to permanent suture and these are then fixed appropriately to the rectus fascia. We have found this procedure useful but have modified it such that we apply heterologous or autologous sling material additionally to the patch.[82] Although comparative studies are not available, this method has several advantages:

1. It uses vaginal mucosa that is discarded during cystocele repair.
2. It leaves the periurethral nerve and blood supply intact as it avoids dissection in the area.
3. The vaginal mucosa patch has virtually no likelihood of eroding the urethra.
4. Vaginal wall is considerably more elastic than fascia or heterologous material such as Marlex®, Mersilene®, or Gore-Tex® and therefore may be less likely to obstruct the urethra.

TABLE 6-5 Summary of Indications, Complications, and Success Rates for Various Incontinence Procedures

Procedure	Indications	Possible Complications	Success Rate, %	Remarks
1. Anterior colporrhaphy (Kennedy-Kelly plication)	Central anterior vaginal wall prolapse (central cystocele) Possibly mild incontinence	High failure rate for incontinence Stenotic vagina	35–90	Not recommended as sole treatment for incontinence
2. Burch, Tanagho (modification)	GSI, mild to severe	Posterior vaginal ridge De novo DI Possible enterocele formation Nerve injury due to retractor pressure	75–95	Does not repair cystocele (Recommend culdocleisis to prevent enterocele)
3. Burch colpo-suspension (Stanton)	GSI mild to severe	Anterior displacement of vagina Posterior transverse vaginal ridge Increased risk enterocele formation Nerve injury from retractor pressure	75–95	Does not repair cystocele (Recommend culdocleisis to prevent enterocele)
4. Ball-Burch procedure	GSI with urethrovesical funneling Low-pressure urethra	Obstructive flow Inadvertant suturing of transurethral catheter	85	Ball procedure never used alone Always in combination with RPU Corrects low urethral pressure, May correct funneling

Procedure	Indications	Complications	Success rate (%)	Comments
5. Marshall-Marchetti-Krantz	GSI mild to severe	Anterior angulation of urethra; urethral obstruction (usually subsides by 3 mo) Osteitis pubis (8%) Rare osteomyelitis De novo DI Enterocele formation	60–90	Same as Burch Many variations reported Placement of sutures lower in pelvis than Burch To avoid enterocele recommend culdocleisis (Moschkowitz or Halban)
6. Paravaginal repair	GSI mild to severe	Obturator nerve and vessel injury Rarely suture pullout from obturator fascia	90–97	Less potential for enterocele formation Probably less potential for DI Success enhanced if suture placed through ileococcygeus fascia or periosteum underlying levator
7. Endoscopic, needle suspension (Pereyra, Stamey, Raz, Gittes, Muzsnai)	Potential incontinence Possibly mild to moderate GSI (some authors)	Suture pullout Ileoinguinal nerve injury Obstruction (usually subsides within 8 wk) Groin and leg pain Bladder penetration and injury	50–85	Must perform cystourethroscopy Variable success rate for GSI

(continued)

TABLE 6-5 (Continued)

Procedure	Indications	Possible Complications	Success Rate, %	Remarks
8. Suburethral sling	GSI with low-pressure urethra *and* urethrovesical mobility (> 30° Q-tip test)	Obstruction. Frequent UTI Vaginal erosion, Urethral erosion, Severe DI.* Peri-sling infection	20–80	Can be taken down after 3 mo for obstruction or severe DI with 15% recurrence rate of GSI*
9. Periurethral bulking agents (collagen, fat)	GSI with low-pressure urethra without urethrovesical mobility (< 30° Q-tip test) Poor surgical candidates Failed surgery with no descent Neuropathic urethra Scarred urethra	Hematoma in fat donor site UTI Obstruction (usually subsides within 24 h)	50–80	Requires only local anesthesia Simple to perform Holds much promise May be repeated 3–4 times or possibly more often High patient acceptance Minimal discomfort
10. Artificial urinary sphincter	Low-pressure urethra without urethrovesical mobility (> 30° Q-tip test)	Leakage of tubing Urethral erosion Mechanical failure	80%	Difficult for patients with poor manual dexterity Expensive

DI, detrusor instability; GSI, genuine stress incontinence; RPU, retropubic urethropexy; UTI, urinary tract infection
*DI is usually more severe and more difficult to treat when caused by obstruction from sling.

COMPARATIVE CURE RATES OF VARIOUS PROCEDURES

Richardson[38] has analyzed and summarized the literature comparing both subjective and objective cure rates of all types of procedures. He discusses a wide range of public health consequences in assessing comparative cure rates. For example, a recent paper reports 30% fewer hospital days, 50% decrease in blood loss, and lower surgeons' fees in patients undergoing needle urethroscopic suspensions compared to retropubic urethropexy.[83] Although complication rates were felt to be comparable, Richardson points out that the paper assumed that cure rates were identical; therefore the authors erroneously concluded that a needle suspension is the procedure of choice in most cases of stress incontinence. If one compares the higher failure rates of needle suspension, one can hardly justify the cost of repeat surgery and the distress to the patient while she awaits another procedure, more than nullifying any initial seeming advantage.

SPECIAL PROCEDURES INDICATED FOR INTRINSIC URETHRAL DEFICIENCY WITHOUT VESICAL DESCENT

Some patients with loss of mobility of the bladder neck present a fixed or "drain pipe" urethra, which is functionless, adynamic, and often scarred. On urodynamic evaluation, most of these people reveal a low-pressure urethra, unless they have a significant degree of surgical scarring or obstruction that may increase the urethral pressure. A neuropathy may be involved. Such cases often present imperceptible, intermittent, or continuous loss of urine, particularly if they have low urethral pressure. Importantly, they typically lose urine without increases in abdominal pressure, without urgency at rest. Frequently, they display worse incontinence when intra-abdominal pressure increases. They are at high risk for secondary surgical failure, and thus the decision for surgery must be carefully weighed before undertaking it. Many of these patients, on more meticulous scrutiny, are found not to be surgical candidates at all. The patient's age and other medical conditions, even in the presence of good tissue quality, must be carefully considered before advocating any surgical procedure. A trial of vaginal estrogen, physical therapy, including vaginal cones, or electrical stimulation should be attempted. The surgical treatments of choice in patients in this category are probably either artificial sphincter or periurethral bulking agents.

Artificial Urethral Sphincter

Experience with the artificial sphincter is somewhat limited in incontinent women. Scott[84] and others[85,86] have had the widest experience and have obtained an 85% to 90% success rate using the artificial urethral sphincter in selected groups of patients. The artificial sphincter is relatively contraindicated in patients with vesical instability.[86]

The sphincter consists of a balloon reservoir, pressure pump, and cuff, which fits around the urethra. The balloon is placed intra-abdominally near the bladder and the cuff (sphincter) is placed around the urethra by a vaginal or a transabdominal approach. The cuff is not activated for 6 to 8 weeks to avoid erosion of the urethra before surgical healing. Saline has been used as the fluid to inflate the cuff because there is minimal tissue reaction to saline if leakage occurs as a consequence of pump, cuff, or tubing connector malfunction. The pressure in the balloon is set below diastolic pressure, usually between 51 and 70 cm water pressure to avoid necrosis of the urethra. Cuff erosion continues to be the worst complication of the artificial sphincter.[84,85] Mechanical malfunction requiring reoperation occurs in 21% of patients with artificial sphincters so, because of erosion and malfunction, it cannot be regarded lightly.

Other Procedures

A technique reported by Ganabathi and colleagues[87] combines a bulbocavernosus (Martius) graft with a Stamey procedure. In their series they treated 40 women who had previous stress incontinence surgery. Although the follow-up ranges from only 4 to 24 months postoperatively, they report an 80% cure rate with 11% poor results. The advantages of the procedure, according to these authors, is low morbidity and a short hospital stay. An increase in urethral pressure in these patients may be seen 3 to 6 months postoperatively. This increase in pressure may be ascribed to an increase in blood flow to the urethra. The use of the Martius graft is certainly worth investigating in combination with other surgical procedures including suburethral slings for incontinence, as many women with recurrent stress incontinence and previous surgery have poor blood supply and atrophic tissue in the area. Since urethral pressure is in part determined by urethral blood flow, this and other procedures combined with a bulbocavernosus fat pad deserve adequate clinical trials in the future with longer clinical follow-up. The Martius graft is also a useful technique in itself to add bulk to the attenuated tissue between the urethra and the vagina.

Glutaraldehyde Cross-linked Collagen and Urethal Bulking Agents

Glutaraldehyde cross-linked (GAX) bovine collagen has been used effectively in patients with a fixed low-pressure urethra. Preliminary clinical trials of collagen have shown much promise. GAX collagen is injected periurethrally at the bladder neck under endoscopic control until coaptation or closure of the urethra is seen through a 0-degree urethroscope. In Appel's clinical evaluation of 68 patients, he injected a mean volume of 14 mL and obtained an 81% continence rate using up to two treatments.[88] He measured an average increase in mean urethral closure pressure of 25 cm water. Patients with vesical instability were excluded from this study. A small percentage of patients developed vesical instability after GAX collagen injections, which spontaneously resolved within 3 months. The GAX collagen is totally absorbed by the body and replaced by the patient's own collagen within a period of 6 to 12 weeks, but patients nonetheless remain continent. Collagen may provide satisfactory treatment for a large number of women who are not surgical candidates or who are not willing to undergo surgery, particularly elderly women. More widespread usage, with reports of clinical efficacy and complication rates, is necessary to elevate more properly this modality in the future.

Before attempting periurethral injections, patients must undergo a small subcutaneous injection as a test for allergy. The rare occurrence of delayed hypersensitivity reaction (myositis) in patients injected with non–cross-linked collagen had delayed release of GAX collagen by the Food and Drug Administration. Finally, in late 1993, sufficient trials convinced authorities of its safety and it has rapidly come into general use. Other bulking agents have been tried, including Teflon,[89] cellulose, and autologous fat.[90] Migration of Teflon to local regional lymph nodes with subsequent granuloma formation has caused safety concerns and discontinuation of its use.[91]

Blaivis and Santarosa[90] reported periurethral injections of autologous fat in patients who are candidates for collagen (low-pressure urethra without mobility). Autologous fat has been used for decades by plastic surgeons to augment soft tissue without any reports of immediate or delayed hypersensitivity,[92] in contrast to collagen, which may produce hypersensitivity in rare instances. Fibroblast proliferation increases and stimulates endogenous collagen production in the area and probably acts in the same fashion as GAX collagen injections. Long-term success is unknown. In our clinical trials with autologous fat, obtained by syringe suction evacuation of the abdominal wall fat layer,[93] we have obtained a 75% success rate with minimal complications in patients with low pressure urethra without urethrovesical descent.

SUMMARY

It should be clear from the above discussion that the choice of surgical or nonsurgical management is as individual as the patient and surgeon and is a complicated formula with multiple variables. New surgical procedures and combinations seem to be evolving in never-ending fashion. Although none is ideal, a select few have emerged as reliable enough to give a 90% or better cure rate over a reasonable time. Because of the complexities involved, no one operation will ever be "perfect," considering surgeon to surgeon differences and patient to patient variations. Yet is is conceivable, with proper training and ultraspecialization, using the correct mix of common sense and intelligent interpretation of sophisticated diagnostic methods, we can develop a growing cadre of adept physicians capable of solving complicated urogynecologic problems at a high rate of cure. This must include the capacity to repair concomitantly all accompanying problems of pelvic relaxation and prolapse by both the vaginal and abdominal routes. As the 20th century comes to a close, looking over the remarkable progress of the past 100 years in breaking barriers in the comprehension and treatment of incontinence, we should be proud of ourselves. Yet, we have a long way to go and the light never stops shining.

REFERENCES

1. Hosking MP, Warner MA, Lobdell CM, et al. Outcomes of surgery in patients 90 years of age and older. *JAMA.* 1989;261:1909–1913.
2. Gillon G, Stanton SL. Long-term follow-up of surgery for urinary incontinence in elderly women. *Br J Urol.* 1984;56:478–481.
3. Suthherst J, Brown M, Shaner M. Assessing the severity of urinary incontinence in women by weighing perineal pads. *Lancet.* 1989;23:1128–1131.
4. Scotti R, Myers D. A comparison of the cough stress test and single channel cystometry with multichannel urodynamic evaluation in genuine stress incontinence. *Obstet Gynecol.* 1993;81:430–433.
5. Borcier A. Conservative treatment of stress incontinence, Abstract presented at American Urogynecology Society annual meeting, Cambridge, Mass. September 1992.
6. Norton P, Boyd C, Deak S. Abnormal collagen synthesis in women with genital prolapse or stress urinary incontinence. *Neurology and Urodynamics.* 1992;11:300–301.
7. McGuire EJ. Urodynamic findings in patients after failure of stress incontinence operations. *Prog Clin Biol Res.* 1981;78:351–356.
8. Sand PK, Bowen LW, Panganipan E, et al. The low pressure urethra as a factor in failed retropubic urethropexy. *Obstet Gynecol.* 1987;69:399–402.
9. Bowen LW, Sand PK, Ostergard DR, et al. Unsuccessful Burch retropubic urethropexy, a case controlled urodynamic study. *Am J Obstet Gynecol.* 1989;160:452–458.
10. Summitt R, Bent AE, Ostergard DR, et al. Correlation of preoperative Q-tip test with success using a suburethral sling procedure for stress urinary incontinence and low urethral closure pressure. *J Reprod Med.* 1990;35:877–880.
11. Bergman A, Koonings PP, Ballard CA. Negative Q-tip test as a risk factor in failed incontinence surgery in women. *J Reprod Med.* 1989;34:193–197.
12. Bump RC, Fantl JA, Hurt WG. Dynamic urethral pressure profilometry pressure

transmission ratio determinations after continence surgery: Understanding the mechanism of success, failure, and complications. *Obstet Gynecol.* 1988;72:870–877.

13. Langer R, Ron-El R, Newmann M, et al. Detrusor instability following colposuspension for urinary stress incontinence. *Br J Obstet Gynaecol.* 1988;95:607–610.

14. Awad SA, Flood HD, Acker KL. The significance of prior anti-incontinence surgery in women who present with urinary incontinence. *J Urol.* 1988;140:514–517.

15. Lindner P, Mattiasson A, Perssons L, et al. Reversibility of detrusor and hyperplasia after removal of infravesical outflow obstruction in the rat. *J Urol.* 1988;140:652–656.

16. Snooks SJ, Swash M, Setchell M, et al. Injury to innervation of pelvic floor sphincter musculature in childbirth. *Lancet.* 1984;2:546–548.

17. Snooks SJ, Swash M, Henry NM, et al. Risk factors in childbirth causing damage to the pelvic floor innervation. *Br J Surg.* 1985;72(suppl):15.

18. Smith ARB, Hosker GL, Warrell DW. The role of partial denervation of pelvic floor in the aetiology of genitourinary prolapse and stress incontinence in women: A neurophysiological study. *Br J Obstet Gynaecol.* 1989;96:24–29.

19. Gilpin SA, Gosling JA, Smith ARB, et al. The pathogenesis of genitourinary prolapse and stress incontinence of urine: a histological and histochemical study. *Br J Obstet Gynaecol.* 1989;96:15–18.

20. Bergman A, Koonings PP, Ballard CA. The Ball-Burch procedure for stress incontinence with low urethral pressure. *J Reprod Med.* 1991;36:137–140.

21. Scotti RJ. The diagnosis and treatment of surgical failures in genuine stress incontinence. *Urogynecologia International Journal.* 1991;5:65–80.

22. Mahoney DR, Laberte RO, Blais DJ. Integral storage and voiding reflexes: Neurophysiologic concept of continence micturition. *Urology.* 1977;10:95–106.

23. Sand PK, Bowen LW, Ostergard DR, et al. The effect of retropubic urethropexy on detrusor stability. *Obstet Gynecol.* 1988;71:818–822.

24. Mendelovici R, Scotti RJ. Funneling of the urethrovesical junction in women with urgency and urge incontinence. Abstract presented at American Urogynecology Society and Urodynamic Society annual meeting, San Antonio, Tex. October 1993.

25. Hilton P, Stanton SL. The use of intravaginal estrogen cream in genuine stress incontinence. *Br J Obstet Gynaecol.* 1983;90:940–942.

26. Rud T. The effects of estrogens and gestogens on the urethral pressure profile in urinary continent and stress incontinent women. *Acta Obstet Gynecol Scand.* 1980;59:265–270.

27. Bhatia NN, Bergman A, Karram MM. Effects of estrogen on urethral function in women with urinary incontinence. *Am J Obstet Gynecol.* 1989;160:176–180.

28. Fantl JA, Wyman JF, Anderson RL, et al. Postmenopausal urinary incontinence: comparison between non-estrogen supplement and estrogen supplement women. *Obstet Gynecol.* 1988;71:823–827.

29. Plevnik S, Janez J, Vrtacnik P, et al. Short-term electrical stimulation: home treatment for urinary incontinence. *World J Urol.* 1986;4:24–26.

30. Olah KS, Bridges N, Farrar D. The conservative management of genuine stress incontinence. *Int Urogynecol J.* 1991;2:161–167.

31. Kegel AM. Physiologic therapy for urinary stress incontinence. *JAMA.* 1951;146:915–917.

32. Peattie AB, Plevnik S, Stanton SL. Vaginal cones: A conservative method of treating genuine stress incontinence. *Br J Gynaecol.* 1988;95:1049–1051.

33. Bhatia NN, Bergman A, Gunning JE. Urodynamic effect of vaginal pessary in women with stress urinary incontinence. *Am J Obstet Gynaecol.* 1983;147:876–877.

34. Russell JK. The dangerous vaginal pessary. *Br. Med J.* December 1991;1595–1597.

35. Schraub S, Sun XS, Maingon P, et al. Cervical and vaginal cancer associated with pessary use. *Cancer.* 1992;69:2505–2509.

36. Vargas I, Scotti RJ. Rectal erosion and fistulization from a vaginal pessary. *J Gynecol Surg.,* 1994. Accepted for publication. In press.

37. Biswas N, Spencer P, King J. Conservative management of stress incontinence with a bladder neck support prosthesis (BSP). *Neurourology and Urodynamics.* 1993;12:311–313. Abstract.

38. Richardson DA. The evaluation of different surgical procedures. In: Ostergard DR, Bent AE, eds. *Urogynecology and Urodynamics Theory and Practice.* 3d ed. Baltimore: Williams & Wilkins; 1991:413–421.

39. Stanton SL, Cardozo LD. A comparison of vaginal and suprapubic surgery in the correction of incontinence due to urethral sphincter incompetence. *Br J Urol.* 1979;51:497–499.

40. Weil A, Reyes H, Bischoff P, et al. Modification of the urethral rest and stress profile after different types of surgery for stress incontinence. *Br J Obstet Gynaecol.* 1984;91:46–55.

41. Walter S, Olesin KP, Hald T, et al. Urodynamic evaluation after vaginal repair and colposuspension. *Br J Obstet Gynaecol.* 1982;54:377–380.

42. VanGeelen JM, Theeuwes AGM, Eskes TKAB, et al. The clinical and urodynamic effect of anterior vaginal repair and Burch colposuspension. *Am J Obstet Gynecol.* 1988;159:137–144.

43. Bergman A, Kooning PP, Ballard CA. Primary stress urinary incontinence and pelvic relaxation: Prospective randomized comparison of three different operations. *Am J Obstet Gynecol.* 1989;161:91–101.

44. Kelly HA, Dunn WM. Urinary incontinence in women, without manifest injury to the bladder. *Surg Gynecol Obstet.* 1914;18:444–450.

45. Kennedy WT. Incontinence of urine in the female, the urethral sphincter mechanism, damage of function, and restoration of control. *Am J Obstet Gynecol.* 1937;34:576–587.

46. Tanagho EA. Colpocystourethropexy: The way we do it. *J Urol.* 1976;116:751–753.

47. Beck RP, McCormick S. Treatment of urinary stress incontinence with anterior colporrhaphy. *Obstet Gynecol.* 1982;59:269–274.

48. Nichols DH. Anterior colporrhaphy. In: Nichols DH, Randall CL, eds. *Vaginal Surgery.* Baltimore: Williams & Wilkins; 1991:254–259.

49. Kujansuu E. Urodynamic analysis of successful and failed incontinence surgery. *Int J Gynecol Obstet.* 1983;21:353–358.

50. Kujansuu E, Kauppila A, Lahde S. Correlation between urethrovesical anatomy and

urethral closure function in female stress urinary incontinence before and after operation: Urethrocystographic and urethrocystometric evaluation. *Urol Int.* 1983;38:19–25.

51. Marshall VF, Marchetti AA, Krantz KE. Correction of stress incontinence by simple vesicourethral suspension. *Surg Gynecol Obstet* 1949;88:509–516.

52. Burch JC. Urethrovaginal fixation to Cooper's ligament for correction of stress incontinence, cystocele and prolapse. *Am J Obstet Gynecol.* 1961;81:281–290.

53. Milani R, Scalambrinos S, Quadri G, et al. Marshall-Marchetti-Krantz procedure and Burch colposuspension in the surgical treatment of female urinary incontinence. *Br J Obstet Gynaecol.* 1985;92:1050–1053.

54. Mainprize TC, Drutz HP. The Marshall-Marchetti-Krantz procedure: a critical review. *Obstet Gynecol Surv.* 1988;43:724–729.

55. Richardson AC, Edmonds PB, Williams NL. Treatment of stress urinary incontinence due to paravaginal fascial defect. *Obstet Gynecol.* 1981;57:357–362.

56. Shull BL, Baden WF. A six-year experience with paravaginal defect repair for stress urinary incontinence. *Am J Obstet Gynecol.* 1989;160:1432–1440.

57. Hall DL, Scotti RJ. A comparison of outcomes in patients undergoing Burch procedures and abdominal cystocele repair: Paravaginal defect repair versus modified colposuspension. Abstract presented at International Continence Society annual meeting, Halifax. September 1992.

58. Stanton SL. The Burch colposuspension procedure. *Acta Urol Belg.* 1984;52:280–282.

59. Wiskind AK, Creighton SM, Stanton SL. The incidence of genital prolapse after the Burch colposuspension. *Am J Obstet Gynecol.* 1992;167:339–405.

60. Drutz HP, Baker KR, Lemieux MC. Retropubic colpourethropexy with transabdominal anterior and/or posterior repair for the treatment of genuine stress urinary incontinence and genital prolapse. *Int Urogynecol J.* 1991;2:201–207.

61. Grody MHT. *Oophoropexy in Residual Ovary Syndrome and Abdominal Cystocele Repair.* ACOG Audiovisual Library 1990; AVL 64.

62. Vancaillie TG, Schuessler W. Laparoscopic bladderneck suspension. *J Laparo Surg.* 1991;1:169–173.

63. Pereyra AJ. A simplified surgical procedure for the correction of stress incontinence in women. *West J Surg.* 1959;67:223–226.

64. Stamey TA. Endoscopic suspension of the vesical neck for urinary incontinence. *Surg Gynecol Obstet.* 1973;136:547–554.

65. Raz S. Modified bladder neck suspension for female stress incontinence. *Urology.* 1981;17:82–85.

66. Muzsnai D, Carillo E, Dubin C, et al. Retropubic vaginopexy for correction of urinary stress incontinence. *Obstet Gynecol.* 1982;59:113–117.

67. Gittes RF, Loughlin KR. No-incision pubovaginal suspension for stress incontinence. *J Urol.* 1987;138:568–570.

68. Kelly MJ, Knielsen K, Bruskewitz R, et al. Symptom analysis of patients undergoing modified Pereyra bladder neck suspension for stress urinary incontinence. *Urology.* 1991;37:213–219.

69. Bhatia NN, Bergman A. Modified Burch versus Pereyra retropubic urethropexy for stress incontinence. *Obstet Gynecol.* 1985;66:255–261.

70. Bump RC, Fantl JA, Hurt GW. The mechanism of urinary incontinence in women with severe uterovaginal prolapse: Results of barrier studies. *Obstet Gynecol.* 1988;72:29–33.

71. Richardson D, Bent AE, Ostergard DR. The effect of uterovaginal prolapse on urethrovesical pressure dynamics. *Am J Obstet Gynecol.* 1983;146:901–905.

72. Bergman A, Koonings P, Ballard CA. Predicting postoperative urinary incontinence development in women undergoing operation for genitourinary prolapse. *Am J Obstet Gynecol.* 1988;158:1171–1175.

73. Henderson ML, Scotti RJ, Albini M. Potential incontinence in patients with severe urogenital prolapse. Abstract presented at International Continence Society annual meeting, Halifax. September 1992.

74. Funt MI, Thompson JD, Burch H. Normal vaginal axis. *South Med J.* 1978;71:1534–1537.

75. Ridley JH. The Goebell-Stoekel sling operation. In: Mattingly RF, Thompson JD, eds. *Telinde's Operative Gynecology.* 6th ed. Philadelphia: JB Lippincott, 1985:623–636.

76. Aldridge AH. Transplantation of fascia for relief of urinary stress incontinence. *Am J Obstet Gynecol.* 1942;44:398–401.

77. Horbach NS, Blanco JS, Ostergard DR, et al. A suburethral sling procedure with polytetrafluorethylene for treatment of genuine stress incontinence in patients with low urethral closure pressure. *Obstet Gynecol.* 1988;71:648–649.

78. Summitt R, Bent AE, Ostergard DR, et al. Suburethral sling procedure for genuine stress incontinence and low urethral closure pressures; a continued experience. *Int Orogynecol J.* 1992;3:18–21.

79. McGuire EJ, Bennett CJ, Konnak JA, et al. Experience with pubovaginal sling for urinary incontinence at the University of Michigan. *J Urol.* 1987;138:525–526.

80. Zacharin RF. Abdominal perineal urethral suspension in the management of recurrent stress incontinence of urine. *Obstet Gynecol.* 1983;62:644–654.

81. Raz S. Surgical therapy for urinary incontinence: sling procedures; vaginal wall sling. In: Raz S. *Atlas of Transvaginal Surgery.* Philadelphia: WB Saunders; 1992:78–85.

82. Scotti RJ, Mendelovici R. Suburethral vaginal patch-sling for low pressure urethra. Presented at Robert Wood Johnson Medical School, New Brunswick, NJ: December 1993.

83. Loughlin KR, Gittes RF, Klein LA, et al. The comparative medical costs of two major procedures available for the treatment of stress urinary incontinence. *J Urol.* 1982;127:436–438.

84. Scott FB. The artificial urinary sphincter: Experience in adults. *Urol Clin North Am.* 1989;16:105–108.

85. Light JK, Scott FB. Artificial urinary sphincter in the treatment of genuine stress incontinence in females. In: Ostergard DR, ed. *Gynecologic Urology and Urodynamics.* 3d ed. Baltimore: Williams & Wilkins; 1991:459–466.

86. Diokno AC, Hollander JB, Alderson TP. Artificial urinary sphincter for recurrent urinary incontinence: Indications and results. *J Urol.* 1987;138:778–780.

87. Ganabathi K, Abrams P, Mundy AR, et al. Stamey-Martius procedure for severe genuine stress incontinence. *Br J Urol.* 1992;69:34–37.

88. Appell RA. New developments: Injectables for urethral incompetence in women. *Int Urogynecol J.* 1990;1:117–119.

89. Politano VA. Periurethral Teflon injection for urinary incontinence. *Urol Clin N Am.* 1978;5:415–418.

90. Blaivas JG, Santarosa RP. Periurethral fat injection for sphincteric incontinence. *Neurourology and Urodynamics.* 1992;11:403–404.

91. Malizia AA, Reiman HM, Myers RP, et al. Migration and granulomatous reaction after periurethral injection of polytef (Teflon). *JAMA.* 1984;24:3277–3280.

92. Nguyen A, Pasyk KA, Bouvier TN, et al. Comparative study of survival of autologous adipose tissue taken and transplanted by different techniques. *Plast Reconstr Surg.* 1990;85:378–381.

93. Scotti RJ, Mendelovici R, Zahreddine N, et al. Periurethral autologous fat injections for minimally mobile low pressure urethra. *Internat Urogynecol J.* 1993;4:390.

Anterior Pelvic Compartment Reconstruction: The Total Vaginal Approach

Marvin H. Terry Grody

As illustrated in the previous chapter, in the latter part of this century, much stress has been placed on the mitigation and elimination of anatomic defects and disabling symptoms associated with the anterior pelvis by surgery through the space of Retzius. Because of anatomic impracticality, however, it is recognized that not all anterior defects can or should be repaired from a suprapubic entry, especially in older women. Most climacteric women present with a multiplicity of impairments relating to the mid-pelvic and posterior pelvic compartments as well, and these generally are best repaired through a perineal approach. Thus, if surgery is planned to correct all lesions at the same time to eliminate a double hospital admission and a double anesthesia exposure, she may become a victim, under the most popular current arrangements, of a single long operation performed through two entries under a single prolonged anesthesia. Certainly older women are more fragile than younger women and they have narrower safety margins. Then, all things considered, menopausal women are truly best served by the shortest possible operation through a single approach, when possible, so long as high quality surgical efficacy can be maintained. In this chapter, such a method is the major theme. These paragraphs represent, in effect, a clarion call to the adept practitioner to return to the vaginal approach as the sole entry

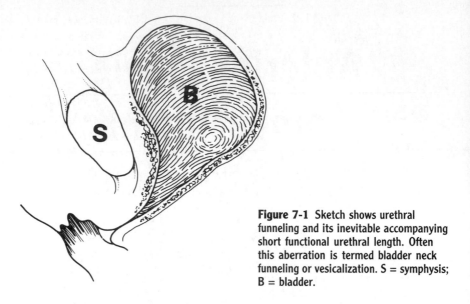

Figure 7-1 Sketch shows urethral funneling and its inevitable accompanying short functional urethral length. Often this aberration is termed bladder neck funneling or vesicalization. S = symphysis; B = bladder.

through which, using anatomically plausible techniques, long-term highly successful outcomes can be routinely anticipated.

CLINICAL DESCRIPTION

The surgery described is designed to correct the three most commonly occurring major anatomic defects of the anterior pelvis—the area anterior to the vagina, cervix, and uterus. For full comprehension of the remarkable efficacy of these methods, the particular impairments, principally three, are portrayed initially in their full-blown manifestations.

The repair of all three of these lesions within the same operating room setting presents one of the most challenging situations that can confront the gynecologic surgeon. As already noted, the current most popular approaches involve combined entries vaginally and suprapubically. The operative plan at Temple University Hospital (TUH) effectively accomplishes total corrections entirely from below, the route tolerated best by the postmenopausal patient.

The first lesion of reference is the intrinsically damaged urethra with marked funneling[1,2] in association with a functional length of only 1 to 2 cm (Figure 7-1) and an abnormally low urethral closure pressure. Most usually a sling of some sort, using either harvested autologous fascia from elsewhere in the body or synthetic material, is prescribed in these cases. This contrasts with the TUH approach, which uses adjacent (paraurethral) fascia.

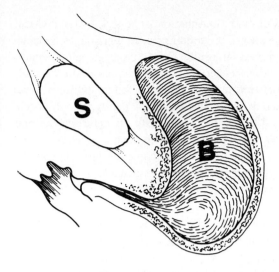

Figure 7-2 Combined rotational descent of the urethrovesical junction (hypermotile urethra) and cystocele. S = symphysis; B = bladder.

Secondly, separation of the proximal urethra, urethrovesical junction, and bladder from their natural bilateral attachments to the obturator internus fascia at the arcus tendineus fasciae pelvis is confronted in this operative plan. This anatomic problem has been termed paravaginal defects.[3–6] The dissociation at the proximal urethra and urethrovesical junction is due to the disruption of the posterior superior pubourethral ligaments in the area of the anterior end of the arcus tendineus. This particular segmental lesion is called rotational descent of the urethrovesical junction or, more simply, hypermotile urethra (Figure 7-2). The paravaginal lesion involving the bladder results in displacement cystocele. Specifically, this abnormality arises from separation of the pubovesicocervical connective tissue layer, which supports the bladder like a hammock, from its normal union with the arcus tendineus ("white line"), extending from the pubourethral ligaments to the ischial spines. This may occur on one or both sides. Added details are found in Chapter 6.

For repair of the urethral rotational descent (hypermotile urethra), currently a wide variety of operations are in vogue, for example, Marshall-Marchetti-Krantz, needle suspensions, and Burch (see Chapter 6). All of these involve suprapubic incisions and usually invasion into the space of Retzius. Of the various suprapubic approaches, only the paravaginal defects repair via the retropubic space, quite different from the three methods above, popularized by Wayne Baden and A. Cullen Richardson, is geared to correct the displacement cystocele. The paravaginal repair is unique; it is the only procedure of this nature that directly restores the normal anatomy (see Chapter 6). At TUH, restitution of this defect to normal is accomplished from below, after the manner presented by White[7,8] with modifications.

The third anatomic deviation of the common anterior compartment lesions and the one enjoying the longest temporal recognition is the distention cystocele or central bladder herniation. Generally this is repaired from the vaginal approach as a proximal extension and continuation of a series of individual midline sutures running from the area of the urethrovesical junction, as popularized by Kelly[9,10] to the anterior vaginal vault. These sutures repair a central defect by reuniting disrupted pubovesicocervical connective tissue in the midline. However, this kind of repair has a high degree of failure (50% to 60%) over the long term (5 years) if the defect is mistaken for a paravaginal cystocele and it really is *not* present at all, or if it coexists with an unrecognized and unrepaired paravaginal (displacement) cystocele. When such erroneous neglect happens, the lateral paravaginal separation may become exaggerated by the constricting action of the centrally placed sutures, especially if no midline bladder herniation exists. Symptoms remain uncorrected and ultimately worsen postoperatively.

A true central bladder herniation can be corrected from above, most usually in conjunction with abdominal hysterectomy, after appropriate dissection, starting at the vaginal cuff, between the bladder base and the anterior vaginal wall down to the natural urethrovaginal union (see Chapter 6). This can then be followed by a suprapubic urethral suspension or a paravaginal repair through the same abdominal wall exposure.

SURGICAL PRESENTATION A—EXPOSURE

After a suprapubic Foley drainage catheter is placed (standard in every case), the actual surgery is initiated in the usual fashion for anterior repair by a transverse incision across the vaginal vault immediately in front of the hysterectomy scar, or just anterior to the cervix in the unusual case where the uterus is retained. A vertical midline vaginal incision is then made from the center of the vault opening to a point 1 cm distal to the external urethral meatus. Vaginal flaps are then created bilaterally by a clean sharp separation of all connective tissue (urogenital diaphragmatic and urethrovesicocervical), displaced or not, and associated scar tissue from the internal surface of the vaginal wall out to the inferior rami of the pubic bones. Dissection is then continued, both sharply and bluntly, up the surface of the obturator internus muscle fascia to the arcuate line ("white line") along its entire length on each side. Occasionally there is such marked disruption at the "white line" that even the levator musculature on one side or the other, rarely both, is torn from its arcuate origin. In these cases, the examining finger can easily wander into the space of Retzius and palpate the superior ramus of the pubic bone on the affected side, with easy identification of the obturator canal and its neurovascular bundle. When this is discovered, the levator muscle is automatically simultaneously reattached in the repair process.

Infrequently an anterior enterocele appears as part of the anterior compartment prolapse. When this occurs, usually the sac is dissected, excised, and closed first before the actual anterior repair begins.

For guidance, a 16F Foley catheter is then inserted transurethrally into the bladder. The balloon is filled only to 4 mL, not more, to gauge better the extent of the elongated abnormally enlarged bladder neck (urethral funneling). Armed in advance with the known urethral length, this permits appropriate designation of the true urethrovesical junction where the so-called key suture will be placed on either side for the best guarantee of its replacement to normal location within the sphere of intra-abdominal pressure. The transurethral Foley catheter also affords precise definition of the total urethral situation.

SURGICAL PRESENTATION B—PARAURETHRAL REPAIR

The first specific portion of this complete anterior compartment repair is called paraurethral fascial sling urethropexy (PFSU). Allis-Adair clamps are placed into the pubovesicocervical layer (PVCL) on either side of the urethra about 3 mm from the midline at the estimated urethrovesical junction site. Additional Allis-Adair clamps are then placed similarly bilaterally 1 cm proximal (under the bladder neck) to the initial or key clamp and 1 cm distal to the key clamp, also 3 mm from the midline. Then, in succession, using Metzenbaum scissors against finger counterpressure, very meticulously PVCL flaps are formed on either side of the urethra, usually inwardly to 2.5 cm and to a length, from proximal urethra through bladder neck, of 2.5, occasionally 3, cm (Figure 7-3). These flaps are thin but of great strength, which is invariably tested before any suturing is begun by tugging on the clamps enough actually to move the patient. If a grasped edge tears, the clamp is simply replaced inwardly about 2 mm and retested to ensure strength. Any torn tissue is always in the medial edge and considered devitalized, thus of no value anyway.

Infrequently the urethra may be entered during the above dissection. In such event, the rent is simply closed by interrupted 4-0 polyglycolic acid sutures and the operation is continued. Even more infrequently an inward-running split may appear in one of the paraurethral flaps. These can simply be ignored and the suturing can be carried out as if the separation were not there; the flaps work just as well even with the disruption.

We feel that nonabsorbable suture of reasonably heavy caliber offers the best insurance for good long-term results in extensive anterior colporrhaphy. More precisely, for all the reasons clearly delineated in Chapter 16, we have chosen CV-0 polytetrafluorethylene (Gore, Inc., Flagstaff, AZ; PTFE) as the stitching material of choice. Except for surface closure, it is used exclusively for all the planned repair work in the three operative segments described in this chapter.

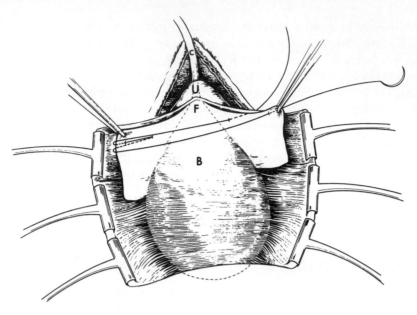

Figure 7-3 Illustration of the fully formed bilateral paraurethrovesical connective tissue flaps. The initial suture placement, starting on the patient's left, depicts the succession of far-near-far-near punctures that leads to the formidable sling described in the text. C=catheter; U = urethra; F = funneling; B = bladder.

Three interrupted stitches are used to create this urethral sling, one in association with each level of Allis-Adair clamp placement, beginning distally. The technique of penetration is in a far-near-far-near order, with the far punctures 2.0 to 2.5 cm from the flap edge and the near perforations just under the grasp of the clamp. In the first two needle entries, far (left side) and near (right side), the needle points toward the patient, while the last two, also far (right side) and near (left side), respectively, point toward the operator (see Figure 7-3). The sutures are tied only after all have been properly positioned. Once tied, a broad sling is dramatically revealed to elevate and relatively fix the area of the urethrovesical junction some 2.5 to 3.0 cm above its original location from the cut mucosal edges (Figures 7-4A,B).

The concept of paraurethral flaps is not new.[11,12] Neither is the fear of necrosis that might be engendered if the flaps are extended more than a few millimeters laterally on each side. Theoretically it has been postulated that any extensive isolation of tissue flaps would so jeopardize their innervation and blood supply that they would die. In 1989, I challenged this hypothesis by deliberately creating the wide and deep flaps already described. As will be related later in this chapter, necrotic disaster has not occurred at all. Contrarily, the effectiveness of paraurethral flaps has been abundantly successful with no evidence of necrosis of any kind. It seems that any disruption that might result

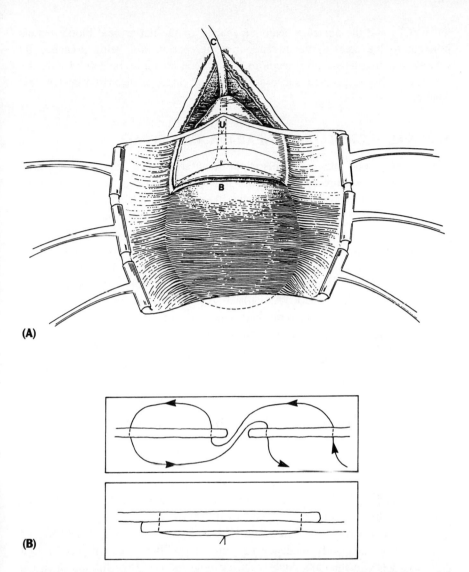

Figure 7-4 *(A)*, The sling is completed, the left flap under and external to the right flap, and the sutures have been tied. The effective elevation and elimination of funneling are easily interpolated. C = catheter; U = urethra; B = bladder. *(B)*, The "double-breasted" formation of the sling is seen in cross section.

from surgical neurologic damage[13,15] and vascular deprivation is compensated by rapid neurocirculatory regeneration. In the end, this "double-breasted" uplifting sling forms a far healthier structural support under the urethra than existed in the preoperative status (see Figure 7-4). Objectively, because of the strength of the nonabsorbable microporous PTFE suture, the innate durability of the PVCL, and the amazing healing capacity of the nerves and blood vessels inherent to the areal tissue, the negative perception *still* being preached by otherwise authoritative urogynecologists has been proven to be entirely false by our new highly respectable successful series of cases, as discussed later in this chapter.

SURGICAL PRESENTATION C—PARAVAGINAL REPAIR

We call the second segment of this tripartite anterior pelvic anatomic correction the WREBS procedure or, more descriptively, paravaginal defects cystocele repair, a vaginal paravaginal cystopexy. The acronym WREBS pays tribute to the surgical pioneers responsible for developing recognition and acceptance of the concept of paravaginal defects as a major cause of cystocele, arguably a more common lesion than the central tissue division leading to the traditionally accepted distention cystocele. These innovators, in line with the acronym, have been George White, Benjamin Word, Tom Walker, A. Cullen Richardson, Paul Edmonds, and Bobby Shull. (Actually only White performed this procedure vaginally as a routine[7,8] and Word had done some of his cases vaginally before we began doing ours consistently from below in 1990. Now Shull is operating paravaginally frequently from the introital entry.) In almost all cases referred into TUH, we find a substantial degree of both types of cystocele, as already implied, in coexistence. Perhaps it is of great significance that 90% of these patients have had at least one attempt at anterior repair of some sort already and many of them have withstood more than two previous operations, ending in symptomatic and anatomic failure.

Preparation for the actual WREBS correction has been accomplished by the dissection into the area of the arcus tendineus as already described. The "key" suture (CV-0 PTFE) is placed initially through the obturator internus fascia (OIF) laterally at the "white line" at a point judged to be about 4.5 cm from the external urethral meatus. It is tugged to demonstrate the strength of the bite. Some surgeons have a misconception that obturator fascia may frequently be weak, with an associated tendency for suture "pull-out" (see Chapter 6). Our extensive work in this area defies such an impression. In the line between the mid-symphysis and the ischial spine, we have found the fascia overlying the medial surface of the obturator internus muscle to be consistently strong. The second part of the stitch is then thrust appropriately through the PVCL lateral to and covering the urethra at the level previously designated as the urethrovesical junction. As with the OIF bite, about 4 mm of tissue is included. Again testing by tugging is done to ensure that the stitch will not pull out. Care is then taken, as the suture is tied, to note that no undue tension results. We tie these sutures as we position them to avoid the confusion of profusion of suture ends occurring when instead one waits to tie them after all have been placed. We find no difference in the end result no matter which course is followed,

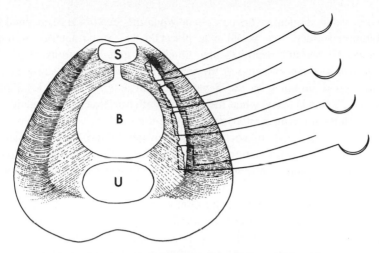

Figure 7-5 Sketch depicts the method of WREBS suture placement in correcting paravaginal defects from the vaginal approach. S = symphysis; B = bladder; U = uterus.

although we have feelings that, by securing the key stitch first, we have a more reliable gauge for placement of the others than we would have if we held off to tie all at once. A similar suture then anchors the residual pubourethral ligament fibers at the level of the proximal urethra to the OIF about 8 mm distal to the key suture. This is followed by a succession of one to four more sutures proximal to the key suture (Figure 7-5), connecting appropriate points of PVCL overlying first the bladder neck and then more of the bladder, depending on the extent of the bladder detachment, to the area of the "white line" on the OIF in the direction of the ischial spine. These 4-mm long stitches are placed about 5 mm apart and are tested for holding strength at each anchoring spot before tying, a point so important we feel compelled to reemphasize it. After one side is completed, the procedure is mirrored in the opposite paravaginal area. Even though the paravaginal defect may be one sided, or the lesion may be of lesser extent on one side than the other, it seems wise, while the operative field is open, to bolster supports as much as possible to give the best odds against future breakdown by always doing both sides.

In instances where the levator seems to be shorn away, we tend to over-correct laterally with the key suture going about 5 mm higher than usual to produce a slightly sharper angle. In such cases we also tend to bite more tissue adjacent to the urethra and bladder to help in the reestablishment of levator attachment to the arcus tendineus. Also, with levator detachment, often no arcus tendineus may be visible or palpable. So it must be reformed by creating an imaginary line between the mid-symphysis and the ischial spine on the involved side with suture placement accordingly. It must be remembered that an arcus tendineus forms when fascial planes meet in one line to form a "white" concentration.

Two possible surgical errors can occur when the levators are separated from the obturator surface. It is possible to place the key stitch anterior enough to penetrate the obturator neurovascular bundle, a truly disastrous event. Less dramatic but very discouraging is the inadvertent creation of a straight line of bladder support proximal to the key suture and anterior to the level of the "white line." This happens when the operator, after an excellent dissection, in a state of enthusiasm, temporarily forgets about the need for a good cystourethral angle and the importance of not straying from the "white line" of attachment and places the paravesical sutures too far anteriorly. Erroneously thinking that "the higher, the better," a postoperative situation of uncontrollable incontinence eventuates.

When the WREBS portion of the operation is completed, the transurethral guidance catheter should be removed in such a way that postoperative urethral length can be objectively measured. This is accomplished by pulling the Foley balloon gently into contact with the bladder neck, then placing a thumb and index finger on the catheter at the external meatus followed by balloon deflation and catheter removal. A measurement from the digital position on the catheter to the point of balloon inflation should measure at least 4 cm to indicate elimination of funneling in conjunction with cystourethral angle elevation into the intra-abdominal sphere of pressure influence. Simultaneously urethral pressure should increase dramatically by virtue of this mechanical correction.

A criticism of the WREBS operation has been leveled at the absence of any attempt to include a corresponding bite into lateral vagina with each corrective suture, as done by White originally. It has been theorized that bilateral recreation of the normal-appearing vagina sulci is essential to success in this method of repair because part of the vaginal wall is included in each bite taken in the suprapubic approach to paravaginal repair. We have perceived no impairment in achieving good results without including the vagina in each suture. To our pleasant surprise, we have noticed automatic uniform sustained reformation of the bilateral anterior vaginal sulcus anyhow in postoperative follow-up examinations. Obviously natural healing processes draw vaginal mucosa adherently into anatomically normal position without need for ancillary inclusive suturing in these areas.

SURGICAL PRESENTATION D—STANDARD MIDLINE REPAIR

We call the third operative component in extensive anterior colporrhaphy "intracardinal imbrication." Although this is not an anatomically totally inclusive description title, it does precisely refer to the closure of the almost invariably occurring midline weak point at the uppermost reaches of the bladder base at the level of the anterior vaginal fornix. Essentially this operative segment eliminates the distention cystocele by imbricating at the midline the anterior extensions of the cardinal ligaments and the disparate supportive pubovesicocervical fascia from each side. This is accomplished simply by placing a series of interrupted PTFE sutures in traditional manner, anywhere from two to five, either simple or horizontal mattress, across the midline under and behind the bladder. The number of sutures used depends on the extent of the distention herniation. Exact attention must be focused on the innermost suture. In the great majority of cases, the uterus has been removed at an earlier operation and the vagina anterior to the hysterectomy scar is more or less shortened. Therefore, for best results, and to present the best prophylaxis for the future, dissection anteriorly should almost always be carried 2 to 3 cm posteriorly beyond the hysterectomy scar, especially since the usually overstretched posterior vaginal wall will not thereby be compromised. This permits this farthest suture to be anchored broadly into this deep level of vaginal wall between its bilateral puncture of the residual cardinal ligament fibers at the innermost level of the bladder base.

In a logical anatomic sequence, the original horizontal vaginal mucosal vault opening, assuming initial liberal wide dissection, is closed longitudinally in synchrony with this deep anchoring point, thereby lengthening the anterior vagina and aiding in the ultimate reestablishment of a normal vaginal axis. When hysterectomy is performed at the same setting, the innermost suture incorporates strands of cardinal ligament running anteriorly together with bites into anterior vaginal cuff.

When both paravaginal and central cystoceles coexist, as in the cases described in this chapter, generally we correct the former one first. However, if the distention cystocele is predominant, we will perform the midline repair initially. When this course is chosen, one must take care not to bring more tissue into the midline than necessary for fear of pulling lateral areas too far medially, thereby preventing effective paravaginal defect closure.

COMMENTARY

In performing the combined anterior repair as described, usually the uterus is already gone or it is removed simultaneously as part of the correction of widespread pelvic prolapse. However, if the uterus is well fixed normally, its removal will not improve the surgical result. When the uterus is prolapsed to any appreciable degree, it represents a weak link in pelvic support and generally, in the postreproductive woman, should be removed for best results. Coincidentally, hysterectomy obviates the need for progesterone accompaniment to estrogen replacement therapy (ERT) and eliminates all annoyance and fear arising from endometrial stimulation in ERT.

Similarly, if the posterior fornix is well fixed in its usual elevated position, in accompaniment with appropriate vesical base repair, no further surgery need be done to support the upper bladder. However, we feel that, if the posterior vaginal vault, as judged preoperatively with accompanying Valsalva in the erect posture, descends more than 3 cm, a sacrospinous ligament fixation of the vaginal vault in juxtaposition to the innermost portion of the bladder base is integral to sustained postsurgical maintenance of support.

Again in the same vein, as is now so widely recognized, even the most expertly performed anterior repair is apt to break down under the distorted strain of an abnormal vaginal axis if that is not simultaneously also corrected. This is crucial since the usually preexisting axis aberration is commonly exaggerated by the anterior corrective surgery. Thus, it is advisable in most cases, after the urethrovesical replacement, to perform at the minimum a perineorrhaphy and, if a posterior defect is objectively deep enough, even though asymptomatic, an appropriate posterior colpoperineorrhaphy. Importantly, such simultaneous supplemental surgery discourages future enterocele development.

A thorough search of the literature reveals no report describing paraurethrovesical flaps anywhere close to the magnitude of the ones we fashion as described in this chapter and as illustrated in Figure 7-3. What is generally presented is reproduced in Figure 7-6. Such flaps have been labeled as pubourethral ligaments,[11,12] but this is difficult to conceive since pubourethral ligaments are found to run from each side of the proximal urethra anteriorly to attach to the symphysis pubis. Disregarding this apparent contradiction in terminology, these reduced slips of connective tissue dissected off the urethra seem much too tiny to be of any good. They consist only of central tissue, not nearly as strong as their more lateral extensions, and they are much too narrow and too short to eliminate any funneling or evoke more than a few millimeters of elevation at best. Thus the sling created is much too limited in both width and length to be of any true value as compared to the slings we construct. Finally, descriptions imply that these minimal repairs work by themselves, requiring no adjunctive support. We find that, even with our markedly large slings, they can *only* be truly effective when combined with a paravaginal repair (WREBS) simultaneously.

Trying to understand operative procedures from verbal descriptions, even with ancillary pictorial aids, often is rather difficult. A video of an operation, especially with accompanying full explanatory audio, can make a world of difference. Such motion pictures of the operations shown in this chapter are readily available.[16–18] Considering the fine results we are steadily compiling at TUH using the techniques described in this chapter, such additional reviews could prove most helpful to the interested gynecologist.

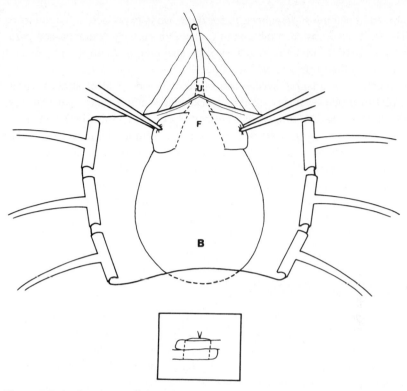

Figure 7-6 Inadequate paraurethral flaps fashioned vaginally. The few millimeters of overlap resulting from inadequate flap dissection are shown beneath in cross-section. C=catheter; U = urethra; F = funneling; B = bladder.

CLINICAL CASES

At the time of this publication, we will have performed over 150 consecutive procedures at TUH on patients presenting with disabling complaints relating to the lesions presented in this chapter.[20,21] A manuscript on this series of patients to include those with follow-up time of 6 months to more than 4 years is being prepared for publication while this book is being completed. Over 95% of the patients are beyond 50 years of age and the range reaches 90 years. Each patient in the group, in addition to the damage in the anterior compartment already noted, revealed symptoms associated with other objective manifestations synchronous with pelvic prolapse in one form or another. Every case displayed hypermotile urethra, displacement cystocele, and distention cystocele. All of them had lesions additionally in the mid-pelvis (uterine prolapse or enterocele) or in the posterior pelvic compartment (perineal defects or rectocele). In our judgment, the mid-pelvic and posterior pelvic lesions were thought to be repaired best or repaired only through the vaginal approach. So we elected to do all surgery entirely from below instead of combining entries, that is, initially vaginally and finishing suprapubically, for the reasons explained at the outset of the chapter. In each instance the opening phase of surgery encompassed paraurethral fascial sling urethropexy (PFSU), paravaginal cystopexy, and standard midline intracardinal imbrication.

Our premise for gauging success is fourfold: (1) absence of stress incontinence, (2) no prolapse of any organs, (3) adequate coital functional capacity, and (4) subjective satisfaction with the operation. On this basis, the results have been running a better than 95% success rate. Admittedly these are select patients all subject to the strict preoperative rules delineated in Chapter 3 and the carefully and repeatedly stressed postoperative standards outlined in Chapter 18. In our minds the most important of these is lifetime commitment to ERT. All but a few of the patients, particularly those with previous recurrent operative failures, had ever taken appreciable ERT, if any at all, before visiting us.

ADDITIONAL CLINICAL POINTS

In completing the discussion of this type of surgery, a few final points are pertinent. In many of the cases presenting to us, the complaint of stress incontinence is absent despite a grossly discernible obvious rotational descent of cystourethral junction, usually with a strongly positive Q-tip test. Without exception, stress incontinence was produced in urodynamic study by alleviating the "kinking" effect of a large cystocele or severe uterine prolapse or both through replacement of the causative defective organ(s) (Figure 7-7). Many of these revealed an earlier history of stress incontinence which disappeared as

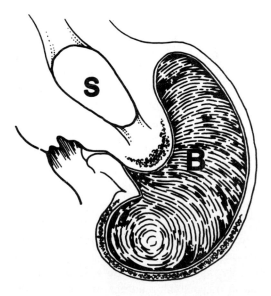

Figure 7-7 "Kinking" effect caused by the compression of the hypermotile urethra by the dominating cystocele. Release of the kinking by correction of the cystocele alone will lead to genuine urinary stress incontinence not present now because of the closure effect of the kinking, as shown. S = symphysis; B = bladder.

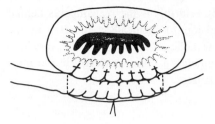 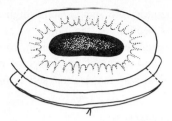

Figure 7-8 On the left, the constrictive effect of imbricating stitches, as in the Kelly method, at the urethrovesical junction and proximal urethra. On the right, the elevating sling described by Grody without luminal impingement on the same areas.

cystocele or uterine procidentia increased and kinking developed. The important point to stress is the need to correct a seemingly asymptomatic hypermotile urethra simultaneously with cystocele repair or almost assuredly stress incontinence will manifest postoperatively.

The PFSU is unique, in its elimination of the enlarged bladder neck (urethral funneling) and elevation of the proximal urethra and urethrovesical junction, by its capacity to increase urethral pressure without constricting the urethra (see Figure 7-4). In combination with the WREBS, it also increases the pressure transmission ratio without overcorrecting it. Even partial urethral obstruction seems almost impossible with the PFSU-WREBS combination, especially when compared to the traditional Kelly sutures[7,8] and probably even to the anchoring urethral sutures of Beck[2] (Figure 7-8). Basically this operation seems to be ideal for the low-pressure urethra. We must also add one other gratifying feature observed by us consistently: the urinary urgency and frequency almost always coexistent with funneling seems almost invariably to disappear after an adequate PFSU.

A singular advantage to performing the PFSU and WREBS procedures together, especially in view of the high success rate, not to mention the single entry and the shorter operating and anesthesia time, is that it is not a last resort. In the small percentage of failures, one can always come back later to do an isolated suprapubic urethral suspension (SPUS). If the SPUS is performed first, in association with other repairs from below, and fails, the options become narrower. Even worse is the primary choice of a sling, using extraneous material, especially if foreign to the body, and it fails. Then reliable alternatives that will satisfy the patient practically disappear. However, in the unusual case where PFSU-WREBS, as described in this chapter, fails, a fascia lata or synthetic sling is still another resort.

Finally, the inclusion of this chapter in this book was not done simply to confuse the reader even more by adding further to the seemingly endless list of kinds of operative sallies into the anterior pelvic compartment. In fact, the three operative components described are truly old ideas that have been modified to work together. What is important to the conscientious and adventuresome operator who sets personal high standards, and this is the real impetus behind this section of the book, is our compulsion to inculcate a mindset in the surgeon, especially if young, to give these ladies a "break," on the very first operative attempt, by doing the most complete operation correctly in the most logical way that is most satisfying to the patient.

REFERENCES

1. Nichols DH. Anterior colporrhaphy. In: Nichols DH, Randall CL, eds. *Vaginal Surgery.* 3d ed. Baltimore: Williams & Wilkins; 1991:252–255.

2. Beck RP, McCormick S, Nordstrom L. A 25-year experience with 519 anterior colporrhaphy procedures. *Obstet Gynecol.* 1991;78:1011–1018.

3. Richardson AC, Lyon JB, Williams NL. A new look at pelvic relaxation. *Am J Obstet Gynecol.* 1976;126:565–573.

4. Richardson AC, Edmonds PB, Williams NL. Treatment of stress urinary incontinence due to paravaginal fascial defect. *Obstet Gynecol.* 1981;57:357–362.

5. Baden WF, Walker TA. Urinary stress incontinence: Evolution of paravaginal repair. *Female Patient.* 1987;12:89–94.

6. Shull BL, Baden WF. A six year experience with paravaginal defect repair for stress urinary incontinence. *Am J Obstet Gynecol.* 1989;160:1432–1440.

7. White GR. Cystocoele: A radical cure by suturing lateral sulci of vagina to white line of pelvic fascia. *JAMA.* 1909;53:1707–1710.

8. White GR. An anatomical operation for the cure of cystocele. *Am J Obstet Dis Wom Child.* 1912;65:286–291.

9. Kelly HA, Dunn WM. Urinary incontinence in women, without manifest injury to the bladder. *Surg Gynecol Obstet.* 1914;18:444–450.

10. Kelly HA. Incontinence of urine in women. *Urol Cutan Rev.* 1915;17:291–296.

11. Nichols DH, Milley PS. Identification of pubourethral ligaments and their role in transvaginal surgical correction of stress incontinence. *Am J Obstet Gynecol.* 1973;115:123–128.

12. Nichols DH. Anterior colporrhaphy. In: Nichols DH, Randall CL, eds. *Vaginal Surgery.* 3d ed. Baltimore: Williams & Wilkins; 1991:254–259.

13. Smith PH, Balentine B. The neuroanatomical basis for denervation of the urinary bladder following major pelvic surgery. *Br J Surg.* 1968;55:929–932.

14. Mundy AR. An anatomical explanation for bladder dysfunction following rectal and uterine surgery. *Br J Urol.* 1982;54:501–504.

15. Benson JT, McClellan E. The effect of vaginal dissection on the pudendal nerve. *Obstet Gynecol.* 1993;82:387–389.

16. Grody MH. *Repair of Paravaginal Defects (WREBS Procedure).* ACOG Audiovisual Library 1991;AVL 67.

17. Grody MH. *Anatomic Surgical Restoration in Extreme Massive Vaginal Eversion.* ACOG Audiovisual Library 1993;AVL 84.

18. Grody MHT. *Complex Procedures and Methods in Pelvic Reconstructive and Urogynecologic Surgery* (video). New York and London: Parthenon; 1993:2,3,4.

19. Grody MHT, Nyirjesy P. *Surgical Correction of Urethral Kinking and Funneling Accompanying Hypermotile Urethra in Massive Vaginal Eversion.* (video). Woodbury CT: Cine Med; 1994 (May). Presented at ACOG Annual Scientific Meeting.

20. Grody MH, Lucyk M, Tinsley WR. Paraurethral fascial sling urethropexy and paravaginal defects repair (WREBS procedure): Pilot study. Presented at annual meeting of American Uro-Gynecology Society, Newport Beach, Calif. October 1991.

21. Grody MH, Lucyk M, Tinsley WR. Vaginal repair of paravaginal defects (WREBS procedure) combined with paraurethral sling urethropexy: Pilot study. Presented at annual meeting of Society of Gynecologic Surgeons, Orlando, Fla. March 1992.

Transabdominal Sacralcolpopexy for Massive Vaginal Vault Eversion in the Posthysterectomy Patient

Stanley F. Rogers

Massive eversion of the vaginal vault following hysterectomy (see Figure 9-5), thought to be relatively uncommon 30 to 40 years ago,[1,2] seems to have increased tenfold in the past decade. Although accurate figures are not readily available, the feedback from gynecologic services across the country coupled with the popularity of discussion of the entity at gynecologic conferences and increased reports on it in the literature indicate that massive vaginal eversion can no longer be considered an infrequent disease.[1–10] In a referral practice at the Woman's Hospital of Texas, for example, we operated on 68 patients with this condition in 1990 while in that same period 1017 hysterectomies were performed. This reflects a steady increase in our own numbers and is quite formidable when compared to Phaneuf's figures of only 7 versus 5554 major gynecologic operations in 1956.[1]

Although vaginal vault eversion exhibits the same defects whether or not the uterus is present, complete posthysterectomy vaginal eversion is more difficult to treat than similar defects occurring in patients suffering only from procidentia

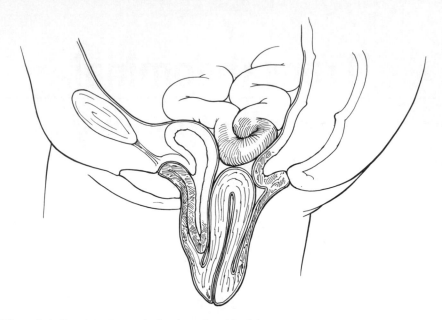

Figure 8-1 Complete uterovaginal prolapse (procidentia).

because the cardinal and uterosacral ligaments are attenuated and all but lost (Figure 8-1). The real chance to prevent vaginal vault prolapse occurs at the time of hysterectomy, when the upper supportive ligaments of Mackenrodt and the utero-sacral ligaments can be used to their fullest extent in both culdeplasty and superior vaginal support.

The large defect of vaginal vault eversion basically begins with the pulsion enterocele, which is always present, and progresses to complete vaginal eversion (Figure 8-2). Specific cases can vary markedly and may also include cystocele, urethrocele, and rectocele defects. Therefore, treatment must be specifically tailored to each case.

We have frequently noted an especially early and dramatic incidence of pulsion enterocele with vaginal vault prolapse within 4 months of combined hysterectomy and urethropexy, particularly when the Burch procedure is used and also following anterior vaginal suspension to the abdominal wall (see Figure 9-5). Addison and coworkers reported data on 21 patients in whom vault prolapse followed soon after high anterior urethropexy or vaginal suspension.[3]

Zacharin has stated "that the upward support of the cervix and upper vagina is the function of the cellular tissues of Mackenrodt, which are held in such position over the levator plate for its support whenever there is an increase in intra-abdominal pressure."[4] For pulsion enterocele and vault prolapse to occur, the upper vaginal supporting ligaments must be weakened or absent and the levator plate deflected by an attenuated levator sling producing a vertical vagina in the standing patient. For proper anatomic repair, the upper vagina must have its new support in

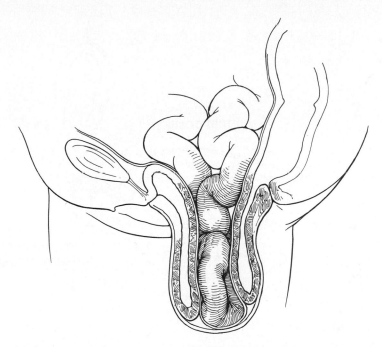

Figure 8-2 Pulsion enterocele accompanying complete posthysterectomy vault prolapse.

the direction of the sacrum using the sacrospinous ligaments, the prespinous ileococygeous fascia or the sacrum itself. Levator and perineal restoration is necessary to prevent recurrence by providing a strong pelvic floor and the proper horizontal vaginal axis in the standing position.

Symmonds and colleagues, whose experience and data have been extensive, prefer the transvaginal approach to correct any enterocele, rectocele, and cystocele defects that may accompany vaginal vault prolapse.[5] They feel that restoration of the levator plate provides adequate support for the vagina. We agree completely that cystocele, rectocele, and enterocele defects must all be repaired when present, along with levator restoration. The real art in this approach, which we have been using over the past 40 years, lies in knowing how extensive the repairs must be to achieve a lasting good result, yet restrictive enough to ensure acceptable coital function. However, when the uterus has been removed, the superior support system is commonly lost, and if we can find a replacement for cephalad support of the vaginal vault, whether by sacrospinous ligament fixation or sacral suspension, it may permit an overall better result.

Ventral slings or fixation techniques to the abdominal wall are apparently performed in some institutions, but we do not condone these techniques because they place the vagina in a more anterior and vertical position in contrast to the desired normal horizontal vaginal axis when the patient is standing. Only when the natural horizontal lie of the proximal vagina is restored is there sufficient protection

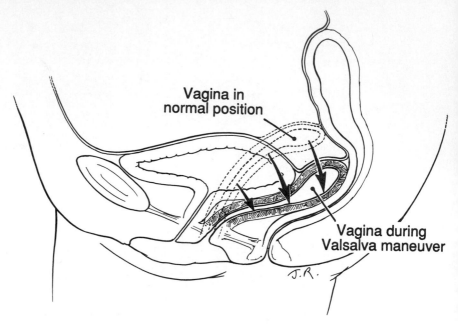

Figure 8-3 Anatomic drawing of normal supportive nulliparous vaginal axis in the standing patient. Produced with help of x-rays. (See reference no. 7, pgs. 5 & 6 fig. 1.3 and fig. 1.4)

from the downward forces on the cul-de-sac (Figure 8-3). Anterior vaginal suspension greatly enlarges the posterior cul-de-sac and commonly leads to enterocele formation.

The sacrospinous ligament suspension of the vagina devised by Sederl,[6] improved by Richter and Werner,[7] and popularized and further improved by Nichols and Randall,[8] and similar techniques by Inmon[9] and Wiser (personal communication, University of Mississippi, 1991) are preferable for elderly or fragile high-risk patients needing repair of complete or partial vaginal vault prolapse (Figure 8-4). The procedure should always include enterocele and rectocele repair along with levator restoration and adequate perineorrhaphy. We use this approach in approximately 20% of our patients. Sacralcolpopexy is our choice in the patient with massive (complete) prolapse and where a premium is placed on vaginal length and a long-lasting result.

TECHNIQUE

The abdomen is opened and adhesions are carefully lysed. The bowel is packed away and a four-way retractor is placed. After the sigmoid colon is retracted to the left, the vaginal hand retractor (a lucite probe with handle) will elevate the vagina to

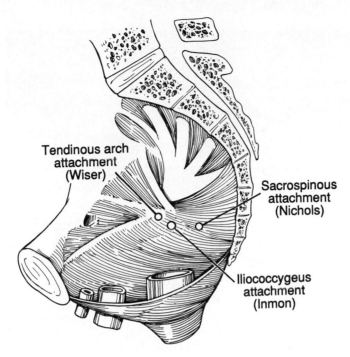

Tendinous arch
attachment
(Wiser)

Sacrospinous
attachment
(Nichols)

Iliococcygeus
attachment
(Inmon)

Figure 8-4 Schematic drawing of transvaginal sites to attach the prolapsed vagina.

its normal position in the pelvis. It is most useful in performing the culdeplasty and sacropexy.[10]

Our usual technique begins with the Halban culdeplasty[11] (Figure 8-5). Interrupted, nonabsorbable monofilament 2-0 sutures are placed as vertical purse-strings, obliterating the cul-de-sac and attaching the upper vagina to the rectum. This is required in most patients because the cul-de-sac defect is quite deep. Whenever the uterosacral ligaments can be retrieved, shortened, and reattached to the lateral angles of the cuff, they may offer additional vertical support in the partially prolapsed vagina.

We frequently perform the presacral preparation first because an extremely vascular sacrum may preclude the use of this technique and alternate modes of suspension may be necessary.

A vertical incision is made in the peritoneum over the sacral promontory and is extended downward to the cul-de-sac. A minimal presacral neurectomy is commonly, but not always, necessary to clear the periosteum. Occasionally, pressure with a moist lap sponge will help to define the periosteum, sometimes without neurectomy.

Much care must be used to identify the right ureter attached under the peritoneum on the patient's right, the middle sacral vessels, and the left common iliac vein beneath and near the mesocolon (Figure 8-6). The presacral periosteum is exposed

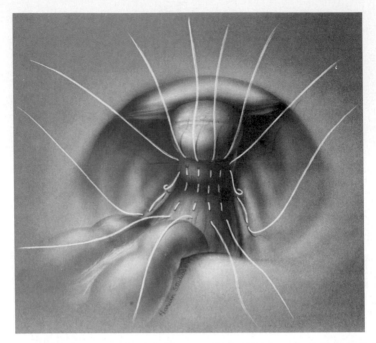

Figure 8-5 Drawing of our modification of Halban culdeplasty using reefing sutures to shorten the sacrouterine ligaments, as well as the more central Halban sutures.

and nonvascular area is cleared of areolar tissue. After the vaginal cuff is prepared by a transverse anterior peritoneal incision, downward dissection of the bladder is accomplished along with denuding the vaginal cuff of its peritoneum.

Many types of patch material have been used for sacralcolpopexy, including fascia lata,[12] dura mater,[13] and Marlex, Prolene, and Mersilene meshes. We prefer to use the 5 × 17, 1-mm thick expanded polytetrafluoroethylene (ePTFE) GORE-TEX Soft Tissue Patch (WL Gore and Associates, Inc., Flagstaff, AZ). It is inert, soft, and quite easy to work with and, postoperatively, its microporous structure allows fibroblasts to become incorporated within the material, giving a strong, lasting support. We trim the patch to fit the vaginal cuff on one end and then attach it to the anterolateral or posterolateral portion of the cuff, avoiding the cuff itself, as it has poor vascularity. Six to eight interrupted 00 monofilament, nonabsorbable sutures are used. The other end is trimmed to fit the hollow of the sacrum to allow for intrusion of the sigmoid colon on the left. It is also shortened just enough still to afford dependable support of the vault, but not so much that rigidity sufficient enough to cause urinary incontinence is produced. Similar sutures attach the upper end of the patch to the prepared sacrum just below the promontory because this favors the desired transverse vaginal axis and is less vascular than the lower sacral hollow (Figures 8-7 and 8-8). The entire area is then reperitonealized using continuous absorbable suture.

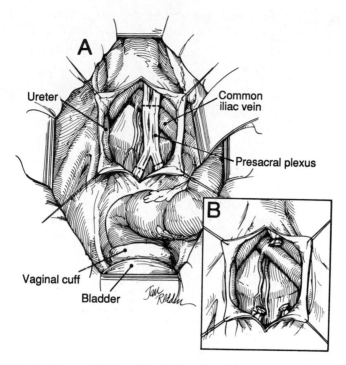

Figure 8-6 Sketch of presacral space and anatomic safeguard areas.

Sacralcolpopexy offers the additional advantage of supporting the anterior vaginal wall when an apparent cystocele is due completely or partially to rotational descent of the anterior vagina instead of the classical bulging central defect of the bladder wall. Not infrequently, by providing adequate cephalad vaginal support, sacralcolpopexy substantially reduces what seems like a large cystocele and eliminates what some consider a moderate defect.

An office examination and preoperative examination under anesthesia as well are needed to ascertain the necessity of performing cystocele repair in these cases by replacing the inverted vagina and determining which support components are lost or compromised. The classical cystocele defect, in which there is marked attenuation of the vaginal muscularis and bladder wall, requires excision of the redundant, weakened vaginal wall and a layered repair of the cystocele defect. This can be done vaginally before performing the sacralcolpopexy or transabdominally by excising the defective central vaginal wedge and performing a two-layered repair using 2-0 Dexon or Vicryl suture. When urinary incontinence is present with the loss of the urethrovesical angle, it is repaired concomitantly either by performing a transvaginal cystourethrocele repair or, preferably, by performing a suprapubic urethropexy of one's choice. We prefer the paravaginal suspension described by Richardson and colleagues[14] and Baden and Walker[15] (see Figure 8-8).

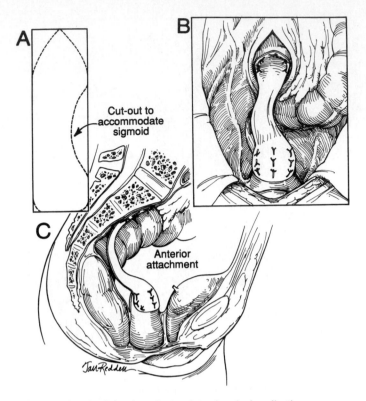

Figure 8-7 Direct and sagittal sketches of anterolateral vaginal application.

After sacralcolpopexy and culdeplasty and the correction of the anterior vaginal wall defects, it is important to correct the posterior vaginal defects. This is crucial in achieving the all-important horizontal vaginal axis.

Complete posterior repair includes correction of the enterocele, which should already have been resolved by the Halban culdeplasty, followed by a fascial plication to eliminate the rectocele. Finally, the levator and perineal restoration are also necessary to reestablishment of a normal vaginal axis and enforcement of the total repair. This also effectively lengthens the vagina by recreating an inclined plane (hypotenuse).

COMPLICATIONS AND VARIATIONS IN TECHNIQUE

Although blood loss is rarely more than 200 to 300 mL, hemorrhage is a possible complication with this procedure. Sutton and colleagues reported a case of massive hemorrhage from an extremely vascular sacral plexus and recommended, very correctly, that this surgery be performed only by surgeons experienced in retroperi-

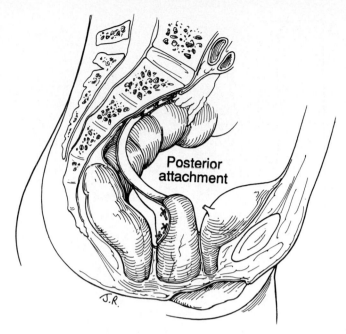

Figure 8-8 Sagittal view of most popular posterolateral vaginal application.

toneal repairs.[16] In our series one patient experienced a blood loss of 3000 mL, which was controlled using sutures and gentle pressure. Because we had to abandon sacralcolpopexy, we used our own uterosacral modification of the Halban culdeplasty, and this has continued to be effective 36 months postoperatively. Special tacks and magnet applicators are now available to help stop hemorrhage if it occurs.[17]

In our experiences, extrusion of the patch material occurred in four patients: three with GORE-TEX and one with Prolene mesh. All occurred from 6 to 18 months postoperatively. The three GORE-TEX extrusions were repaired transvaginally by removing the lower half of the patch material by sharp dissection, then trimming and repairing the scarred vaginal opening. If there is a recurrence of the extrusion, it should be removed transabdominally. The Prolene mesh was removed transabdominally at another facility. All four patients returned to strong, high vault support without further repair.

One patient who had previously elected to delay surgery in favor of a pessary for treatment of a massive prolapsed vagina presented with a ruptured enterocele that required emergency surgery. We feel that the graft extrusions and ruptured enterocele were due primarily to the relatively poor vascularity of the vaginal cuff itself, which can cause the cuff to atrophy with time. Therefore, we currently favor the use of the posterolateral and occasionally the anterolateral vaginal sites for attaching the prosthetic patch, according to where the thickest, most vascular area is found (see Figures 8-7 and 8-8). If the posterior vaginal attachment is used and the entire

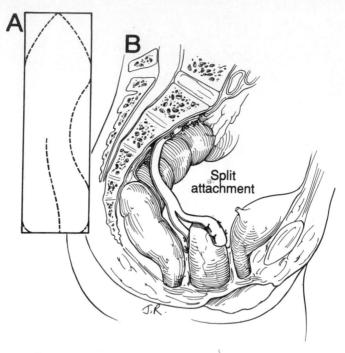

Figure 8-9 Sagittal view of split patch on vaginal end (A) for anterior and posterior application (B).

pelvis can be extraperitonealized, the culdeplasty may be omitted. Alternatively the vaginal end of the patch may be cut vertically to allow an anterior and posterior cuff application (Figure 8-9).

Failures of support are rare. Snyder and Krantz reported data of 147 patients using expanded Dacron or ePTFE with a 93% success rate over 5 years.[18] Addison and colleagues reported only 1 in 143 cases and emphasize the use of nonabsorbable sutures and a broad area of application to the vagina.[19] We concur with these conclusions and have experienced no failures.

Incontinence occurs postoperatively when it is unrecognized beforehand or not corrected during surgery. It also may occur if the vaginal suspension is overly tight. With any history of bladder instability or the appearance of an untreated defect, urodynamic study should be performed, especially when the bladder is displaced upward, similar to patients who experience urinary stress incontinence when a cystocele is corrected by pessary, or when repair is done without consideration of the urethrovesical angle. The patch material or mesh used must always be loosely placed with adequate length to preserve the mobility of the anterior vaginal wall for normal function.

Other complications including ileus or thromboembolic phenomena may occur with the same frequency as in other types of major abdominal surgery.

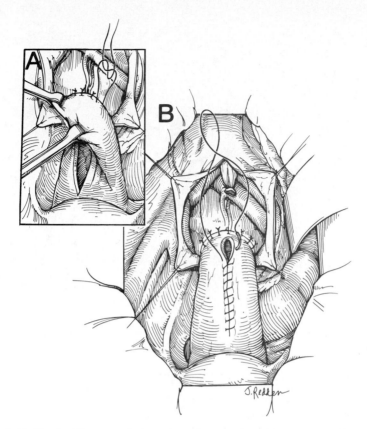

Figure 8-10 Sketch of direct sacralcolpopexy; rare but possible with short pelvis and long vagina.

When the vagina is very long and the pelvic diagonal conjugate is short, a direct attachment of the vagina to the sacrum is possible and desirable if the vagina is not stressed by the attachment (Figure 8-10).

Occasionally, when a wedge of the anterior vaginal wall is to be removed to correct a moderate cystocele transabdominally, as is convenient at the time of sacropexy, a flap can be created by incising the vagina from the urethrovesical junction backward to the cuff (Figure 8-11) and turning the flap backward, instead of removing it, for a direct sacral attachment, as illustrated in Figure 8-12. Again, this is only feasible if the lengthened vagina is long enough to attach without tension.

SUMMARY

Posthysterectomy vaginal vault inversion has become an increasingly common lesion that demands correction because of its associated disability. Unquestionably

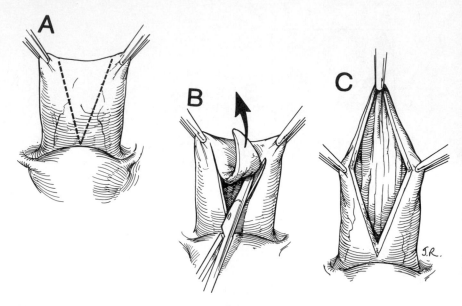

Figure 8-11 Drawing of transabdominal cystocele repair using the usually excised portion to extend the vagina. Bladder and ureters are shown below schematically.

the concomitantly increasing number of anterior vaginal suspensions and urethropexies without culdeplasty has promoted its incidence. The best opportunity to prevent its development is at the time of hysterectomy and/or urethropexy, when culdeplasty and levator restoration should be prime considerations.

Transabdominal sacralcolpopexy is our preferred procedure in patients with complete vaginal vault prolapse because it provides maximum functioning vaginal length and a very low failure rate when correctly performed.

Excellent results are also possible using the transvaginal sacrospinous attachment site popularized by Nichols and Randall[8] as will be discussed in a later chapter, as well as the prespinous iliococcygeus fascia proposed by Inmon[20] and the tendinous arch near the spine by Wiser (personal communication). We also frequently use these sites of attachment, especially on the very obese or fragile patient or when the vaginal vault prolapse is partial, situations where we consider the vaginal route preferable.

We began performing transabdominal sacralcolpopexy after the publication of Birnbaum's report in 1973.[21] Before that time, we repaired all cases transvaginally using techniques similar to those described by Lee and Symmonds.[22] Between 197? and 1981, we performed 95 cases: 86 using Marlex mesh and 9 using Prolene mesh From July 1987 to July 1991, we performed 65 procedures using the GORE-TEX Soft Tissue Patch. There have been no deaths and no recurrences of vaginal vault prolapse in any of the 160 cases, although we experienced an occurrence of postoperative anterior enterocele in 3% of patients.

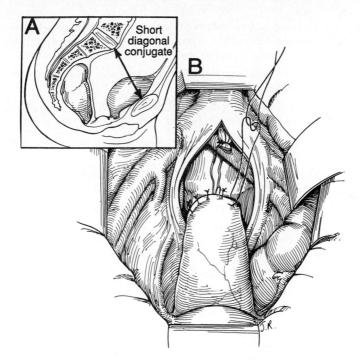

Figure 8-12 Sketches of sacralcolpopexy technique using lengthened vagina in a direct sacral application.

We currently prefer to use the strong, soft, inert ePTFE GORE-TEX Soft Tissue Patch because it affords dependable, long-lasting support and allows tissue in-growth into the material while resisting the formation of adhesions.

Our experience with transabdominal sacralcolpopexy has been excellent. We continue to feel that it is a superior method of obtaining a long-lasting, well-supported, functioning vagina. The procedure should be performed only by surgeons adequately trained in this effective technique. The excellence of the procedure dictates the need for training more young gynecologists in the technique. The complete gynecologic surgeon should be adept at both transvaginal and transabdominal approaches.

REFERENCES

1. Phaneuf LE. Inversion of the vagina and prolapse of the cervix following supracervical hysterectomy and inversion of the vagina following total hysterectomy. *Am J Obstet Gynecol.* 1952;64:739.

2. Symmonds RE, Pratt JH. Vaginal prolapse following hysterectomy. *Am J Obstet Gynecol.* 1960;79:899.

3. Addison WA, Livengood CH, Sutton GP, Parker RT. Abdominal sacralcolpopexy with Mersilene mesh in the retroperitoneal position in the management of posthysterectomy vaginal vault prolapse and enterocele. *Am J Obstet Gynecol.* 1985;153:140.

4. Zacharin RF. Pulsion enterocele: Review of functional anatomy of the pelvic floor. *Am J Obstet Gynecol.* 1980;55:135.

5. Symmonds RE, Williams TF, Lee RA, Webb MJ. Posthysterectomy enterocele and vaginal vault prolapse. *Am J Obstet Gynecol.* 1981;140:852.

6. Sederl J. Zur operation des Prolapses der blind endigenden Scheide. *Geburtshilfe Frauenheilkd.* 1958;18:824–828.

7. Richter K, Werner A. Long-term results following fixation of the vagina on the sacrospinal ligament by the vaginal route. *Am J Obstet Gynecol.* 1981;141:811.

8. Nichols DH, Randal CL. *Vaginal Surgery.* 3rd ed. Baltimore: Williams & Wilkins; 1989.

9. Inmon WB. Pelvic relaxation and repair including prolapse of vagina following hysterectomy. *S Med J.* 1963;56:577.

10. Vaginal Hand Retractor, Medi-Sharp, P.O. Box 1604, Sugar Land, TX 77478.

11. Halban J. *Gynakologische Operationslehre.* Berlin: Urban and Schwarzenberg; 1932.

12. Ridley JH. A composite vaginal vault suspension using fascia lata. *Am J Obstet Gynecol.* 1976;126:590.

13. Lansman HH. Post hysterectomy vault prolapse: Sacralcolpopexy with duramater graft. *Obstet Gynecol.* 1984;63:577.

14. Richardson AC, Edmonds PB, Williams N. Treatment of urinary incontinence due to paravaginal fascial defect. *Obstet Gynecol.* 1981;57:357.

15. Baden WF, Walker TA. Urinary stress incontinence: Evolution of paravaginal repair. *Female Patient.* 1987;12:89.

16. Sutton GP, Addison WA, Livengood CH III, Hammond CB. Life-threatening hemorrhage complicating sacralcolpopexy. *Am J Obstet Gynecol.* 1981;140:836.

17. Timmons MC, Kohler MF, Addison WA. Thumbtack use for control of presacral bleeding, with description of an instrument for thumbtack application. *Obstet Gynecol.* 1991;78:313.

18. Snyder TE, Krantz KE. Abdominal-retroperitoneal sacral colpopexy for the correction of vaginal prolapse. *Obstet Gynecol.* 1991;77:944.

19. Addison WA, Timmons MC, Wall LL, Livengood CH III. Failed abdominal sacralcolpopexy: observations and recommendations. *Obstet Gynecol.* 1989;74:480.

20. Inmon WB. Suspension of the vaginal cuff and posterior repair following vaginal hysterectomy. *Am J Obstet Gynecol.* 1974;120:977.

21. Birnbaum SJ. Rational therapy for the prolapsed vagina. *Am J Obstet Gynecol.* 1973;115:411.

22. Lee RA, Symmonds RE. Surgical repair of posthysterectomy vault prolapse. *Am J Obstet Gynecol.* 1972;112:953.

Posterior Pelvis I:
Analysis and Findings
in Enterocele and
Massive Vaginal
Eversion

Marvin H. Terry Grody

Enteroceles, as well as rectoceles and cystoceles, are true hernias. Hernias are abnormal pouches resulting from disruption of fascial or muscular septa. These protrusions, usually lined with endothelium and containing soft tissue, primarily hollow organs, invade into adjacent areas where they do not belong and progressive disability results.

Generally, hernias are associated with weaknesses in abdominal cavity enclosure and thus the lining of these sacs consists of peritoneum. When this type of lesion is mentioned, one automatically thinks of inguinal, femoral, umbilical, diaphragmatic, and incisional hernias. An enterocele, lined by expanded peritoneum and filled with loops of small intestine, certainly genuinely qualifies as part of this group but seems never to be included. Also not included, most probably because they are not direct peritoneal extensions, are rectocele and cystocele. But these anatomic deviants are in truth herniations of hollow organs that have broken through a natural boundary, in these cases the vaginal wall, because of supportive or suspensory weakness. The disability produced by these sacs, as they progress, ultimately may reach a point where surgical correction becomes a reasonable answer for relief and is requested by the patient.

Enterocele and its big sister, vaginal eversion, are the chief subjects of this chapter and the next in which the main concern will be vaginal reduction and repair of these lesions occurring most often in the aging estrogen-deficient woman. Vaginal eversion and enterocele are not synonymous. The former is simply a descriptive term for a vagina that has partially or completely turned inside out. At the least, the upper paracolpium, which should maintain the proximal vagina in its natural elevated position, and probably a considerable amount of the mesoparacolpium, have been destroyed. When the eversion represents total loss of all or almost all vaginal supports and attachments, the correct terminology is massive vaginal eversion. In essence, the vagina has literally peeled off fairly completely in these cases and is totally outside, hanging on circularly around the rim of the introitus.

In posthysterectomy situations, usually there is at least some degree of enterocele in this kind of severe detachment but not always. In such cases any combination of severe perineal defects, rectocele, cystocele, and hypermotile urethra can fill the bulging sac. A severe vaginal eversion can also occur in the presence of a uterus which will be extruded more or less in the center of the huge defect where the vagina has separated circumferentially from the pelvic walls. Similarly, an enterocele may or may not coexist, but it must always be suspected and certainly must be surgically eliminated if present.

Although many anatomic nuances are described,[1] basically an enterocele as we most commonly encounter it is, in truth, an exaggeration of the cul-de-sac. Obviously this pouch of Douglas, situated at the lowermost point of the abdominal cavity, between the uterus and the rectum, is subjected to the highest degree of intra-abdominal pressure in the erect woman. A significant number of women are born with inherent weakness in this area. Also the depth of the cul-de-sac naturally may vary greatly from one woman to the next. It follows that the weakest and the deepest are those most prone to develop into a symptomatic deformity depending on the degree of stress, over time, placed into such a vulnerable locus. Unquestionably the labor of childbirth plays a key role in promoting anatomic infirmity in and around this pouch, as it does in all other pelvic herniations, for most uncommonly is an enterocele seen in nulligravida women. In these unusual cases, it is most likely congenital.

However, our concepts are beginning to change regarding causative influences. Breakdown in pelvic support has always been thought to occur almost exclusively as a steady ongoing process related to combinations in varying degrees of aging, hormone deficiency, denervation, physical stress, and general atrophy. Ultimately, over a period of years, deterioration would be extensive enough to produce symptoms, primarily well into the climacteric. Such detrimental impairment has, in the past, only uncommonly been linked to a single sudden severely traumatic event, similar to the rupture of an Achilles tendon. Yet cumulative data from accurate histories seem to reveal a significant number of cases that time the onset of symptoms precisely with a single injurious or severely jolting incident such as harsh impact in an automobile accident, a bad fall, or a jump from a height. Until recently we readily dismissed such stories on suspicion that the patient was merely attempting to enhance her chances for a larger insurance liability reimbursement. She would be told that most likely the aggravating condition had already been there for some time and the accident simply directed attention to it. We are no longer so certain—witness other tales of symptom onset that highlight a vigorous tennis match featuring leaps to make difficult plays or a hard pounding day of mogul-jumping on the ski slopes. Both tennis and skiing today are common recreational activities of menopausal women and must be reckoned as factors in pelvic suppor-tive and suspensory injury, perhaps as the "last straw." The most compelling evidence toward credence of the negative potential of these sudden singular dam-aging events arises through the astonishing accounts coming to light of sympto-matic pelvic stresses in young nulliparous women. Nothing could be more striking than accumulating documented reports of pelvic prolapse in women paratroopers in our armed forces trained to hit the ground with tremendous force. Many quit the service because of this development, often with the associated symptom of stress incontinence (AC Richardson, personal communication, 1992). As a corollary, we face with alarm the consequences of pavement-hammering by women jogging addicts. This activity, in the quest for health, ironically is already accepted by many as an interference with persistence of normal pelvic integrity.

Further compounding the issue is the progressive increase in enterocele forma-tion in the years subsequent to isolated suprapubic urethral suspension (SPUS), of all kinds, in the attempt to cure genuine urinary stress incontinence.[2,3] Figures currently are quoted in the range of 15% to 25% of patients who later require posterior surgical correction of enterocele. The obvious explanation for this se-quence of events is the distortion of the normal vaginal axis, probably already borderline, or of the early but still symptomatic abnormal axis, in the afflicted cases, by the perhaps overcorrective forward pull of the SPUS on the lower urinary tract suspensory system. This surgery draws the lower and middle, and sometimes the upper also, anterior vaginal wall forward, thereby widening the vaginal aperture in the anterior-posterior direction, tending to "straighten out" the vagina. This substantially negates the supportive effect of the levator plate or pelvic platform as it simultaneously overstretches the delicate interpendent network of endopelvic fascia designed to maintain the pelvic structures in a state of balance and natural position. Thus strained and weakened, previously probably already compromised cul-de-sac and posterior pelvic connective and elastic tissues further deteriorate, leading ultimately not only to enterocele but rectocele and perineal defects also. The same situation is duplicated in isolated anterior repairs performed from below. In my referral status, I see numerous women presenting with disabling posterior pelvic disintegration subsequent by months or years to an anterior repair, most usually in association with a hysterectomy, in many of whom most likely perineal defects or rectovaginal septal tears were either too minimal or were ignored then because of absence of directly attributable symptoms. I strongly suggest that consideration be given, in all instances of SPUS, to simultaneous appropriate posterior repair from below after completion of work through the abdominal incision. Even more strongly, I feel that any anterior colporrhaphy done in the lithotomy position should be accompanied by a suitable posterior procedure, which may only need to be a perineorrhaphy sufficient to maintain the anterior edge of the levator plate well in front of the vaginal vault, as will be discussed in Chapter 11.

Enterocele is depicted as either traction or pulsion in origin. Precise descriptions in the literature become confusing. Actually there seems to be at least some element of each mechanism in all these lesions although one usually predominates in any given case.

Traction enterocele is most often identified with an associated prolapsed uterus. The prolapse has occurred as a direct result of progressive attenuation of the cardinal-uterosacral complex, the posterior extensions of which help form the anterior wall of the cul-de-sac before they meld into the fibers of the rectovaginal septum. This cardinal complex weakness not uncommonly leads to enlargement of the Douglas pouch, which increases as the descending uterus seems to pull it progressively downward. Actually, the prolapsing uterus is not an active traction source but really a dragging anchor because it is victim to the disabled support at the level of the isthmus, cervix, and vaginal vault.[4,5] So, whether acquired or congenital weakness or both, a true sliding effect may deepen the cul-de-sac and drop the uterus simultaneously. However, it must be emphasized that a prolapsed uterus does not automatically imply an accompanying enterocele, although that patient may very well be more prone to posthysterectomy enterocele in the future than one without the previous prolapse.

Often arguments arise as to the point at which a deepened cul-de-sac becomes an enterocele but, really, who cares? When surgical intervention is indicated, as in prolapsed uterus, eradication of this abnormal peritoneal extension, regardless of its size, is absolutely obligatory at the time of the hysterectomy else a prelude to certain future pulsion enterocele is left behind. I have operated on extreme cases, from time to time, wherein the entire uterus has descended entirely outside the introitus, creating a huge traction enterocele above it measuring from 15 to 25 in^2 of peritoneal surface. Certainly the cul-de-sac can develop into a true enterocele without associated uterine prolapse, but this phenomenon is either uncommon or not well recognized, especially when congenital. When it does occur, usually it is associated with a rectocele. In cases of posterior vaginal repair, it behooves the surgeon to recognize this coexistence, either preoperatively or intraoperatively, and effect complete correction, else recurrent breakdown is likely at a later date.

In passing, also uncommonly, we must make note that an enterocele may quietly worm its way down behind the posterior vaginal wall and not be recognized until surgery occurs to correct an apparent large rectocele. In such cases, on examination, the posterior vault or posthysterectomy cuff may appear to be normally positioned. This appearance is a consequence of the position of this uncommon enterocele behind the rectovaginal septum. It rarely may descend enough to overlie a coexisting low rectocele resulting from a rectovaginal septum ruptured only above the perineal body. The run-of-the-mill enterocele lies anterior to the rectovaginal septum, if the septum is intact at all, but generally speaking, this concept is merely academic. Most often, by the time patients present themselves with eversion or large posterior prolapse, the rectovaginal septum is already torn linearly in the midline or on either side of the midline.

Only brief mention is made at this point of anterior enterocele, an uncommon lesion but one demanding recognition, as opposed to the much more common posterior enterocele, the expanded cul-de-sac, as already described. Although some dispute the existence of this deformity, it is an undeniable fact that it may be stumbled on during surgery, lying either between the bladder and the uterine isthmus or between the bladder and the old hysterectomy scar, appearing preoperatively as a part of a cystocele. This matter will be discussed further under the details of enterocele excision and repair in Chapter 10.

Posthysterectomy pulsion enterocele, considered rare or at the least, uncommon some 30 to 40 years ago,[6-8] in studies which a few of us in retrospect feel were not necessarily accurate appraisals, seems to be an entity that can no longer be considered uncommon. Hardly a week goes by in any major medical center without at least one corrective procedure, whether by the vaginal or abdominal route, for this lesion being listed on the operating room schedule. Because enterocele is primarily a deformity of the aging woman, a significant increase in occurrence is easily understandable in view of changing population figures. In 1960, women over 50 years of age in the United States numbered 21 million and at the time of publication of this book, more than 30 years later, the conservative estimate is 43 to 44 million. Add to this other factors such as concomitant significant increase in life expectancy, a more educated female population about the role and logic of surgical correction, and accompanying intolerance for both long-term pessary usage and a "learn to live with it" attitude, and we end up with a swelling demand for reconstructive repair. Coincidentally, through sophisticated improvements, we have erased most fears about anesthesia; blood banks offer insurance if hemorrhage should occur, including having autologous blood on standby; and infection can be overcome with appropriate antibiotic regimens. Perhaps as major a factor as any other, because these problems primarily afflict the postmenopausal aging woman, professional tolerance for surgery for this age group, especially vaginally, all things considered, currently is far superior from what it was a few decades ago. Internists previously hesitant to grant approval for anesthesia and surgery are much less prone today toward a negative and noninvasive attitude. Instead, with a minimum of distinct exceptions, medical clearance, with attentive coverage both before and after surgery, is generally readily available and applicable. As a result it is no surprise to note a startling increase in both interest in and performance of surgery aimed at correction of enterocele and massive eversion.

However, at this juncture, we are today confronted with a most alarming fact: capable and competent surgeons well trained in what has aptly been termed "a dying art," except for a very few experts, simply are not available. This scarcity applies generally to all phases of pelvic reconstructive and vaginal surgery, a recurrent observation throughout this book, and it is most certainly true in surgical management of vault eversion and enterocele, whether accomplished by the abdominal route or from below. Dr. Stanley Rogers, in Chapter 8, has aptly described a most acceptable and workable suprapubic approach that should serve as a sufficient model, with variations to suit the individual patient and the particular desires of the doctor, to enable the average practitioner to tackle and cure these enormously disabling lesions from above when so applicable. This section and the next should fulfill the same goal via the vaginal pathway.

How does one choose whether surgical correction should be performed abdominally or vaginally? I find great difficulty in being totally objective in responding to this question, as you will readily perceive, but basically the majority of authorities will declare that the route of choice depends on what is most applicable for the particular case. It follows, then, that accomplished gynecologic surgeons should be capable of performance both ways. However, I find that most operators willing to undertake this problem at all lean overwhelmingly to only one of the two methods in practically all cases, that choice being the one at which they are most adept, with minimal regard for what pragmatically may be the best route for a particular patient. In defense of this statement, because most cases can probably be done with equal success by either approach, the best one for the patient is the one at which the doctor is most skillful. This is precisely why, in a publication such as this, wherein expression of personal opinion by each author is encouraged, both viewpoints are presented.

The confusion created by the above paragraph is deliberate because it truly reflects a professional divergence of attitude where the long-term outcomes are probably the same. In my experience of over 40 years dealing with a vast multitude of both private and service patients requiring pelvic reconstruction, learning and changing and hopefully improving along the way, I have quite some time ago concluded, with good reason, that the vaginal approach is superior by far to the abdominal route.

All reconstructive surgery actually begins with the outpatient examination, a time when muscle tone has not been negated by anesthesia. Preoperative delineation of exact defects in a particular patient is vitally necessary to effect the best ultimate repair. Although alteration in a preoperative plan must necessarily be made in some cases during the actual surgery, as in unfortunate situations requiring compensatory ingenuity when dissection reveals fascial remnants deteriorated beyond redemption, precise definition of lesions, I repeat, must be detailed beforehand so as to lead to a more accurate surgical delineation than one of "posterior repair." As already discussed, in so many such instances, lacking advance strategy, each patient is subjected to the same operation regardless of variations in lesions, and this cannot be considered acceptable.

Ultimate accuracy in blueprinting any form of reconstructive surgery can never be attained by examination limited to one in the lithotomy position. Symptomatology, with rare exception, is related to the erect posture. It follows, logically, that detection of anatomic lesions that contribute to complaints is best achieved by manual evaluation of the standing patient. Yet, after 40 years of clinical practice, the last 10 of which have centered on referrals, including case after case with histories of one to four previous reparative operations that have failed, I have yet to see one where preparatory examination has been done previously in the upright attitude. Years of practice have also taught me that older women often have great difficulty in producing a satisfactory Valsalva effect in the lithotomy position where this becomes no problem once they stand. Thus, frequently, blatant tissue defects are missed entirely in the absence of standing examination.[9]

Patients invariably note that distress due to structural imperfections is at its worst at the end of a day replete with activity. Obviously tissue strains are at a maximum after the longest taxing periods. So equally obvious should be the desire, wherever possible, to see patients so afflicted in the later afternoon when defects will become far more apparent than at first thing in the morning after a night of recumbency.

Perceptions vary on the correct method of examination in the erect stance. Several years ago I determined that perhaps the best analysis could be achieved when the patient stands elevated some 8 to 10 inches off the floor on the stool at the end of the examining table with her legs stretched wide apart. Then she is asked to bend her knees slightly bilaterally in an outward direction to provide adequate access for examination. The doctor, kneeling on the floor on the right knee, slightly to the patient's left, will then perform not the traditional limiting bidigital examination with one hand but a bimanual examination to allow for digital opposition and broad and deep analysis not attainable by one hand. This most revealing method occurs with the index and middle fingers of the left hand in the vagina while the index finger of the right hand is inserted into the rectum. At this point the patient is asked to bear down with all her might for several moments to display the maximum level of structural imperfection before the examiner starts to make judgments (Figures 9-1 and 9-2).

In analyzing vault support, if the uterus is still present, in the standing position, a simultaneous assessment of degree of uterine prolapse, if any, or descent of the cul-de-sac is made. More importantly, in the absence of the uterus, so often the case in these situations in older women under consideration, any tendency to vault eversion must be ascertained and not missed, together with its total extent. Whether or not it stretches anterior to the old hysterectomy scar, behind the bladder, and whether or not the hysterectomy scar itself descends must be noted initially because the scar may form the leading point of the eversion. The bulk of most eversions usually lies posterior to the vault scar, regardless of the level of descent of the scar, and its total extent and contents can best be assessed by determining how much of it literally peels off the pelvic wall in all directions. Although enterocele can exist as an isolated lesion as the only component of an eversion, especially when early and asymptomatic, containing only small intestine and perhaps omentum, as the

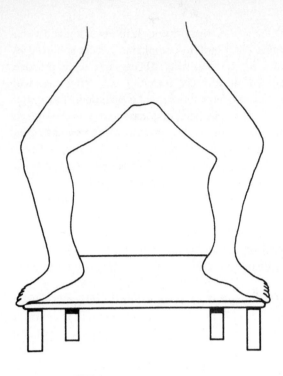

Figure 9-1 Sketch demonstrates stance for examination of the erect patient.

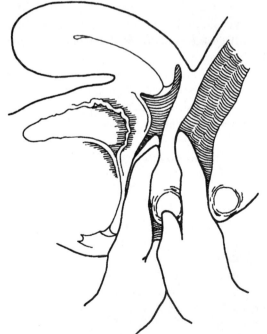

Figure 9-2 Sketch of examiner's fingers, using both hands, in the standing patient. The two vaginal fingers, after posterior compartment assessment, may be rotated 180 degrees to judge anterior compartment defects under Valsalva conditions.

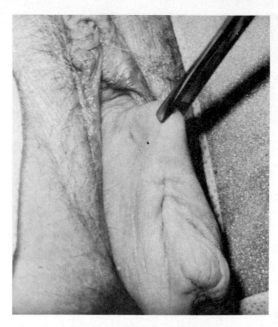

Figure 9-3 Distorted prolapse with complete eversion. Forceps are at the urethrovesical junction.

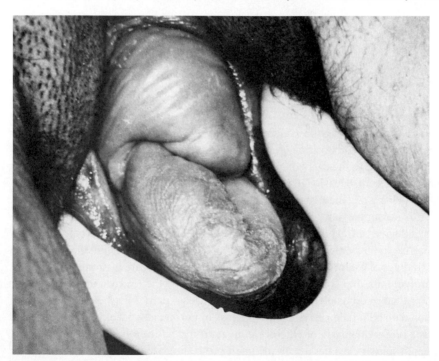

Figure 9-4 Examiner's hand frames a well-scarred everted vagina in a case previously subjected to four pelvic procedures.

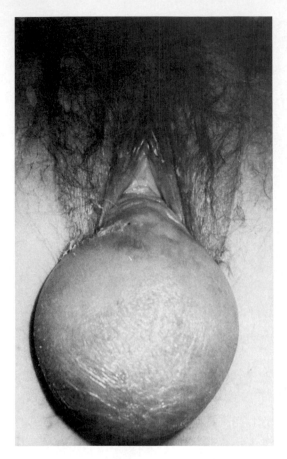

Figure 9-5 Severe total eversion in its worst form. The thin vaginal mucosa signifies rapid progression in recent months.

eversion grows and produces such symptoms as pressure, feeling of protrusion, and dyspareunia, its composition almost invariably augments to include rectum. Further disruption of the eversion can then encompass cystocele, rotated urethra, and empty perineum, occasionally to the point where eversion is so great that the vagina seems to hang out, in full circle, attached only to the introitus (Figures 9-3, 9-4, and 9-5). The examiner must constantly be sensitive to the varying contents of the sac in lesser degrees of eversion, as when an enterocele and prolapsed bladder alone comprise the lesion without significant rectocele contribution. Finally, regarding the findings of examination, by the time the patient seeks care of protruding organs, I rarely do not find some degree of disintegration of the rectovaginal septum, the lesion that precipitates rectocele, and also at least partial perineal defects, associated with both fallen levator plate and loss of normal vaginal axis.

Making a diagnosis of enterocele apart from rectocele is not always easy. In cases of massive eversion with the vault protruding well below the introitus, the palpation of small intestine in the sac while the patient bears down in the erect stance is a diagnostic giveaway. In less obvious cases, when the organ descensus seems not so remarkable, the question initially always rises as to whether one is dealing with merely a very large rectocele, or a smaller rectocele and a superimposed medium-sized or early enterocele. Using the two-handed examining method described previously, the presence of an enterocele can almost always be determined by the Valsalva-produced "double-hump" effect. In such a case, the right index finger in the rectum can roam the rectocele but cannot fit into the upper hump, the enterocele, which is defined by the opposing vaginal fingers of the left hand. Such a maneuver also indicates the level for later exploration in location of the enterocele sac.

Once appropriate detailed assessment has been made and the patient and family have been fully informed, after necessary medical apprisal and adjustment have been completed, corrective surgery is the next step.

REFERENCES

1. Zacharin RT. *Pelvic Floor Anatomy and the Surgery of Pulsion Enterocele.* New York: Springer-Verlag; 1985:77–101.

2. Burch JC. Urethrovaginal fixation to Cooper's ligament for correction of stress incontinence cystocele, and prolapse. *Am J Obstet Gynecol.* 1961;81:281–290.

3. Burch JC. Cooper's ligament urethrovesical suspension for stress incontinence. *Am J Obstet Gynecol.* 1968;100:764–774.

4. Nichols DH, Randall CL. *Vaginal Surgery.* 3rd ed. Baltimore: Williams & Wilkins; 1989:64–81.

5. Nichols DH. Types of genital prolapse. *Postgrad Med.* 1969;46:183–187.

6. Symmonds RE, Pratt JH. Vaginal prolapse following hysterectomy. *Am J Obstet Gynecol.* 1960;79:899–909.

7. Phaneuf LE. Eversion of the vagina and prolapse of the cervix following supracervical hysterectomy and inversion of the vagina following total hysterectomy. *Am J Obstet Gynecol.* 1952;64:739–745.

8. Parsons L, Ulfelder H. *An Atlas of Pelvic Operations.* 2nd ed. Philadelphia: WB Saunders; 1968:280–283.

9. Nichols DH. Enterocele. In: Nichols DH, Randall CL, eds. *Vaginal Surgery.* 3rd Edition. Baltimore, Williams and Wilkins, 1989; 319–320.

Posterior Pelvis II:
Deep Pelvic
Reconstruction—
Enterocele Repair and
Sacrospinous Fixation

Marvin H. Terry Grody

This chapter describes two interdependent sequential operations of great importance: (1) the dissection of the enterocele sac, followed by its peritoneal closure,
excision, and reinforcement, and (2) the sacrospinous ligament fixation (SSF).
The goals of the surgery involved in this deep pelvic area are (1) destruction of
the enterocele and prophylaxis against its recurrence, (2) the establishment of the
vaginal vault high and deep in the recess of the sacral hollow far posterior to
the anterior edge of a normally situated levator plate, and (3) the initiation of return
to a natural pelvic interorgan balancing network of effectively repositioned fibrous,
elastic, and muscle tissue. The corollary benefits of this restoration surgery are
unquestionably the elimination of symptoms caused by the preoperative deformi-
ties and the restitution or maintenance of normal function and comfort.

INSTRUMENTS

Although no one can deny that the ultimate prerequisite for this exacting type of
meticulous surgery demands manual dexterity and skill, the best results are

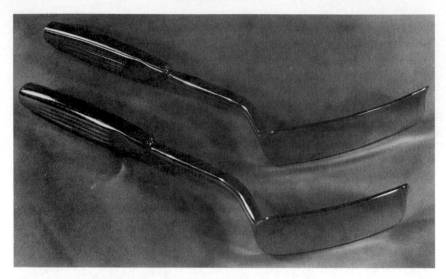

Figure 10-1. Modified Breisskey-Navratil retractors. The handles are angled to increase the operative field of approach. The standard Breissky-Navratil retractors look like a garden hoe.

achieved most efficiently and with the least risk by using instruments particularly adapted to these procedures. Although not denying the old analogy that the magic lies in the hands of the magician and not in the wand, the magic of the good surgeon reaches highest perfection when accompanied by the correct use of the most efficiently helpful and versatile instruments.

In the deep recesses of the posterior pelvis, I strongly feel that Breissky-Navratil retractors offer the best and certainly the safest form of exposure. The blade is straight and slightly convex on its inner surface, allowing for the widest unimpeded view into the operative area, i.e., the sacrospinous ligament locale. The dull heavy ends, even under great pressure, will displace but not cut into adjacent organs. The useful size range of the blade of this instrument, which resembles a garden hoe in its factory issue form, is 3.5 to 5 inches in length by 1 to 1.5 inches in width. A variety of sizes should be available. As shown in Figure 10-1, these instruments become ideal after the handles have been angled backward through a special metal heating process. This keeps the assistants' hands from impeding operative access.

The traditional Deaver retractor, primarily developed for intra-abdominal exposure, is not only inappropriate for use in deep pelvic penetration but can be downright dangerous. Unfortunately, in centers where Breissky-Navratil retractors have not been available, the Deavers have often been substituted, leading occasionally to disastrous results. The curve of a Deaver intrudes into the desired zone of operative visibility, provoking assistants to use strong centrifugal retraction which can force the thin relatively sharp ends to act as cutting edges. Such action can easily lead to adjacent soft tissue invasion, particularly

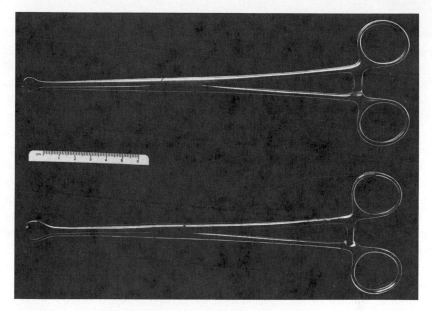

Figure 10-2. The much larger grasping volume of the Grody-Babcock clamp (bottom) is compared to that of the standard Babcock clamp (top).

bowel, at very deep levels in the lowermost areas of the abdomen. Although such episodes have not been documented in medical literature, there are multiple bona fide occurrences of this nature that have been related anecdotally and have most certainly been recorded in the offices of attorneys. However, exceptionally, in reversion to its originally designated raison d'etre, a narrow Deaver retractor is most effective later in the repair in maintaining a clear view during the course of the enterocele neck closure high in the pelvis.

Many surgeons feel it is good practice to grasp the sacrospinous ligament both for identification and for guidance to suture placement. A special instrument for this purpose, the Grody-Babcock clamp (Figure 10-2; George Tiemann Co., Plainview, NY) has been devised for this purpose. The standard long Babcock clamp is generally too small to encompass the heavy ligament and slips off, occasionally snapping and breaking in the attempt to do so. In contrast, the Grody-Babcock grasping tip offers 2.5 times the volume of the ordinary Babcock clamp. Thus, if applied correctly, it can identify and encompass firmly even the thickest ligament without slipping. The dull edges of the tip have no cutting potential, so the inferior gluteal vessels, coursing posterior to the coccygeus muscle, are not endangered.

Some surgeons grip the sacrospinous ligament with a long Allis clamp. This can be deleterious and lead to shredding of the ligament because of the sharper jagged tips and may possibly also induce uncontrollable bleeding if placed too deeply for the same reason.

Three different instrument approaches to the placement of suture through the sacrospinous ligament are most commonly used. I think the safest, simplest, and most manageable of these is the Deschamps suture carrier as modified by Nichols.[1] He has narrowed the caliber of the original relatively thick curved tip and added some 7 cm to the length of the handle to attain a total of 28 to 29 cm. However, many times, in particularly deep pelves, especially those with associated restricted operative access, awkwardness results, impeding correct placement of suture. I have overcome this problem easily by manually bending back the shaft of the Nichols-Deschamps suture carrier about 15 degrees at 6 cm from the pointed tip (Figure 10-3). The facility thus afforded has made this instrument ideal. When the ligament is exposed, even deeply through a narrow approach, it allows for excellent manual control, using the convex aspect of the curved tip itself for soft tissue displacement posteriorly, as it penetrates the ligament from posterior to anterior precisely as desired. The Nichols-Deschamps carrier is strong, controllable and relatively inexpensive.

The Miya hook[2] is popular in many operating rooms. A not inexpensive instrument, it works by trigger mechanism that is activated when the desired position is attained to force penetration of its suture-loaded curved tip in an anterior to posterior direction through the ligament. Many of us feel this poses some degree of danger because it penetrates from front to back rather than the reverse and because the snapping of the release pin does not afford the same level of control as the slow steady hand-directed movement used with the Nichols-Deschamps suture carrier.

Still other surgeons feel too much fuss is made over special tools to be used in suture placement through the sacrospinous ligament. Instead they use a standard long needle driver armed with a free needle through the eye of which runs the desired suture. The dangers inherent in using this technique are implicated in the potential for the needle to shift in the holder or for the needle to break while piercing this very tough, thick, deeply situated, accessibly limited structure. A search for a fragmented needle, especially if the field is obscured by blood, could become harrowing.

A long nerve hook (see Figure 10-3) is almost universally the choice for drawing the suture out from the ligament after penetration has been completed. A simple readily available instrument, it will not fray or crush the suture as might forceps or a clamp.

HAZARDS

Before describing the precise surgical steps involved in accurate correction of enterocele and subsequent ligamentous suspension, precautions and dangers deserve attention. An enterocele sac may contain, although not frequently,

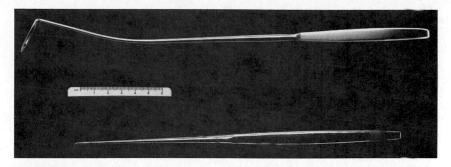

Figure 10-3. Ordinary nerve hook (bottom) and the modified (functional end bent at 15 degrees) Nichols-Deschamps suture carrier (top).

adherent small bowel or omentum. Both possibilities must be considered after the sac has been dissected free and isolated before entry. A large posthysterectomy enterocele may extend well forward and might impinge directly on a bladder displaced posteriorly, especially in situations of previous repair. Ureters similarly could pass under the distended enterocele peritoneum. Obviously, dissection and suture closure must be conducted with these anatomic aberrations in mind.

Surgery deep in the posterior pelvis involving the sacrospinous ligament is fraught with terrible potential hazards. A clear understanding of the immediately adjacent anatomy easily explains why this is so. Just under and slightly lateral to the ischial spine run the internal pudendal vessels and nerves and, in frighteningly close proximity, the sciatic nerve. The inferior gluteal artery, quite a substantial vessel, flows contiguously under the posterior border of the coccygeus muscle. Impinging directly from above are loops of small bowel while rectum bulges into the operative space medially. If this delicately situated field is not threatening enough in itself, one must assess the compounding perils when the pelvis is particularly deep, or the patient is obese with excess fat infiltrating throughout the pelvic tissues, or multiple previous operations in the area have contributed scarring and distortion. Add to this the frequent ventures into this type of surgery by operators without adequate experience or natural skill who might be the slightest bit careless or who might thrust blindly under the presumption that structures are where they should be or where the surgeons think they are. Such situations have produced a substantial record of serious, often permanently disabling, and sometimes tragic episodes subsequent to piercing or severing nerves, blood vessels, or bowel.

Although multiple relevant discussions throughout the literature offer dire warnings of the risks and hazards encountered in the performance of SSF,[3–7] no precise comprehensive accounts tabulating data of complications in this operation have surfaced, at least at the time of this publication. Of course, no one likes to report mistakes, and the obvious medicolegal overtones are a sufficient additional deterrent to keep the matter quiet. Yet cumulative anecdotal tales related by various authoritative gynecologic surgeons and multiple malpractice case records over the past two decades from reliable insurance sources (St. Paul Fire and Marine Insurance Company, Physicians Insurance Association of America, and the Aetna Insurance Company) indicate a significant and substantial number of complications.

Through my frequent participation in conference faculties and grand rounds programs across the nation, I hear a new sad story almost weekly. Even while I write this chapter, I am hearing from two different sources of a case at a nearby hospital wherein, as part of total repair, SSF was included in the operative plan and attempted with serious consequences, i.e., "24 units of blood and a probable permanent colostomy." At a local medical meeting a resident from that hospital has since told me that neither he nor any of his coresidents would ever in their lifetime consider doing "that terrible operation." In the March, 1990, issue of *St. Anthony's Coding for OB/GYN Reimbursement,* at that time the billing standard for the United States, mailed out to every practicing gynecologist in the country, it was bluntly stated that "The sacrospinous ligament suspension is a 'blind procedure'. The physician must perform this surgery by touch, not sight." How utterly misleading and discouraging! In consideration of such ominous warnings[8] plus the verbal reproaches rampant in hospital locker rooms and from lecture podiums, it is no wonder that many capable gynecologic surgeons do not perform SSF in lieu of more tedious and lengthy alternative operations deemed by many "safer and easier," usually through abdominal entry, as described earlier in this book.

One of my major missions in this volume, after a personal experience of over 500 cases, since 1976, without a single major complication, is the display of this procedure in all its remarkable capability of making life worth living for myriads of afflicted and potentially afflicted women, the number of whom seem to be multiplying daily. Trained surgeons, with reasonably natural talent, working under direct vision and using the correct instruments, should be able to perform this type of surgery, when called for, as a routine, with confidence, self-assurance, and conviction.

CHOICE OF SURGICAL APPROACH

Before delineation of safe and practical operative methodology in correction of vault prolapse, including elimination of enterocele combined with SSF, the rationale for choice of this route over the abdominal portal must be presented. To begin with, vault eversion, with or without a uterus, is essentially a problem of the postmenopausal and elderly woman. Rough estimates place the age level of those asking for amelioration of this lesion at 80% to 90% in the 55 years or over category. A significant and ever-growing percentage of these are septuagenarians.

Burdened already in many cases with a variety of cardiovascular, pulmonary, and digestive tract ailments, and beset with aging erosion in function generally, the systemic assault is far greater in an abdominal approach than one from below, magnified progressively with increasing years. A vaginal operation avoids all the displacement packing and manipulation and diaphragmatic pressure that accompanies the suprapubic laparotomy, especially one that requires the extensive exposure of the abdominal sacrocolpopexy. Additionally, elderly women today seem to tolerate vaginal surgery amazingly well, significantly better than that done from above when designed for the same purpose.

Ironically, the great majority of vault eversions are associated with posterior pelvic breakdown which demands simultaneous repair to recreate a normal vaginal axis as insurance for long-term satisfactory outcome. Because correlation of rectocele and perineal body defects cannot adequately be accomplished from above, it behooves the operator who refers abdominal sacrocolpopexy, once that part of the surgery is completed, to place the patient in the lithotomy position and finish the work vaginally. In the end, the patient is subjected to the trauma of two operative entries when one could have sufficed, not to mention the increased operative and anesthesia time.

Arguments are posed in favor of laparotomy when the lesion complex includes anterior pelvic breakdown, especially if genuine urinary stress incontinence is a factor, real or potential. In an abdominal approach, a suprapubic urethrovesicocolpopexy can be performed in immediate sequence to the sacrocolpopexy. However, because the anterior lesions can all be repaired adequately vaginally by current techniques, as described in Chapter 7, especially if a central (distention) cystocele is present, all things considered, I cannot find this argument valid by itself.

Finally, in completion of my disputation favoring vaginal versus abdominal repair of the lesions in question, the single entry, from below, avoids the threat of dehiscence, curtails anesthesia time and depth, reduces operative duration, causes less postoperative discomfort, and engenders faster recovery.

Admittedly, in certain specific circumstances I will opt for abdominal sacrocolpopexy over a vaginal enterocele excision. These occasions arise when I discover the uncommon combination of anatomically and functionally intact perineal body and lower rectovaginal septum coexisting with a symptomatic everting vaginal vault. In such instances, the levator plate is in good position and the normal vaginal axis is fairly well or well sustained. Jeopardizing the integrity of these supportive structures by deliberate surgical disruption just to create an operative field for correction of the defective vault must be considered bad judgment. Even if some degree of anterior compartment breakdown is present, the abdominal approach is preferable in these cases. I find that most often the anterior defect, if one is detected, is rotational descent of the urethrovesical junction. This can easily be corrected on the way out, after the colpopexy is completed and before the abdominal wall is closed, by a suprapubic urethral suspension such as a modified Burch procedure, or by a paravaginal defects repair. Even if a central (distention) cystocele or an upper rectocele accompanies the disabling everting vaginal vault, these are automatically corrected by extending wide enough anterior and posterior arms of prosthetic material deep enough (as should be done in any event) onto the front and back vaginal walls, respectively. Thus, there is no escaping the need for the fully qualified pelvic surgeon to be adept at both the vaginal and abdominal routes.

ENTEROCELE SURGERY: VAGINAL APPROACH

Preparation for the actual surgery follows the lines described in Chapter 3. My initial surgical depiction will center on the posthysterectomy pulsion enterocele rather than on that encountered at the time of hysterectomy, to be discussed afterward. The sequence will then be continued in this chapter by a full disclosure of the mechanics of SSF.

After the posterior vaginal wall is dissected free and opened in the midline to the area of the vaginal vault, as detailed in Chapter 11, the process to isolate the enterocele sac begins.[9,10] Its identification is generally not a difficult task, but in significantly enough instances, especially in cases of one or more previous posterior repairs, even veteran operators become hard-pressed to find it. If an enterocele is present, it must be found and eliminated, not simply stuffed back up and oversewn, for it most certainly will one day reappear and break down the other segments of the posterior repair regardless of the quality of the balance of the surgery. Usually, when previous pelvic surgery has been limited to hysterectomy, as posterior dissection progresses and the rectovaginal space is opened, the enterocele literally pops out at the operator. In tougher situations, it may not be located until exposure posteriorly is complete, including midline vaginal wall division to the posterior vault and full-length clearing out to the sidewalls. If a peritoneal fold is then not readily visualized, without hesitation, after a second glove is placed over the nondominant hand, a rectal finger can explore the extent of any rectocele, defining its upper limitations so as to ease trepidation in the pursuit of the enterocele.

This simple concept, born of common sense, seems so natural, yet all of us, in our stubbornness, including myself in more times than I would like to admit, occasionally persist in tedious dissection without rectal examination until, having missed the telltale vertical bowel striations, enter the rectal lumen. Although thus chagrined, do not make a big deal over this truly slight mishap. The worst thing to do at this point is to close the hole at once. Instead, having made the error, use it to advantage. Lavage the area thoroughly with the Vital-Vue (Davis and Geck, Inc.) propelled fluid stream and keep it open, using the inadvertent aperture as a further guide in discovering the enterocele. If it is closed immediately, in one's embarrassment, the guessing game simply begins all over again. The open hole at least tells you where you are and helps make the search easier. Once the enterocele is finally located, the rectal opening can be closed in any standard manner, always transversely, with continuous or interrupted sutures, with edge inversion into the lumen or with through and through stitching. It really does not matter because, properly closed, it always heals readily and, when the area is adequately lavaged, I have never seen it impede the healing process. Because of natural tissue resistance in this area to coliform bacteria, I have not found additional antibiotic coverage to be necessary because no increase in postoperative infection rates have been noted. After closure, simply get on with the operation as though the rectal entry had never happened.

If one anticipates difficulty in detecting enterocele peritoneum, in the same routine manner as used in laparoscopic procedures, the abdomen can be inflated with gas after the posterior vaginal wall has been divided and cleared. Then, a reasonable Trendelenberg position should produce ballooning of the defect and aid considerably in directing delineation.

On more than a few occasions even the most experienced of diagnostic gynecologic surgeons, in cases of moderate to severe vaginal eversion, will be convinced preoperatively that a true pulsion enterocele is present only to learn during the operation that none exists. In these cases either the rectocele or an associated cystocele or both are so huge that an illusion of enterocele is created, even to the extent that one thinks small bowel is felt in the protrusion, most likely only convoluted feces in the enlarged rectal lumen. Most often a large full-length rectovaginal septal separation has allowed a rectocele to assume extensive dimensions, filling the vagina from the perineum to the top of the vault with associated vault descent and some degree of external protrusion on Valsalva, especially when erect. Such occurrences, when the expected is not uncovered, although a source of embarrassment, especially if associated with pomposity or arrogance, humbling as they may be, serve best as reminders of the need for thoroughness in on-the-scene surgical decision-making. A good surgeon, after clean dissection to the vault, with a rectal finger placed at the uppermost forward point of the rectocele, followed by the dropping of a metal catheter into the bladder, has all the requisites necessary to make a quick assured decision about the prospective surgical plan. Although no enterocele is found in these instances, an associated SSF, as will be mentioned again later, is imperative for lasting correction.

Defacography has enjoyed a certain degree of recent popularity in ascertaining preoperatively the presence or absence of enterocele. It is beside the point that this method, in my brief experience with it, yields enough false positive and false negative results, to mislead a too trusting operator, especially a neophyte. It is of no more use than the intravenous pyelogram, which can even be dangerous, in preoperatively locating markedly displaced ureters due to huge fibromyomatous masses, telling you what you know anyhow and not obviating the need to avoid the ureters or to find them in exactly the place you expect them to be without radiographic help. Besides being expensive and exposing the patient to unnecessary irradiation, defacography in no way negates the job of the capable operator to search and discover, whether or not the procedure is done. So I do not do it and advise against it.

Anterior enterocele, less common as compared to the posterior or combined posterior and vault enterocele of our main discussion, lying posterior to the bladder and anterior to the hysterectomy vault scar, or anterior to the uterus if it is still present, must be recognized. This is generally an intraoperative discovery but must be suspected preoperatively in any situation of large distention cystocele that seems to reach the vault and bulges inordinately with Valsalva. Unusually anterior enterocele is an accidental finding uncovered during thorough dissection of anterior vaginal flaps when an open space is inadvertently entered. Initial anguish over possible vesical penetration is quickly replaced by relief when bowel or omentum is visualized. Most often such a fortuitous event does not occur, and the anterior peritoneal defect will be unnoticed unless it is suspected; a metal catheter is then dropped transurethrally into the bladder to reveal a bulging gap between the most posterior descent of the catheter tip and the hysterectomy scar. This is not necessary when simultaneous hysterectomy is being performed and an enlarged anterior pouch is noted after uterine removal. Such a bulge must be explored and opened, with dissection and repair as done posteriorly. Simple oversewing, without excision, of this peritoneal redundancy, whether discovered or not, increases future prolapse potential because of its vulnerability to intra-abdominal pressure.

Although on many occasions one cannot precisely identify the peritoneal herniation of an enterocele without making an entry into it, generally the sac is found first, sooner or later, and entry is best delayed until a reasonable amount of separation of the lesion is attained. Safely identified, it should then be opened. There is no question that the ultimate complete dissection and isolation of the sac is best accomplished when a counterpressing finger is placed inside, against the peritoneal lining. The actual separation is accomplished by a judicious blending of both sharp and blunt dissection, the former via Metzenbaum scissors and the latter using fingers and wet gently applied sponges. When cutting is called for, sometimes best results are obtained when the surgeon, especially if one finger is in the rectum, offers bimanual countertraction and counterpressure while a first-rate assistant sharply separates tissue under the surgeon's guidance.

Emphasis cannot be placed strongly enough on the need to isolate the lesion in toto before closure (Figure 10-4) and then to excise the freely dissected peritoneum up to the closure tie. Only thorough eradication provides the best prophylaxis against recurrence in the future. This can be accomplished by peritoneal clearance up to the "yellow line" posteriorly and to the bladder anteriorly, plus corresponding clearance bilaterally to imaginary lines connect-

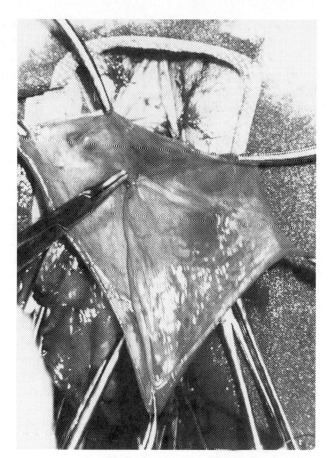

Figure 10-4. Purse-string closure at the neck (level of "yellow line" posteriorly) of a very large pulsion enterocele. The total peritoneal surface of this sac measured 29 in².

ing these two areas. The yellow line is a level of easily visualized retroperitoneal fat that anatomically demarcates abdominal peritoneum from cul-de-sac peritoneum, and this line fixes the upper limit for separation. Meticulous effort must be exercised in stripping the peritoneum cleanly, principally to avoid blood vessels, but also to bypass ureters that might have wandered lower than usual due to previous attenuation from prolapse. A truly rare finding, which I have seen but twice in 40 years of reconstructive pelvic surgery, both occasions in elderly women, is a single isolated ovary attached only to an upper posterolateral surface of enterocele peritoneum. Positive tissue verification was made later by microscopic inspection. One can only postulate on the evolution of this residual phenomenon.

The neck of the enterocele is designated as the ring formed by the level to which dissection has been carried as noted above. Using a narrow Deaver retractor for good exposure, rotating it progressively opposite to the point of each successive needle puncture, I close this neck in purse-string fashion (Figure 10-6). I find a curved Heaney needle driver most convenient for this job, as I do for all my vaginal suturing. Peritoneum is a thin delicate membrane of tissue with no tensile strength, which heals and seals rapidly. It reacts readily to irritation and trauma to form adhesions. We understand this so well that most surgeons avoid a sutured peritoneal approximation in abdominal operative wound closure because the peritoneum will heal without sutured closure. The only reasons for closing the peritoneal opening after vaginal hysterectomy are for (1) directing any untoward postoperative bleeding extraperitoneally both as tamponade and for earlier awareness of bleeding and for (2) helping in obliterating the cul-de-sac. Because the enterocele neck must be closed, the most logical purse-string material, as reasoned in Chapter 16, is a narrow-gauge rapidly absorbable polyfilament synthetic coated suture. I use 2-0 coated polyglycolic acid (Dexon II; Davis and Geck). I compromise on the caliber slightly because 2-0 is less likely to tear through the tissue than is 3-0 or 4-0. Catgut is too reactive. However, we must discuss the incomprehensible trend by so many capable gynecologic surgeons who currently use nonabsorbable, sometimes wide-gauged, material for closing enterocele neck peritoneum. Common among these are, amazingly, silk, the worst, and various forms of polyfilament and monofilament synthetic sutures, such as polyester and polypropylene. For underlying connective tissue and fascial support, perhaps, but for peritoneum, decidedly not! Although not an exact analogy, the classic comparison can be made to hitting a thumb tack with a sledge hammer. If there is a good reason at any time ever to use heavy or nonabsorbable suture on peritoneum, it surely escapes me.

Although some experienced pelvic operators feel that a good deep colporrhaphy is sufficient to lend adequate support to the enterocele neck closure, many of us feel an additional intervening buttress is more reassuring against recurrence. (Certainly this makes more sense than the use of powerhouse sutures in the peritoneum, users of which claim such closure negates the need for this buttress.) Accordingly, I currently now invariably place four to six successive interrupted 0 polyglyconate (Maxon) or 0 polytetrafluoroethylene (Gore-Tex) sutures to accomplish this end. Running in a line from front (bladder area) to the back (rectovaginal area), deep endopelvic fascia, almost always readily available and elastic enough, is drawn from the sides to the midline in a series of bites that usually forms a surprisingly formidable floor for the closed enterocele neck. One should not be self-duped into bringing perirectal connective tissue, which is closely adherent to the rectum, to the center to do this job; it will not work. The desirable tissue is more lateral, and usually slightly more anterior, on each side. These fibers are part of the intricate connective tissue network of the pelvis that holds all the structures together in balance between the peritoneum above and the levator muscle floor below.

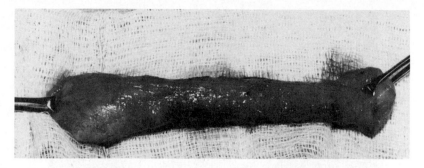

Figure 10-5. Typical specimen of extirpated postmenopausal uterus that was prolapsed totally outside perineum, accompanied by deep cul-de-sac large enough to classify as a moderate-sized enterocele sac. Corpus on left; cervix at right.

Restructuring this uppermost connective tissue into the total posterior repair can make the difference between long-term success and failure.

A final word on enterocele correction must cover the management of peritoneal herniation accompanying the presence of a uterus. A severely prolapsed uterus may coexist with a shallow cul-de-sac, especially if the bulk of the prolapse consists of elongated cervix. At the other extreme, a postmenopausal uterus can be found entirely outside the introitus, literally lying in a large sac of peritoneum with accompanying small bowel. In the latter instance, mere obliteration is unacceptable. Tedious and precise dissection to free up and excise the redundant peritoneum, exactly as in instances of pulsion enterocele corrected months or years after hysterectomy, must be followed by closure of the raw surface left behind as an imperative component for laudatory surgery (see Figures 10-5 and 10-6). Whether obliteration by any technique (McCall, Moscowitz, or Halban) or peritoneal excision should be used depends, in these incidences of simultaneously preceding vaginal hysterectomy, on the size of the pocket and the judgment of the operator. When there is doubt, despite its greater time consumption, I always advise peritoneal excision.

SACROSPINOUS LIGAMENT FIXATION: DISCUSSION

Turning now to the procedure, SSF, how does one know whether or not it should be included as part of any reparative operation? Occasionally this is a difficult decision to make because no woman should ever be subjected to any more surgery than that necessary to ensure full correction of defects. However, neither does the doctor have a right to shortcut the surgery and deprive a patient of the best guarantee possible against recurrence of breakdown and prolapse that will necessitate a further restorative procedure later.

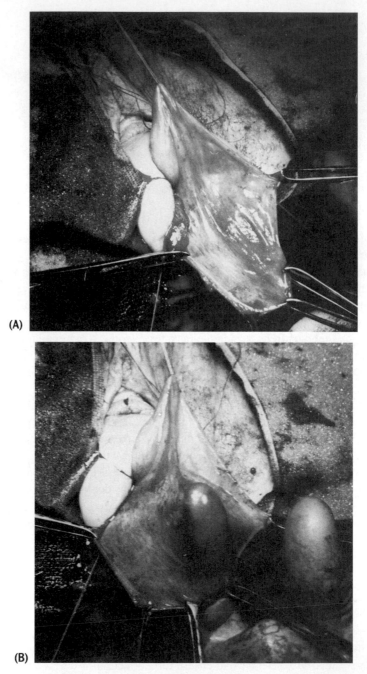

(A)

(B)

Figure 10-6. (A) Enterocele sac associated with uterus of Fig. 10-5. Peritoneal lining almost totally stripped free from cuff edge (bottom) to "yellow line" (top) where it is still attached. (B) Same as (A) with an index finger from behind revealing its translucency. The prolapse is so extreme that even the abdominal peritoneum has shifted down into it posteriorly (top).

Obviously guidelines are necessary, particularly for those newly embarking in the field of pelvic reconstruction who, possessing both adequate training and native skill, lack the experience requisite to comprehensive decision-making. I cannot begin to recount the number of instances of referral to our service in which, within years or months, sometimes even weeks, after a vaginal hysterectomy for prolapse, with or without a posterior repair of some sort, a posterior eversion has occurred. We see similar cases in situations of posthysterectomy posterior collapse wherein attempts at correction, with or without enterocele eradication, have failed. Do unfortunate circumstances such as these, given otherwise favorable factors toward success, develop because of poor surgery initially, as many critics contend, or because, despite acceptable technique, the one additional ingredient, the bottleneck, an SSF, was omitted? Certainly, the fixation, a procedure not without potentially serious hazard, as already pointed out, cannot be advocated as a routine procedure and must be reserved for special but precise indications. How does one make the right determination?

Generally, with minimal exception, a resolution to include or not to include SSF in an operative plan is formulated during the preoperative examination of the patient. The conclusion must be definitive, rarely equivocal, at that time. In this respect, I must interject the subject of persistent debate revolving about the idea of prophylactic SSF. I think there is no such thing. Either the patient needs it or she does not. If the calculated judgment of the doctor, based on findings and concepts I will outline, determines that SSF is indicated, then it becomes an integral part of the total operation. Strong voices state vehemently, for reasons beyond my comprehension, that in association with a hysterectomy, a sacrospinous suspension operation is unnecessary, while, at best, others unkindly term it "prophylactic," if done. On the other hand, some claim it should be included as an essential unit of a multifaceted operation routinely in *every* case where vaginal hysterectomy for prolapse is performed. The same people make similar claim for routine SSF in all cases of full vaginal length rectocele, called essential by some and prophylactic by others. They are all wrong. Neither a vaginal hysterectomy for whatever reason nor a full-length posterior vaginal repair is the determining factor in the question of associated need for SSF.

Very simply, while the patient is in the erect posture, under Valsalva influence, as described in Chapter 9, the doctor must evaluate the support of the posterior fornix. If it hardly budges, or remains fixed in an elevated posterior position, no matter how great the uterine prolapse or how large the rectocele, SSF is superfluous. Conversely, if the posterior fornix is markedly everted, literally sliding downward, then SSF becomes vital to prolonged corrective operative success. In between these two extremes, an astute assessment of a multiplicity of determining factors should be carefully weighed before an ultimate decision is reached. Some of these deserve discussion to illustrate how one decides.

Arbitrarily, my experience of 40 years in this business has taught me that an

SSF is indicated when the posterior fornix falls more than 3 cm in association with the combination of full-length rectocele, prolapsed uterus, and severely attenuated cardinal-uterosacral complexes. If the patient is relatively young, as in the perimenopause, and needs surgery because of a multiplicity of symptomatic supportive defects of moderate nature of both the anterior and posterior pelvis in association with a moderate prolapse of the uterus, I feel SSF is an integral necessity to the success of the surgery. Under such conditions, I cannot consider it prophylactic, especially if the patient presents a concomitant history of prior herniations elsewhere in the body, i.e., inguinal or umbilical, perhaps indicating general fascial weakness. In anticipation of a long life ahead, the obligation to offer the best opportunity for the greatest length of time in successful outcome is a moral responsibility of the surgeon. Therefore, brushing aside the semantic arguments over the adjectives "prophylactic" and "indicated," in my opinion SSF is crucial in the total management perspective of these tenuous young perimenopausal cases. Again, when previous reparative procedures of the pelvis have failed and reoperation is indicated, stabilization of the vaginal vault posteriorly by SSF may be the key link for reassurance of final achievement of lasting success. In some instances of severe major defects of the anterior pelvic compartment, as in severe cystocele, with some degree of accompanying apex invagination, even though the posterior defects alone might not be sufficient indication, SSF may be the best way to anchor the bladder base to reinforce the repair. This makes sense because the innermost lateral attachment of the pubovesicocervical fascia is at the level of the ischial spine, the most posterior point of the arcuate line and starting point of the sacrospinous ligament.

Although generally preoperative determinations should not be altered regarding a plan of repair, because loss of muscle tone under anesthesia renders a false picture of relaxation, on occasion this rule must necessarily be broken. These critical times arise whenever disrupted fascial and ligamentous tissues intended for surgical reunification are so deteriorated that they are beyond reliability to sustain long-term adequate support. Such a discovery and conclusion can only be made during surgery after dissection is completed and corrective surgery is attempted. In my extensive experience, posteriorly this occurs when only fragments of rectovaginal fascia can be found on each side and even levator fascial extensions are bilaterally too fragile for enduring dependability. In these circumstances, a full-length rectocele under repair is doomed to recurrence unless ancillary help is provided. In such situations, where vault mobility preoperatively was thought not enough to warrant SSF, that procedure, combined with approximation in the midline of deep endopelvic or residual posterior cardinal ligament extensions from each side may well compensate, at least in the upper vaginal area, for the unanticipated weak tissues below. Although this additional thought will be expanded in the next chapter, I must add here that concomitant meticulous rebuilding of the perineal body, attaching its uppermost portions to rectovaginal septal remnants, in conjunction with the SSF balancing effect above, as described, usually leads to surprisingly satisfactory results. In effect, the weak area in between, i.e., in the middle, is balanced by compensatory strength above and below.

SACROSPINOUS LIGAMENT FIXATION: PROCEDURE

When enterocele is present, it should always be repaired before SSF is attempted. Once again, as mentioned earlier in this chapter, pursuit of the sacrospinous ligament may begin only after dissection, as described in Chapter 11, is complete to the level of the posterior fornix or the vaginal vault and out laterally equally to both sidewalls.

At this point, through the right pararectal septum, I identify the right ischial spine by palpation with my right middle finger. The sacrospinous ligament, lying in the posterior border of the coccygeus muscle, is attached to the posteroinferior surface of the ischial spine so that the same examining finger, moving posteromedially, falls directly onto the ligament, tracing it to the sacrum. Then, bluntly, digital penetration of the lateral pararectal barrier opens up the area, allowing for sweeping of areolar tissue off the anterior and inferior surfaces of the ligament over as much of its extent as possible. Clearing only these aspects for at least 2.5 to 3 cm is all that is necessary to provide adequate visualization. Attempting more ambitious exposure is not only unnecessary, but might lead to aberrant anterolateral entry into the greater sciatic foramen (notch) containing sciatic nerve, or posterolateral intrusion into the lesser sciatic notch, which provides passage for the pudendal vessels and nerve. The dangers are obvious. I rarely resort to sharp dissection in this deep paraligamentous space, and when I do, I exact extreme care. The key to averting trouble is the certain identification of the tip of the ischial spine, which always projects medially beyond both sciatic portals. Damage to the inferior gluteal blood vessels, which enter the coccygeus muscle region behind and inferior to the sacrospinous ligament, can be avoided, by locating, grasping, and elevating the ligament to allow for puncture to remain anterior to the vasculature.

A salient feature of the sacrospinous ligament is its incorporation into the posterior border of the coccygeus muscle, not anterior, as is often erroneously preached. In younger women, the ligament, though very strong, is relatively small and well covered by muscle fibers. Ironically, as women age, the ligament generally becomes progressively thicker and more prominent and identifiable as dense connective tissue steadily replaces muscle at the coccygeal posterior border.

The absolute primary key to successful surgery and to the escape from calamitous catastrophe in this deep relatively narrow operative field is constant unrelenting direct vision during any type of sharp penetration of tissue.[11,12] Sutures placed by touch alone can wander a few too many millimeters laterally and involve pudendal or sciatic nerve fibers with obvious dire consequences, sometimes rendering lifetime crippling. In the same area, severe hemorrhage uncontrollable by direct access might occur via unintended injury to the pudendal artery. When the suture-carrying instrument or needle under only finger control rather than guidance by sight inadvertently encircles the ligament instead of piercing through it, a similar hemorrhagic danger surfaces, courtesy of the inferior gluteal artery. Because this sudden frightening life-threatening event has been recorded in the past and undoubtedly will recur, prudence dictates the need for awareness of the solution of the problem at this point of the discussion. All attempts to control hemorrhage by a direct approach to either the pudendal or the inferior gluteal artery are mechanically impossible, all things considered, and any attempt to do so will prove totally fruitless while the patient's life hangs in the balance as transfusion blood is pumped into her. Perception that this vascular misfortune is happening must be immediate, followed by emergency repositioning of the patient as the abdominal wall is opened and the bifurcation of the common iliac artery is identified bilaterally. The internal iliac artery is the parent source of supply for both the pudendal and inferior gluteal arteries. There is no time to search for the posterior parietal branch of the internal iliac to get closer to the offending vessel. Instead, the ipsilateral internal iliac artery must be ligated first at once, followed by ligation on the opposite side. Control of both sides is necessary because of the rich anastomotic vascular network of the pelvis and because, if the original surgery is continued, it may be necessary to go to the opposite sacrospinous ligament where a similar mishap just might occur.

Proximity of small bowel above and large bowel medially relative to the operative area of present concern has already been mentioned. Unless there is proper direct visual access accompanied by appropriately correct retraction, these precariously close intestinal components may easily be entered by the needle intended only for the sacrospinous ligament. Once the ligament is grasped and brought into sight, usually the easiest part of what can be, in some cases, a difficult procedure, the bowel can be safely retracted out of the danger zone. The operator must watch the target zone without lapse. The horrible consequences of unwitting and unknowing bowel penetration can easily be imagined.

Although either the right or the left side is usually essentially equal in the capacity to afford support, almost without exception the right side is chosen as the anchor. The simple reason for this option is the presence of the distal sigmoid colon and upper rectum on the patient's left, thereby narrowing the safety zone on that side. Coincidentally the majority of operators are right-handed and the procedure of ligament fixation can be more comfortably performed by them on the patient's right side. There are exceptions. For reasons not always explicable, rarely may right-sided ligament access be so difficult or so technically impractical that one must use the opposite side to achieve satisfaction. Also, on occasion, the right ligament may seem weak or insubstantial. In such instances, a switch to the left is logical and sensible.

Some proponents of this operation insist that the most effective course is a bilateral fixation to provide a better balanced and more secure result. Most surgeons feel that the minimum deviation at the vault to one side is of no lasting consequence and that using both sides at the least doubles the risk factors and may add too much tension where it is least desirable. Also, bilateral SSF may open the top of the vagina and weaken the vault. Analyses of long-term case follow-ups bear out the opinion that one side is more than adequate for long-term success.

Having cleared the right sacrospinous ligament bluntly as described (sharp dissection is dangerous, as already mentioned) both superiorly and anteriorly, it must then be exposed to sight. This is best accomplished by the correct placement, ever gently, of the Breisskey-Navratil retractors (Figure 10-7). The depth of the ischial spine from the perineum determines the length of the retractor to be chosen. The first is placed anterolaterally, the second anteromedially, and the third, offering countertraction, is positioned posterolaterally barely external to the ligament and the ischial spine. This accomplished, in "virgin fields," the ligament may easily pop into view and be appropriately grasped (see Figure 10-7).

For beginners, exposure of the ligament is always the most difficult step in this surgical enterprise, but even veterans may be challenged to the utmost in cases of previous repairs (the more, the worse) that have attempted to reestablish posterior pelvic and vault support. In these latter cases, excessive scar, tissue distortion, and fatty impingements can be extremely unnerving and taxing, sometimes driving surgeons to gamble by driving the sharp-pointed suture carrier blindly through a ligament they think they can feel but do not see. The perils are obvious.

However, when such formidable circumstances are encountered, I have devised a simple time-saving technique that avoids trouble. As soon as difficulty becomes obvious, with no success at exposure after some 2 minutes (an arbitrary time limit) of blunt clearing anteriorly and inferiorly adjacent to the palpable but still invisible ligament, the middle and index fingers of the left hand are inserted along the medial surface of the right lateral pelvic wall until the tip of the middle finger contacts the ischial spine. The ligament is then again briefly palpated where it begins just posterior to the spine for absolute identification. Next, with the middle fingertip replaced on the spine, the closed Grody-Babcock clamp is passed medially along the finger to its tip and, opened fully, at a 45-degree angle with the horizontal level, it is thrust vigorously at the ligament to close around it in firm grasp just medial to the spine. Often, it is necessary for the operator, if sitting, as I usually am, to rise slightly to a

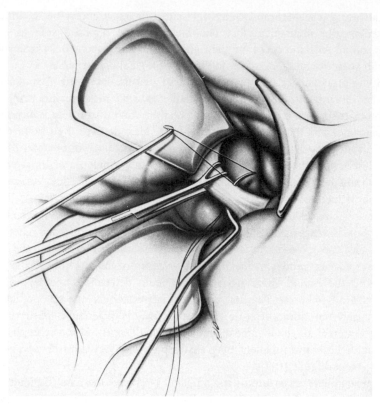

Figure 10-7. The right sacrospinous ligament as it is seen in the lithotomy position (coccygeus muscle omitted from the sketch so as to reveal the proximity of the bowel above). The Breissky-Navratil retractors are in good position, the ligament is grasped by the Grody-Babcock clamp just medial to the ischial spine, the Nichols-Deschamps suture carrier is piercing the ligament in a safe manner, and the nerve hook is pulling the suture through.

semisitting posture to do this. Tugging on the clamp moves the whole patient, proving its correct placement. Vascular damage is not a problem because the ends of the clamp are dull and they fit snugly against the ligament. The three retractors, which were removed during the grasping maneuver, are then repositioned, after which it is but a matter of seconds before the ligament, now clearly identified, is stripped easily to bring a substantial segment of it into view. Using this technique, the average time we consume now for visualizing, grasping, and piercing the sacrospinous ligament, starting from penetration of the pararectal pillars, has been cut to 3 minutes. If there is exasperating time delay in cases of correction of massive vaginal eversion, all reports indicate that it most likely occurs during the pursuit of the enterocele or the sacrospinous ligament, usually relatively proportionate to the number of preceding reconstructive endeavors in the area and to the experience of the operator.

Although I am blatantly repetitive, I cannot emphasize enough the obligatory maxim of total visualization, the handmaiden of thorough wide deep dissection, for all aspects of reconstructive surgery, but particularly for those centering on the deep posterior pelvis. Blind surgery is cousin to incompetence and it can lead to serious complications and charges of malpractice, but more importantly than all else, it is perilous for the patient. When the maneuvers described herein become too difficult for you in any given case, or you are tempted to take a chance, by all means, quit right there and choose a lesser and safer course within your capabilities. The end results may not be quite what you and the patient had hoped for, but better to endure some disappointment than a major calamity.

The crux of the SSF is the correct penetration by appropriate sutures through the ligament followed by precise placement of the same sutures into the vaginal wall at the vault. If the Grody-Babcock clamp is attached to the ligament, in juxtaposition to the ischial spine, or as close to it as is feasible, and at least 1 cm additionally, usually more, of the ligament is easily visible, insertion through the ligament well medial to the clamp and therefore also medial to the greater and lesser sciatic notches which are lateral to the spine, should guarantee safety. The stitch should capture at least half the thickness of the ligament, preferably two thirds, especially if it seems slightly narrower than expected. In postmenopausal women it is often as thick as a fifth finger. Never should it be passed completely around this tough structure, where it can strike the inferior gluteal artery to produce disaster. Figure 10-7 reveals a simple sketch of an isolated right-sided ligament, as seen in lithotomy position, with the balance of the coccygeus muscle deleted. All the instruments described above are illustrated at work, including the nerve hook pulling the loop beyond the puncture site.

Two sutures are recommended, one for each side of the vaginal vault. Several available choices are manufactured in 60-inch lengths so that only one thrust through the ligament is necessary because the pulled loop can be cut to form two segments. When suture lengths of 30 or 36 inches are used, two separate sharp perforations, each pulling individual sutures, must be made because unworkably short lengths remain if these are severed in half.

The precise points of placement of the sacrospinous sutures into the raw dissected surface of the wall of the posterior vaginal vault is crucial. The calculated spot must allow for direct contact with the ligament without tension. However, inadvertent tension should not be placed on the anterior vaginal wall either, for this may produce postoperative lower urinary tract symptoms that were not present preoperatively. Even worse, if anterior pelvic disruption has been simultaneously repaired, and it should always be done first, undue tension from the SSF may nullify the effectiveness of a good anterior repair. Conversely, correctly selected vaginal suture placement points in an SSF, neither too tight nor too lax in the ultimate effect anteriorly, can help restore and ensure bladder base support at an anatomically normal deep level contiguous with the innermost extent of the arcus tendineus or "white line."

I feel very strongly that any indicated anterior pelvic repair must precede the SSF. Restoring the supportive and suspensory apparatus of the urethra first and then of the bladder followed ultimately by fixation of the innermost area of the bladder base at the vaginal vault by the SSF is a logical and workable sequence. Reversing the order, i.e., performing the SSF initially, not only might make anterior technical accessibility difficult but it might compromise natural anatomic replacement in the urethral and vesical areas as well as introduce undesired tension. Conversely, when preceded by thorough dissection, no such jeopardy is introduced when either the SSF itself or the posterior repair is done after the anterior pelvic compartment has first been reestablished. This argument is interjected at this point because some proponents of SSF feel that a concomitant anterior repair should be done only following the SSF. Obviously, I cannot see the logic to this.

Allowance for mild longitudinal laxity of the posterior wall, rarely a problem if associated with very wide and deep dissection of vaginal mucosa, is desirable. Such laxity will disappear as the vaginal length increases while the normal vaginal axis is restored, as described in the next chapter.

The vital points of sacrospinous attachment can be selected best not by guesswork but by an assessment using a long Allis clamp grasping various loci and thrusting them into contact with the ligament until the most ideal suture placement spot is found. The two chosen vault placement points are usually about 5 to 8 mm from the midline, one on either side. In accordance with the suggestion of Nichols,[5] a single throw or half-knot is made in the right-sided SSF stitch at its junction with the vagina, as seen in Figure 10-8. Thus fixed, a pulley effect is created that allows one to pull on the other end to test effectiveness before tying and, more importantly, to give assurance of direct contact, for "suture gap," as I call it, would render the entire SSF exercise a waste of time. Because the suture slides at only one juncture point, fixation is easy to accomplish. A pulley knot is mechanically unnecessary on the second side because contact fixation will already have been established when the first suture is completely tied. However, it is important not to tie the SSF sutures at this time, only to have them in place ready for tying.

If the SSF sutures are knotted now, elevating the vaginal vault deeply posteriorly, it may become impossible, or certainly very difficult, to start the closure of the posterior vaginal wall, previously divided in the midline during the opening dissection up to the top of the vault. Simultaneously, access to the deepest endopelvic recesses may be so compromised as to obviate placement of at least two innermost colporrhaphy sutures. I feel this deep initiation of colporrhaphy closure in almost all cases is vital as a substantial underpinning to buttress the SSF, for this vaginal fixation should not stand alone without underlying connective tissue enforcement. So the two colporrhaphy sutures are placed, as will be described in the next chapter, and held, not to be tied until after the SSF sutures are tied. In turn, the vaginal vault mucosal closure must be

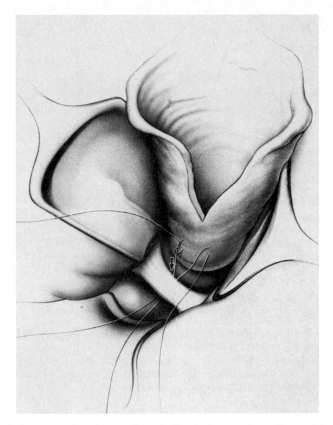

Figure 10-8. The two suture lengths through the right sacrospinous ligament have been attached to the raw posterior surface of the vaginal wall on either side of the midline near the vault (dotted line). The "pulley stitch" (single knot throw) is shown, ready for contact with the ligament (arrow).

carried for at least five or six suture bites while it still is in view. Then, and only then, the two SSF sutures first and next the two colporrhaphy sutures are tied in succession. Of incidental note, if enterocele excision has been performed before the SSF, its neck closure and underlying supportive sutures are coincidently carried posteriorly into well-protected location as the SSF is completed.

Occasionally, one may be confronted preoperatively with the problem of so shallow a vaginal depth that, after digital replacement of the eversion, quite obviously the vault will not even come close to the sacrospinous ligament. The first step in overcoming this dilemma is preoperative estrogen replacement therapy for a minimum of 6 to 8 weeks, necessary anyhow in all of these cases before any surgery is attempted. This will restore a significant elasticity and flexibility to the vaginal wall. Often this will be adequate enough if combined with the next step, at the time of surgery, namely, thorough wide and deep

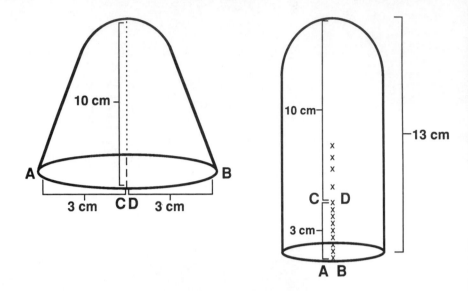

SIMPLE TRANSFORMATION

Figure 10-9. The cone, whether everted or still inverted, must be transformed into a cylindrical shape. Points A and B represent the lateral corners at the outset of surgery; C and D designate either side of the original fourchette as the posterior vaginal wall is bisected toward the vault. After thorough dissection, the reparative process moves C and D inward as the vagina is reshaped and lengthened while A and B meet at the new fourchette.

dissection out to the pelvic sidewalls bilaterally and up to the peritoneal cavity, beyond the uppermost reach of the replaced vagina. This problem usually happens in vaginas that have lost their normal axis and are more conical than cylindrical, yet have good surface area. Thus, after making a full-length midline posterior wall incision, between the rejuvenated mucosa and the very wide dissection, enough shifting of tissue, converting cone to cylinder, is often possible to allow contact of posterior raw vault surface with the ligament (Figure 10-9).

If foreshortening is so great as to raise doubt about this method working, the diligent use of silicon vaginal dilators, lubricated with Premarin cream, two to three times a day, 3 to 5 minutes at a time, for 1 to 3 months will often create a pliant, adequate surface. These dilators (Milex, Inc., Chicago, IL) are graduated both in width and length to cover all possible diminution in measurements.

When even then it still seems likely that the vaginal length will fall short, the usual posterior straight line vaginal wall incision should be shunned in favor of a zig-zag opening (Figure 10-10). Stretched out, such a cut can increase the linear dimension by as much as 50%. If none of this works, but at least some degree of closer proximity has been attained, a final solution will certainly be

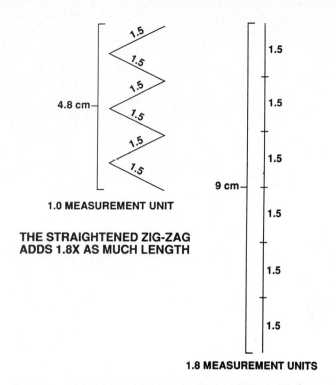

1.0 MEASUREMENT UNIT

THE STRAIGHTENED ZIG-ZAG
ADDS 1.8X AS MUCH LENGTH

1.8 MEASUREMENT UNITS

ZIG-ZAG POSTERIOR VAGINAL INCISION

Figure 10-10. When the posterior vagina has been freely dissected to the pelvic sidewalls and to the vault, a zig-zag incision, when anchored at the top, allows for a substantial increase in vaginal length.

realized with the use of a small segment of Mersilene mesh or a Gore-Tex patch to bridge the gap, rarely necessary.

Any gynecologic surgeon who performs a significant number of full posterior compartment repairs, including SSF and deep posterior colpoperineorrhaphy, and who is considered an expert, sooner or later has to wonder, at the immediate conclusion of the surgery, why some cases seem so much more satisfactory both in depth and axis than others. In no way is this the fault of the surgeon. The variation in end result is simply a reflection of the particular bony architecture of each individual pelvis (Figure 10-11). The osseus pelvic configuration determines the location of the sacrospinous ligament. Reverting to obstetric terms, the longer the birth canal, the deeper will lie the ligament. Conversely, in a shallow pelvis, the reconstructed vagina will be necessarily shorter. Similarly, the deeper the sacral curve and the more it rotates backward, the greater the vaginal depth and the better the axis, and vice versa.

Before leaving this chapter, a discussion of suture choice for the SSF is

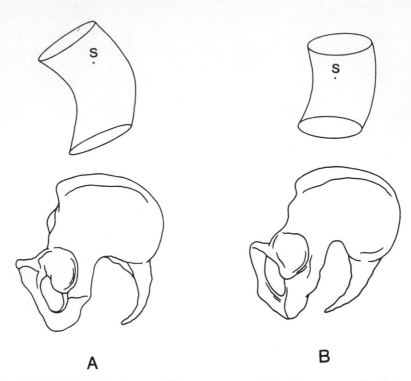

A   B

Figure 10-11. Pelvis A is deeper and its sacrum more posterior than corresponding features in pelvis B. The ishial spine (S) lies more posteriorly in pelvis A than in pelvis B. Hence, a more mechanically efficient result is possible in A than in B.

pertinent. Originally, as the SSF was gaining early prominence in the field of reconstructive surgery, rapidly absorbable material, such as catgut and polyglycolic acid, both polyfilaments, were most commonly used. It was reasoned that catgut, a highly reactive natural substance, would provoke considerable inflammation and, therefore, a stronger scar would result. The idea of rapid absorption seemed most acceptable as prophylaxis against permanent or serious damage in the event of errant suture entrapment, as with nerves. Most operators felt also that, regardless of suture choice, ultimate lasting good outcomes, assuming good surgical technique in general, depend primarily on postsurgical strong scar formation. The reports in the literature would seem to support this concept.[4,5]

However, over time, more and more of these SSF procedures are being performed with nonabsorbable suture.[11,12] The reason for this is that, despite reports of a very high percentage of good long-term results so far, many of us feel this is not good enough. Thoughts pervade that SSF is one operation that, under the best circumstances, should yield close to 100% in excellent outcomes over the very long term, at least relative to posterior support, especially important because female life expectancy continues to rise. Those of us who use nonabsorbable ("permanent") suture feel strongly that a small but significant gain in positive statistics is a likely and important expectation in the future.

I began performing SSF in 1976, using nonabsorbable suture from the outset. I worked first with a very satisfactory suture, number one caliber polypropylene (Surgilene, Prolene). In 1986 I changed to an improved suture, number one gauge polybutestor (Novafil) and 3 years later, I changed still again to the material I feel will be the best of all for this particular operation. For all the reasons thoroughly elaborated in the chapter in this book on suture selection, since 1989 the only suture I have used for SSF is zero caliber polytetrafluoroethylene (Gore-Tex). The primary compelling feature of this material is its capacity for suture incorporation into the scar, from the start of the healing process, because of its physical property of microporosity. All other nonabsorbable sutures are only encapsulated by scar formation and slide as a result.

REFERENCES

1. Nichols DH, Randall CL. *Vaginal Surgery*. 3rd ed. Baltimore: Williams & Wilkins; 1989;341–342.

2. Miyazaki FS. Miya hook ligature carrier for sacrospinous ligament suspension. *Obstet Gynecol.* 1987;70:286–288.

3. Nichols DH, Randall CL. *Vaginal Surgery*. 3rd ed. Baltimore: Williams & Wilkins; 1989:338–342.

4. Morley GW, DeLancey JOL. Sacrospinous ligament fixation for eversion of the vagina. *Am J Obstet Gynecol.* 1988,158:872–881.

5. Nichols DH. Sacrospinous fixation for massive eversion of the vagina. *Am J Obstet Gynecol.* 1982;142:901–904.

6. Drutz HP, Cha LS. Massive genital and vaginal vault prolapse treated by abdominal-vaginal sacropexy with use of Marlex mesh: review of the literature. *Am J Obstet Gynecol.* 1987;156:387–392.

7. Zacharin RF. *Pelvic Floor Anatomy and the Surgery of Pulsion Enterocoele*. New York: Springer-Verlag; 1985:102–133.

8. Wall LL, Stanton SL. Alternatives for repair of post-hysterectomy vault prolapse and enterocoele. *Contemp OB/GYN.* September 1988:32–48.

9. Grody MHT. *Complex Procedures and Methods in Pelvic Reconstructive and Urogynecologic Surgery* (Video). New York and London: Parthenon; 1993:2–4.

10. Grody MHT. *Anatomic Surgical Restoration in Extreme Massive Vaginal Eversion with Hugh Pulsion Enterocoele* (Video). Washington: ACOG Audiovisual Library; 1993.

11. Kettel LM, Hebertson RM. An anatomic evaluation of the acrospinous ligament colpopexy. *Surg Gynecol Obstet* 1989;168:318–322.

12. Wheeless CR. *Atlas of Pelvic Surgery*. 2nd ed. Philadelphia: Lea & Febiger; 1988:56.

Posterior Pelvis III: Rectocele and Perineal Defects

Marvin H. Terry Grody

THE VAGINAL AXIS

During the decade preceding the publication of this book, certain terms and concepts relative to the supportive and suspensory apparatus of the posterior pelvis have come into prominence. Perhaps the most all-encompassing, most graphic, and most important of these is the *normal vaginal axis*. To the anatomically knowledgeable gynecologist, such a term should instantly draw to mind a vagina the most distal third of which is almost vertical while the upper two thirds lie almost horizontally. The innermost portion, the posterior vault, should lie deep in the posterior pelvis, projecting into the most recessed point of the sacrococcygeal bony curve.[1,2] This hollow organ, the vagina, should be envisioned as the central core of the pelvis, with the uterus above, the bladder and urethra in front, and the rectum behind, held in a delicate functionally adjustable balance by a composite of connective tissue, elastic tissue, smooth muscle, and striated muscle in an interdepen-

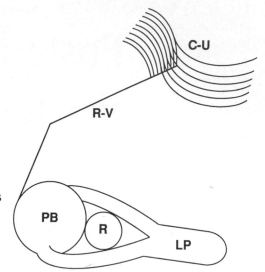

Figure 11-1 Mainstays of vaginal axis integrity. C-U, cardinal-uterosacral ligament complex; RV, rectovaginal septum; PB, perineal body; R, rectum; LP, levator plate with connecting arms on either side around the rectum.

dent pelvic network.[3] It is now well understood that progressive weaknesses or defects in any of these tissues in any area of the pelvis can lead to a disturbance in this normal axis which ultimately might produce symptoms requiring attention. It is equally accepted that the bottleneck for vaginal stability lies primarily in the posterior pelvis, i.e., damage in this anatomic region is most apt to disturb the vaginal axis.

The principal elements in this crucial organ security begin at the top with the posterior inferior extensions of the cardinal-uterosacral complex that suspend the upper vagina posterosuperiorly[4] and also both help form the anterior wall of the cul-de-sac and blend into the next vital part of maintenance of axis, the rectovaginal septum. The suspensory fibers are contiguous with the cardinal-uterosacral complex above, which form the lowermost para-metria (Figure 11-1). This long strong connective tissue band is called the upper paracolpium, which slings the proximal vagina to the posterolateral pelvic walls and to the sacrum. Together with their anterior extensions, they form the cephalad portion of the endopelvic fascia, already described as a network, that distally terminates in the perineum posteriorly and the urogenital diaphragm anteriorly.

THE RECTOVAGINAL SEPTUM

After many years of debate as to the existence at all of a rectovaginal septum (the fascia of Denonvillier) as a separate entity, not to mention its precise boundaries and function, it has now become recognized as an important finite constituent of normal posterior pelvic integrity.[5,6] It begins superiorly as noted above, at the pouch of Douglas and runs down to join into the perineal body distally (see Figure 11-1). Laterally its fibers blend into the fascial coverings of the iliococcygeus muscles. It lies in direct proximity to the posterior vaginal wall in the normal status, and this is why, until relatively recently, it had been considered part of the vagina, but it can be bluntly separated from the vagina. It forms the anterior border of the rectovaginal space and probably, together with the fibromuscular bands that extend bilaterally from the vaginal wall itself to the pelvic diaphragm at the sidewalls, should be considered part of the mid-paracolpium. This relatively thin but remarkably strong, when intact, structural sheet histologically consists of dense collagen fibers, mostly lateral, smooth muscle, similar to perivaginal muscle, lying primarily in the midline, and dense elastin distributed evenly. Nowhere else in the entire pelvis are the elastic fibers so dense as they are in this unique membranous layer.

The rectovaginal septum deserves special attention because it is so critically important to understand its anatomy and function to accomplish a correct repair. Until recently, few of us were taught anything about it. For years, in every operating room across the country, and we still hear it in many places, gynecologists about to embark on what has been called "a posterior repair" would say, "Now we'll finish up quickly with a glorified episiotomy." Generally there was no idea of any role or existence of particular tissue, and thus, coupled with inadequate and limited dissection, excessive mucosal excision, and suturing together into the midline inconsequential perirectal fibers, a most unsatisfactory result was common and unfortunately still is.

Ruptures, detachments, and tears involving this somewhat trapezoidal layer of tissue are responsible for rectoceles, one of the most common structural herniations. In the nulliparous woman, or in women with a normal vaginal axis, the location and strength of the rectovaginal septum can easily be assessed, but few practitioners really pay attention to these points of anatomy. Therefore, it is only logical that they will likely incorrectly or insufficiently evaluate a rectocele in a multiparous woman whose rectovaginal septum was damaged many years before in childbirth. The limits and extents of injury to this fascial sheet can easily be apprised by a gentle but thorough rectal examination. Only thus armed with definite information can the surgeon proceed with an operation designed specifically for that patient, in contrast to the operator who, unaware of the anatomic fine points, performs essentially the same procedure on everyone, particularly in the absence of examination with the patient in the erect posture.

Defects in this septum can occur in a variety of locations. Perhaps the most common, at least the type we are most often called on to repair because a rectocele is bursting through it, is linear, or vertical, either midline or to one side or the other. These tears can be complete, from top to bottom, or they may be partial, usually described relative to the lower third, middle third, or upper third of the vagina. Again, the most prevalent seem to be those in association with the lower half of the posterior wall of the vagina, and they are, in my long experience, rarely not accompanied by some degree of perineal disintegration (Figure 11-2). Thus,

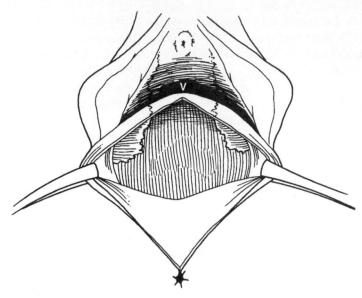

Figure 11-2 Linear disruption of rectovaginal septum above a markedly disintegrated perineal body.

although rectocele and perineal defects are truly different lesions occurring in entirely different structures,[7] they frequently exist together (Figure 11-3). Under these circumstances, if one or the other is repaired inadequately, the long-term outcome may be poor because of their adjacent interdependence. Such deficient correction absolutely precludes restoration of a normal vaginal axis.

It is my distinct impression that a high percentage of rectoceles are progressive, not just in the amount of outward protrusion over time, obvious to all of us, but in the extent of the tear. I have observed patients coming to me over many years, initially with an asymptomatic lower third rectocele that has steadily developed into a full-length symptomatic rectal protrusion for which the patients ultimately request correction (Figure 11-4). Many come in for the first time with a full-length lesion and large external herniation, describing a steady development from either an annoying pressure or a small *ball* some years ago that has steadily grown to the present disabling situation. Whether or not the beginning tear was small and slowly extended or it was large from the start hardly matters. What does matter is that, when the patient is brought to the operating room for correction of defects any-where in the pelvis, this posterior imperfection must be simultaneously amended in its entire extent. By the same token, patients may present for correction of symptomatic anterior pelvic defects or uterine prolapse, but examination reveals addition-ally a "silent" linear separation in the rectovaginal septum. We know that almost certainly such a lesion is destined to foster later herniation despite current absence of posterior pelvic symptoms.[8,9] Appropriate simultaneous repair of this anatomic

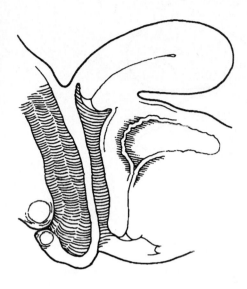

Figure 11-3 Coexisting defective perineal body and low rectocele with associated vertical vagina.

flaw is imperative and should be thoroughly discussed with the patient in advance. The situation becomes even more tenuous if overt perineal defects are also present, thereby already distorting the vaginal axis by widening and straightening it. The patient should be fully informed that a correction of the symptomatic defects alone, surgically pulling the anterior vaginal wall forward, will exaggerate the axis deformity, thereby certainly accelerating deterioration of the known weakened but asymptomatic posterior and vault areas. By apprising her thoroughly that subsequent need for further surgery will be almost inevitable, the doctor is conforming to the highest professional standards and the patient's best interests are being served. Obviously the ideal plan includes repair of all lesions, symptomatic or not, simultaneously.

The most dramatic type of rectocele one can see, although I think they are the most infrequent, are those breaking through the mid-third area only (Figure 11-5). An examining rectal finger can sharply define the exact boundaries of such lesions. This information can lead to relatively simple but satisfying, to the doctor, and gratifying, to the patients, surgical experiences that result in a very high rate of long-term surgical cure.

When rectocele occurs in the upper third of the vagina, it probably very rarely is an isolated lesion. Most often it is part of a full-length rectocele, and I always assume, erring perhaps in some cases, but playing on the safe side, that there must be at least some degree of disruption from the posterior descending extensions of the cardinal-uterosacral complex. Certainly there is no question about this abnormal circumstance when the posterior fornix descends at least 2 to 3 cm on Valsalva when the patient is examined in the erect position. Such awareness obviously

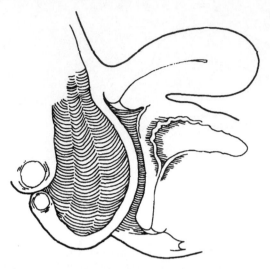

Figure 11-4 Full-length rectocele continuous with severely defective perineal body and abnormal vaginal axis.

should lead to more thorough surgery. An associated enterocele must never be out of consideration.

Although linear septal separations are not necessarily in the midline and may well be off center quite a bit to one side or the other, this does not matter as long as the surgeon becomes more directly cognizant during the dissection and places the sutures correctly. This will be described later in this chapter.

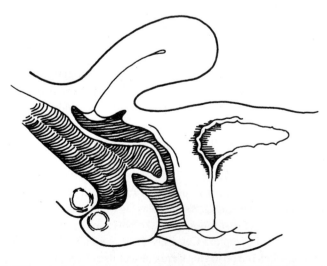

Figure 11-5 Mid-vaginal rectocele as an isolated lesion. Vaginal axis is fairly normal.

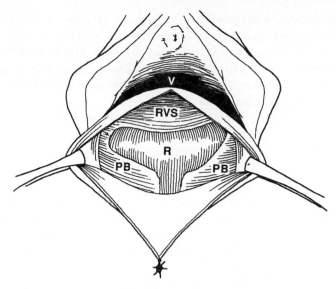

Figure 11-6 Transverse separation of rectovaginal septum (RVS) from disrupted perineal body (PB) in low rectocele. R, rectum; V, vagina.

Detachment of this fascia of Denonvillier transversely from its natural juncture with the superior extents of the perineal body is common and logically creates the weakness for a horizontal type of low rectocele. One can absolutely count on such a lesion when perineal body disruption itself coexists to any extent (Figure 11-6). This situation is often overlooked during surgery and consequently crucial sutures to reestablish the natural septal-perineal body connection may not be placed. Looking further posteriorly, adequate correction of levator plate descensus may literally hang on recognition and repair of this transverse defect because of the interdependent connecting nature of endopelvic support. Especially is this so if the integrity of the perineal body is not what it should be.

THE PERINEAL BODY

In my opinion, in assessing the roles played by various pelvic elements in maintaining the balance necessary for a normal vaginal axis, the perineal body is the most fascinating and yet enigmatic structure of all. It is often called the focus, the core, the bottleneck of all pelvic support in its situation between the lowermost vagina and introitus in front and the distal rectum and anus behind. In such a strategic position, directly and indirectly, all the elements of pelvic support from all directions, above, lateral, front, back, feed into it much as spokes of a wheel connect to a hub, or control center. When impaired by attenuation, detachment, or degeneration, sooner or later, given enough time in the aftermath of childbirth trauma to the general pelvis,[7,10–12] it may well set off a sort of domino effect as other elements successively break down. From another viewpoint, to emphasize its importance, an intact perineal body may entirely block the appearance of symptoms from other supportive tissues already weakened.

Questions regarding the pivotal role of the perineal body must be carried further, particularly since so rarely is its full clinical impact explained or discussed to the adequate satisfaction of practitioners. Quite often our examinations will reveal it to be in a state of marked deterioration, but the patient will remain entirely asymptomatic, even though the normal vaginal axis may be thereby somewhat compromised, as already mentioned. Yet, in cases of major pelvic reconstruction, we leave ourselves open to strong criticism if we neglect doing a good perineorrhaphy, and we all have witnessed ultimate breakdown of the entire procedure because of failure to do this. Then again, a well-accepted doctrine today is the need to accompany every anterior pelvic repair with at least a perineorrhaphy, if not a low colpoperineorrhaphy, to compensate the forward alteration of the vaginal axis.[8,9] Without some sort of associated posterior buildup, we have observed a significant later incidence of enterocele. And then, again, if the perineal body is truly such an important link in the total chain of stability, why does not the rest of pelvic support steadily disintegrate in cases of chronic fourth degree perineal laceration, where a perineal body is nonexistent? Surely this is an oddity, a paradox. So, why?

Consider basically that the perineal body of the young primigravida with an unrepaired complete perineal laceration and that of the postreproductive woman with severe perineal defects are anatomically essentially the same, vanished and functionless. In the former, curiously the balance of pelvic support remains undisturbed, whereas in the latter the endopelvic musculofascial apparatus has progressively deteriorated.

In the young healthy female patient, the single delivery is not likely to reflect any significant lasting weakening of the uterosacral complex suspending the lower uterus and vagina well above the pelvic diaphragm. Even more importantly, the rupture through the perineum takes the bulk of the stretch and strain of delivery off the pelvic floor, primarily the levator plate and the levator ani, which exert their influence principally behind the anus, so no lower level disturbance is apparent.[13] Full natural estrogen stimulation has maintained a high level of general texture, tone, collagen content, and vascularity throughout the pelvis. Perhaps the most significant factor, according to recent neuromyographic research, is the rapid recovery of pelvic nerve damage after the first delivery almost to normal levels.[14] So, except for absent sphincter control of fecal excretion, the reproductive woman's pelvis appears otherwise untouched despite the destruction in the perineal body.

Opposite circumstances coexist with the decimated perineum in the older woman. More often than not the pelvis has been subjected to the general trauma of multiple deliveries.[15,16] Denervation of both striated and smooth muscles increases, and recovery is more minimal with each vaginal delivery. This factor is compounded by the now well-recognized serious neurologic deterioration of the pelvis that accompanies aging.[17,18] The resultant progressive muscular atrophy is markedly augmented by hypoestrogenism. Multiple other negative influences, not prominent in younger people, such as chronic coughing, poor nutrition, and constipation, have taken their toll over time. Lastly, the fascial-ligamentous network, chronically afflicted by all of the aforementioned detrimental elements, has become attenuated and lost elasticity, no longer capable of providing the structural strength needed to prevent herniations from popping through.

An interjection here of a pertinent clinical point is explicitly appropriate. Prophylactic perineorrhaphy should be considered in all cases in which vaginal hysterectomy alone, for whatever reason, is planned. Such women, parous, otherwise healthy, ranging usually from 35 to 50 years in age, frequently also have asymptomatic but significant perineal defects that may sit seemingly silently for several years. Then, suddenly, led on by the deficient perineum, somewhere in the menopausal state, the rest of the pelvis begins to come apart. When such a potential is recognized, prudence dictates the need for full discussion with the patient of the benefits of a combined procedure in an effort to persuade her to agree to the low posterior repair also. I routinely pursue this approach, where applicable, in all such hysterectomy cases and make note of it in the patient's record. About one in five thus apprised respond positively and none has ever regretted the decision. I predict, without reservation, that time will reveal a significantly lower incidence of later supportive lesions in such cases.

To a surgeon, the microscopic anatomy of a particular organ or structure is of less concern than both the gross anatomy, normal and abnormal, and the malfunction or disease the correction of which is the goal of the planned surgery. Nonetheless, at least general perceptions of the intrinsic nature of a structure are necessary to choose the best method and materials in a surgical repair. In this regard, the ignorance of gynecologic surgeons about the perineal body is appalling. Therefore, it is incumbent that this subject is discussed, albeit briefly, before the presentation of the surgery itself.

The basic histology of this somewhat pyramidal pelvic centerpiece approximately 3.5 to 4.0 cm high, situated midway between the ischial tuberosities, consists of fibrous, elastic, and muscular cells. Because of its concentration of elastin and smooth muscle, it is flexible and functionally mobilizes in cohesion with activities of the vagina in front and the rectum behind, to both of which it is attached. This motility and compliance are controlled from within by a substantial concentration of nerve fibers and ganglia which seem to work in rhythmic cohesion directly with the muscular-elastic activity of the rectovaginal septum above and the levator complex laterally and posteriorly.[19] Although the size, shape, and tone of the perineal body and its precise cellular composition vary from one individual to the next, its attachments to, and its fibromuscular cellular interspersions with, adjacent structures are relatively constant. These include, in addition to those mentioned above, fibers of the sphincter ani (from behind), Colles fascia (from above), and the urogenital diaphragm (from in front). With all these factors in mind, it is not difficult to comprehend the problems that develop when the perineal body becomes victim to deleterious circumstances. These include not only direct laceration, linear or diffuse, with no repair, or poor repair and poor healing, but traumatic detachments from adjacent organs and structures, general deterioration from aging, and denervation. Obviously operative planning and expectations depend considerably on preoperative comprehension of the nature and composition of the perineal body as well as its exact defective condition at the time of surgery.

THE LEVATOR PLATE

The midline confluence of the levator ani musculature forms a strong relatively thick band of connective tissue which essentially runs from the anorectal junction to the lowermost spinal segments. This structure is commonly called the levator plate. In its normal anatomic state it lies almost horizontally as the fundamental pelvic floor support for the rectum, the vagina, and the cul-de-sac.[3,7,20,21] Because levator plate fibers actually loop around the anorectal area (middle external sphincter) and extend into the perineal body, we consider its anterior boundary to be anterior to the anus at the perineal body.

Hardly ever is the status of the levator plate precisely defined in the evaluation of conditions of defective pelvic support. Rather, if it is considered at all, it is by conceived implication rather than by direct examination. In fact, it is easy to evaluate. Except in cases of marked obesity, the lowermost borders of the levator musculature, medial to the inferior rami of the pubic bones, can be traced as they slant centrally, from anterior to posterior, to meet behind the rectum to form their conjoined dense collagenous union so vital to the integrity of the pelvic floor.[3,7,22,23] This information is gleaned by the lateral pressure of two fingers inside the introitus in association with opposing pressure against the perineum by the thumb of the same hand. Analysis is best achieved, as usual, by examination with the patient in the standing position, and this is most dramatically enhanced by pressure of an examining rectal finger downward and backward. Thus, the clinical significance of a fallen levator plate, tilted downward from its posterior lower spinal attachment, enlarging the rectogenitourinary hiatus, can be more easily understood. As illustrated graphically in Figure 11-7, pelvic structures can easily slide down the abnormal incline to a position of prolapse, a condition easily exaggerated in the presence of concomitant cardinal ligament weakness.

The descent of the levator plate generally is a reflection of attenuation of levator musculature. Effective surgery in posterior restoration is directed at overcoming this weakness, which cannot be accomplished for the long term without accompanying estrogen replacement therapy. Less commonly, as described in Chapter 7, the

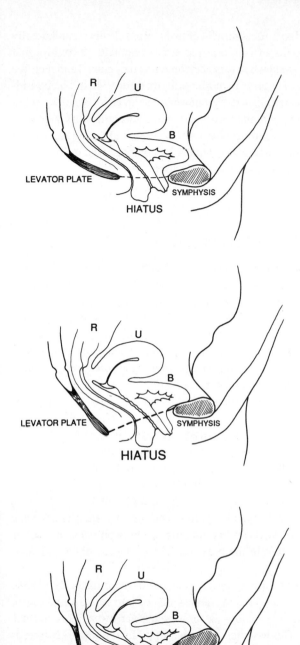

Figure 11-7 Alterations in rectogenitourinary hiatus with progressive rotational descent of the levator plate. B, bladder; R, rectum; U, uterus.

levator plate may fall secondary to detachment of levator muscle fibers, unilaterally or bilaterally, from their points of origin at the arcus tendineus. It follows that surgical results are best rewarded when this detachment is recognized and rectified during anterior compartment surgery. Its correction, therefore, should be considered crucial and can be accomplished by suturing the muscle bundles, either suprapubically or vaginally, back to the arcus tendineus as described in Chapter 7.

It must be remembered that, when atrophy is severe, especially in the presence of marked denervation, the results will unfortunately be compromised despite one's best efforts, even with adequate estrogen replacement.

COLPOPERINEORRHAPHY: DISSECTION

The operation for repair of rectocele is called colporrhaphy and should be qualified by its location as high, mid, low, or full length. Operations designed to correct perineal defects are known as perineorrhaphies and should be described as minimal, moderate, or total, depending on the magnitude of the lesion in the perineal body. The combined procedure is a colpoperineorrhaphy and the popular locution is simply posterior repair, which is too nondescriptive to be acceptable today. The current third-party coding systems are of no help, lumping all these repairs under one code number regardless of the extent of the operation.

I consider it judicious, as soon as the patient is anesthetized, before applying the sterilizing preparation fluid, to conduct a bimanual examination with the index finger of the right hand in the rectum and the first two fingers of the left hand in the vagina (see Figure 9-2). Thus, visual and tactile sensations can quickly reassess both the extent of the lesions of the rectovaginal septum and the perineal body and the danger points for dissection where scarring, especially in previously failed cases, may have caused direct apposition of vaginal and rectal walls with no intervening tissue. In the perineal area, in addition to noting how much and to what degree tissues have dispersed laterally, the integrity of the sphincter ani can be evaluated, particularly important in the presence of any degree of loss of fecal control.

I begin posterior corrective surgery in a rather traditional manner by placing Allis clamps at the mucocutaneous junction of the widened introitus at either side of the fourchette in such a way as to allow for an ultimate narrower, more normal, loose three-finger introitus. This assumes a totally longitudinal midline closure, as will be described, throughout whatever the length of the vaginal wall incision may be, with continued central unification over the perineum, to structure the introital diameter to the desired three fingers. However, occasionally, when the perineum is fairly intact or the fourchette area is well scarred, such a placement of clamps may leave too small an area in between to allow for a workable entry for accomplishment of the wide dissection above. In such cases, the Allis clamps must simply be

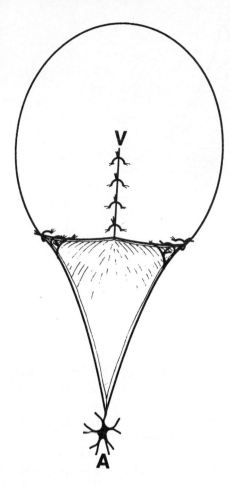

Figure 11-8 Transverse sutures at the corners to prevent introital constriction from a purely midline closure in posterior vaginal repair.

positioned as far laterally and anteriorly as necessary to provide unrestricted work space, anticipating two or three interrupted horizontal closure sutures at each corner at the end of the operation to avoid too narrow an introitus and to keep the vagina fully functional (Figure 11-8).

In either case, the mucocutaneous junction between the two clamps is then incised across the fourchette in one line. In the presence of perineal defects of any magnitude, an inverted isosceles triangle of perineal skin (Figure 11-9) is then excised to allow for the ultimate placement of a wide perineal suture described later in this chapter. This eliminates redundant attenuated skin which would only bunch and wrinkle on closure after correct midline perineal body reunification. When perineal skin is minimal, i.e., the distance between anus and fourchette is less than 2 cm, this is not done. After hemostasis of the raw triangular bed by cautery, the edge of the vaginal mucosa is grasped in the midline by a Pratt clamp (T clamp). Using a Mayo scissors, while pulling directly outwardly with tension on the Pratt, the internal surface of the posterior vaginal wall can be rapidly stripped of all scar

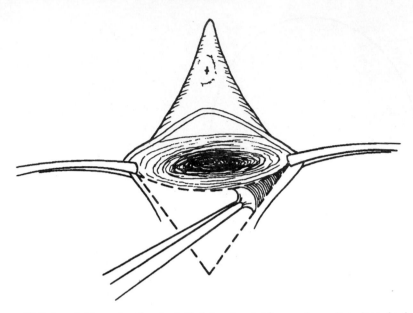

Figure 11-9 Inverted isosceles triangle of skin being denuded from perineum in perineorrhaphy.

tissue, displaced fascia, and rectovaginal remnants. Pressing the tips of the scissors against a counterpressing index finger of the nondominant hand, and armed with the knowledge of scarred danger points learned from the completed preoperative bimanual rectovaginal examination, a skilled operator can usually dissect the vagina totally free in a matter of seconds, a minute or two at the most, without buttonholing the vagina or entering the rectum. This dissection must be carried out to the lateral sidewalls and to a point above the upper limit of any linear rectovaginal septal disruption. In full-length rectoceles, the clearing must be carried to the vault. Untraditionally, I rarely ever incise the posterior vaginal wall until the dissection is at least almost complete. The unusual occasions when I will transect it as the dissection progresses occur in these cases in which the scarring is excessively dense from one sidewall to the other and extends upward more than the usual 3 to 5 cm. Maintaining an intact vagina as a solid sheet under strong outward tension evens out the scarred areas and allows the movements of the scissors tips to be followed easily both by index finger touch and indirect vision. No attempt should be made to elevate the edge of the vaginal wall to allow a direct peek at the scissors. If one does this, almost certainly the tips will inadvertently point toward the rectum, auguring entry.

Unquestionably the reader will have difficulty picturing enough of the details of my verbal operative descriptions and thus will come away somewhat confused. Sadly no sketches or drawings adequately portray some of these techniques I describe enough to relieve the hazy mental image my words create. The solution for correction of this dilemma is direct live visualization of the technique in the

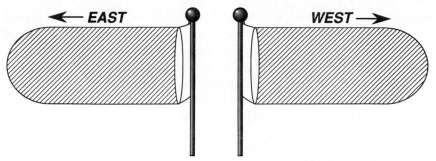

**IT MATTERS NOT WHICH WAY THE WIND BLOWS:
THE BAG IS JUST THE SAME**

Figure 11-10 Airport windsocks illustrating in analogy that an everted vagina is most likely the same size as a normally inverted one, obviating the false concept that eversion automatically dictates need for excision of nonexistent "excess" mucosa.

operating room; that failing, there are several operative videos available that vividly illustrate these techniques (see Chapter 10 references). It is time for surgeons to learn more directly from operating room situations, including live closed circuit television at the least, and from conferences with strong audiovisual themes.

In my 40 years of experience I have been first puzzled, then annoyed, and finally ultimately thoroughly aggravated by the ridiculously illogical automatic assumption, in situations of prolapse, even by the best operators, of the presence of "excess vaginal mucosa." In brief, false postulation accepts that, if something sticks out that should be inside, it must be in excess; therefore some of it should be chopped off. Such distorted thinking ignores simple mathematics: no excess develops until what sticks out becomes larger than what originally, and naturally, was "stuck in." Universally, almost without exception, because it seems that we were all taught so by revered elders, like sheep we immediately, on opening posteriorly, in any case of prolapse, take out an "ample" triangle of vaginal mucosa. My most exasperating moments come when I hear one after another of our leading gynecologists state to idolizing audiences at major conferences that they are satisfied at the conclusion of a posterior repair with a vagina of 6 to 7 cm in length. The very moment vaginal mucosa is sacrificed to any extent the operation becomes doomed to a less than satisfactory result and often, in time, to failure. Not only is such a short vagina coitally dysfunctional, but reconstitution of a fully normal vaginal axis is beyond possibility.

Figure 11-10 draws dramatic allusion to the airport wind sock, which remains the same size whether the wind blows east or west. Figure 10-9 reveals a misshapen vagina, in sketch, somewhat widely conical, next to its reconstructed elongated cylindrical shape of the same volume and surface after adequate wide and deep dissection without tissue wastage and with meticulous readjustive surgery. Figures 9-3 and 9-4 reveal respectively a severe uterine prolapse and a marked posthysterectomy prolapse, both of which should have no mucosal excision. Figure 9-5, however, shows protrusion well beyond any normal measurements of vaginal length and width and requires precise trimming to attain a reconstructed and restored vagina of natural full dimensions and normal axis.

Although the most common presentation in situations of prolapsed organs is an amply sufficient surface of vaginal mucosa, as already discussed and illustrated, not so frequently but often enough to demand attention, cases crop up with severe support defects and ironically grossly insufficient tissue to allow for restitution of a deep vagina and a normal vaginal axis. The corresponding complaint invariably echoes, "We know that a sacrospinous ligament fixation is indicated in this case, but it is impossible for the available vaginal mucosa to reach the ligament, not to mention inadequate amounts to reestablish a normal vaginal axis and functional vaginal measurements."

This problem and its solution are thoroughly discussed in Chapter 10, including reemphasis on the fact that estrogen not only will thicken and vascularize the mucosa, it also will prepare and maintain it in a healthy compliant state not only by reviving collagen production but by restoring the natural elasticity.

When judgment deems a maximum benefit from this preliminary approach, surgery should be initiated with a distinct plan in mind to increase significantly the longitudinal measurement of the vagina as it becomes converted from its state of eversion to an internal position, again as discussed and illustrated in Chapter 10.

When still more posterior vaginal length is required, again referring to Chapter 10, vertical transection of the posterior vaginal wall should be fashioned zig-zag rather than straight. When this healthy elastic tissue is then placed under stretch, an astonishing increase in length can be realized (see Figure 10-10) in much the same way, but not quite so startling, as would the incredibly jagged coast of Rhode Island, if straightened out, run most of the length of the eastern seaboard.

Having thus made possible the attachment of vaginal vault to the sacrospinous ligament without anterior or posterior vaginal tension and simultaneously converting width into length so a normal vaginal axis can be recreated, the crucial posterior colpoperineorrhaphy must be appropriately engineered. This consists of the meticulous and precise placement of a succession of interrupted sutures, from the innermost endopelvic connective tissue underlying the peritoneum to the most caudal perineal body layer in the pelvic floor, as described later in this chapter. However, because of the factor of initial paucity of surface tissue rather than the usual overabundance, the surgical closure intensity is much more demanding to lend maximum support and stability to the widely shifted new fixation configuration.

A corollary thought, of necessity, must be inserted to cover the dilemma that arises in those rare cases in which, despite all efforts, the sacrospinous ligament cannot be reached and its attachment is deemed vital to any potential for sustained vault support. In these situations less remote points of fixation can be used, as described in Figure 8-4. The skillful surgeon should then resort to every compensatory device using any connective tissue within reach, to attain a satisfactory reconstructive result.

Correct dissection is crucial to long-term success in posterior repair. As an operating room witness and nonparticipant, I have observed countless cases of grossly inadequate dissection in various forms of attempted posterior pelvic reconstruction. I have seen failures come to my office that cannot help but conjure images of insufficient tissue exposure at previous surgery. I exercise incredible restraint when I hear operating room phrases, during dissection, such as, "We've gone far enough; we'll be in trouble if we go further," or "There is so much bleeding; I think we have sufficient tissue for repair already," or "There's no need to go deeper; after all, her problem is at the introitus, anyhow." Such attitudes are the death knell of this surgery; the operation will not work. Without clear dissection to the pelvic sidewalls, there is no way that the operator can comfortably reach out bilaterally to grasp the shorn rectovaginal septal fragments to reunite them over the rectum and eliminate the rectocele. What usually has happened in these cases of inadequate dissection is the suturing of perirectal fibers, usually the outermost parts of the rectal wall, or connective tissue just external to the rectum, together in a way that is totally ineffective for any purpose. As for the bleeding, it must be expected and, though annoying, a competent surgeon can adequately squelch it in short order. Additionally, in most cases, the bleeding, which originates usually from the middle hemorrhoidal vessels, extends only to the upper limits of the heavily scarred areas of old episiotomies and previous repair attempts in the perineal area. Above this level tissue planes are generally easily established with negligible bleeding.

Because of the close approximation of the rectovaginal septum to the vagina, it is of utmost importance that the dissection of the vagina leave it as thin as possible. In no other way can one be certain that all available strands of the disrupted rectovaginal septum are adequately cleared so as to make possible the most effective repair. For best results there is no place for carelessness or waste; because one begins with tissue deficiency, one must use whatever still remains in the restoration process. I cannot repeat strongly enough the absolute need to sever cleanly all tissue attached to the posterior vaginal wall completely out to the pelvic sidewalls. Every bit of it will be needed to help constitute a successful repair over the rectum.

Because none of us is perfect and because residents in training lack the dexterity of experience, buttonholes happen in the course of dissection. When they are made in the vaginal wall, often enough they are in or near the midline and can simply be incorporated in the ultimate vertical vaginal incision that is essential for visual access in adequate reparative suturing. When further lateral, usually one or two stitches may be used to close them but, if very small, they can be ignored because they will heal most readily. However, if the buttonhole is made into the rectum, it absolutely must be recognized. If unnoticed, the consequences could be disastrous. If rectal entry is made, adequate lavage is called for immediately, but closure should be delayed. Having made the hole, the operator can use it as a guide through the balance of the dissection until the rectal wall is completely cleared. Then it should be closed in routine fashion. If the operator, in this state of chagrin, immediately repairs the hole, he or she is back at the beginning and may well make another entry higher up, especially if scarring is dense, having been blinded to the importune opportunity for guidance. Having "been there" myself enough times during my 40 years in gynecology, I have long ago learned that rectal holes, properly closed, with associated adequate lavage and hemostasis, cause absolutely no disruption in the healing process and should not change the usual planned postoperative regimen. However, I would discourage rectal thermometers and insist that enema nozzles point posteriorly when used postoperatively.

Although somewhat repetitive, I suggest that none of us, in the more difficult cases, do rectal examinations during the course of the actual surgery as often as we should. If we did, certainly the extent of residual intact rectovaginal septum could be reassessed, thereby defining precisely correct limits of upward dissection but, more importantly, we could dissect over the rectal finger, thereby augmenting speed, safety, and efficiency.

COLPORRHAPHY: RESTORATION

Again sounding repetitive, but necessarily so in the interest of producing the best prophylaxis against recurrence, the issue of any role for a sacrospinous ligament fixation (SSF) in association with high rectocele repair must be discussed. Whether or not the deep colporrhaphy is performed in association with vaginal hysterectomy, if one desires additional vault support at the top of the repair, I feel the cardinal-uterosacral complex often is far too deficient in cases of genital prolapse for the expected reliability many operators attribute to it. In every phase of surgery we are issued the most remarkably ambiguous warning, "Never do more surgery than is absolutely necessary." Exactly how such dogma, with its morally responsible implications, should be interpreted sparks seemingly endless controversy, especially in such instances as to when and when not an SSF should be done beyond the crystal-clear indication of massive vaginal eversion. To confuse the issue even more, I feel strongly that this wonderfully supportive surgical adjunct (SSF) is not used often enough, yet far too few operators are adept enough at doing it with safety, and therefore they should skip it. Specifically, I think the SSF plays a strong role in selected cases of repair of full-length or high rectocele repair, even in the absence of enterocele. Many will disagree with such a posture and call it unnecessary surgery. I counter by stating that omission of it in the circumstances I will describe constitutes inadequate surgery not in the best interests of the patient. Of course, I infer a competent operator. Circumstances that I judge deserving of consideration of associated SSF are those that, individually or in combination, (1) include a descending posterior vault secondary to rectovaginal detachment from the cardinal-uterosacral complex, (2) involve extensive loss of support throughout the pelvis with severe disruption of the normal vaginal axis in a relatively young woman, (3) record two or more previous rectocele repair failures, and (4) reveal in the course of dissection minimal or negligible available rectovaginal septal remnants to afford satisfactory suppression of the rectocele bulge. In the latter instance, for example, a posteriorly fixed vault combined with a firm perineorrhaphy and an associated reelevated levator plate may compensate for an unavoidably weak colporrhaphy. Regrettably, I must agree that unquestionably there are capable surgeons who perform SSF procedures in cases where I, among others, feel it is superfluous.

Choosing the correct suture is critical to the enduring benefits of colpoperineorrhaphy. Catgut, with its marked temporal limitations in tensile strength and its pronounced reactive nature in adjacent tissue, has no place in any kind of reconstructive surgery today. Although commonly used currently, the popular polyfilament synthetic relatively inert sutures such as Dexon (Davis and Geck, Wayne, NJ) and Vicryl (Ethicon, Cincinnati, OH) are poor choices also for this surgery. Their tensile strengths are about 5 to 10 days longer than catgut, still far short of the needed long term for fascial and connective tissue healing in the demanding pelvic floor. Also, bacteria can hide in the polyfilament interstices, which are inaccessible to protective scavenging white blood cells. There remains, then, the choice between monofilament delayed absorbable and nonabsorbable materials. A rising debate simmers at present among the experts as to which should be used in a posterior reconstructive procedure. Most operators remain leery of using nonabsorbable suture because of the proximity of the rectum, fearing either undetected penetration into rectal lumen during the surgery or erosion into it during the recovery phase. So the majority have opted for the former and use either Maxon (Davis and Geck) or PDS (Ethicon). Both of these retain significant tensile strength for 40 to 60 days, are essentially inert, and discourage infection because they are monofilaments. Arguments in favor of nonabsorbable material cite the need for long-term support to cover the 115 to 120 days necessary for maximum healing of the fascial and connective tissues of the pelvis. However, all the synthetic nonabsorbable sutures currently in vogue, for example, polypropylene or polybutester, except for one, polytetrafluoroethylene (PTFE; see Chapter 16), leave stiff prickly ends when cut. These ends, if they should protrude through mucosal surfaces, can cause lasting coital discomfort vaginally and enduring fissures rectally. I have chosen a position of compromise. In those cases of one or less previous failures and fairly strong tissues to work with, I use Maxon. In instances of two or more recurrent posterior breakdowns, especially if the fascial and connective tissue is well-compromised, I use PTFE (W. L. Gore and Associates, Flagstaff, AZ), which is soft and very flexible.

The caliber of suture to be used is still another matter of controversy. Because the weight of the entire torso rests on the pelvis, I think one must use material of substantial bore to help resist such stress, especially because narrow-diameter sutures are apt to cut through tissue under pressure. Also, as one would expect, the tensile strength lasts longer when the suture is thicker. Therefore, as opposed to that still large group which recommends 3-0 and 2-0 sutures, I work only with, and recommend, zero caliber Maxon or PTFE.

When the rectovaginal septum has separated from the posterior descending fibers of the cardinal-uterosacral complex above it, something that should have been determined preoperatively, interrupted sutures must be placed transversely and diagonally as necessary to effect a reunion. In cases of full-length rectocele, suturing should begin at the level of the vaginal vault at its designated deepest hindmost point of fixation so as to guarantee its location ultimately well posterior to the anterior edge of the levator plate below in the pelvic floor. Depending on the particular anatomic bony configuration, this initiation of repair might lie behind the interspinous line.

Repair should then progress by a series of interrupted transverse sutures 8 to 10 mm apart that rejoin the torn septal fragments from each side, over the rectum, working from above toward the perineal body. The operator should be certain to depress the rectum in the midline with the index finger of the nondominant hand as each stitch is taken. The progressive suppression and disappearance of the rectocele should become more obvious with the completion of each suture. Proficient assistance for effective exposure is necessary. Great caution must be exercised as each bite is placed, first on one side and then the other. They should consist of broad but shallow traverses of available connective tissue at each lateral aspect of the operative wound. This will ensure inclusion of all segments of disrupted rectovaginal septum at that level while avoiding digging into levator muscle. Text after text, including a major atlas published in 1992,[24] speak of grasping the levator muscle from each side and bringing it to the midline. Including muscle in the stitch is most undesirable; not only is it unanatomic, for only rectovaginal septal sheets and connective tissue constitute the rectovaginal barrier, but sutures through the soft muscle will simply cut through it and the stitch will ultimately lie limp and ineffective.

Many experts and texts on this subject describe a "dashboard" effect if sutures are placed improperly. Why the term dashboard is used is beyond my comprehension when the true intended descriptive analogy for an uneven surface resulting from sutures placed irregularly or too far apart is "washboard." The latter comparative term conveys an image of a corrugated bumpy surface and this is really what is meant. Some operators contend that a continuous suture is more conducive to both regularity and proximity of suture but I, as do others, disagree with this approach. Because the lesion is irregular to begin with, as is the distortion from scarring, it is felt that individual sutures, carefully evaluated after each bite to avoid vaginal stricture, are superior because they avert tissue bunching and better accommodate the irregular tear. The adequacy of each bilaterally completed stitch should be tested before tying by tugging on the ends together to demonstrate the strength of the tissue grasped. Also to be noted, even when pulling on the innermost strands, is the elevation of the levator plate. This is illustrated by the upward puckering of the perineal floor behind the anus during such tugging. Again the continuity of the entire pelvic connective tissue network is exemplified.

Some special pointers can help lead to the most desirable result. If a particular completed suture seems to be less effective than one desires, it should be removed and redone. This also applies to any suture positioned overzealously, thereby narrowing the diameter at that particular level, a forerunner to later vaginal stricture of that area. To check on such potential impingement on width, after every two connective tissue stitches have been tied, the vaginal mucosal edges should be correspondingly united and then a two finger examination can readily assess vaginal capacity. Because the longitudinal rectovaginal tears are irregular anyhow and not apt to be precisely in the midline, frequently more tissue is available on one side than the other. This explains why the knots often do not end up in the midline. I find in some cases of especially deep disruption, especially as the perineal body region is approached, two smaller overlying stitches serve better than one larger one. This may avoid both leaving too much tension on one suture alone or undesirable roominess of the vagina at that point. Occasionally, after the placement of two successive seemingly satisfactory supportive sutures and the accompanying corresponding mucosal closure, the associated vaginal segment seems a bit too roomy, as mentioned above. Correction is easily remedied by swinging a submucosal stitch perpendicular and anterior to the others, using an adequate sized needle, bringing just enough additional rectovaginal remnants together from each side to effect sufficient tightening.

If these suturing instructions are followed, always beginning at the deepest extent of the rectovaginal defect or the rectocele, inevitably the upper two thirds of the vagina will resume an almost horizontal pelvic lie. Not only is this proof of restoration to the normal configuration but, assuming a subsequent reestablishment of a full normal perineal body, it guarantees that the innermost vaginal recess will occupy a site well posterior to the most anterior edge of the levator plate.

Isolated high or mid-rectoceles are corrected according to the suturing principles already outlined. However, as mentioned, to best ensure lasting results, the correction should start slightly above the uppermost extent of the rectovaginal lesion and end slightly below the lowermost point of the rectovaginal disruption.

PERINEORRHAPHY: RESTORATION

Reestablishment of full perineal body mass and integrity follows a somewhat different pattern from that of the colporrhaphy.

A true perineorrhaphy begins approximately 3.5 to 4.0 cm internal to the perineal floor contiguous to the anus. A correct restoration will add as much as 3 to 5 cm to vaginal length (Figures 11-11 and 11-12) as it simultaneously creates an almost vertical lower one third of the vagina, thereby guaranteeing return of a normal vaginal axis.

Rather than reuniting a tough but thin membrane as in colporrhaphy, the surgical goal in perineorrhaphy is the recreation of a solid sideways "A-frame" tissue

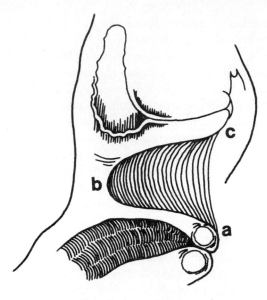

Figure 11-11 Posthysterectomy case with severe perineal defects exaggerating an abnormally shaped conical vagina marked by points a, b, and c.

structure that is relatively thick, particularly at its base inside the perineal skin where it should separate the anus from a reestablished fourchette by an average of 4 cm. Although the individual bites still come from one side to the other, they are taken at different angles and different depths to suit the extent of the particular disruption and to accommodate the amount of available tissue, because the size of perineal bodies varies from one patient to another. Precise methods of reconstructing a perineal body are important because the success of an entire repair may hinge on how well it is done. Excellence in this surgical phase arises from a combination

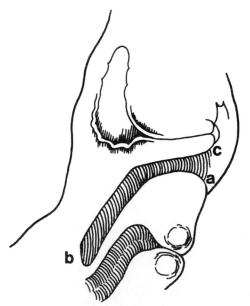

Figure 11-12 Posthysterectomy postperineorrhaphy illustration revealing restored curved cylindrical vagina, marked by a, b, and c, with functional measurements and normal axis after repair.

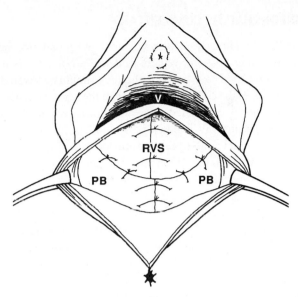

Figure 11-13 Repaired perineal body (PB) rejoined by separate sutures to a restored rectovaginal septum (RVS). Linear tear of RVS was not in same line as vertical PB disruption. V, vagina.

of good teaching and experience. I have never performed any two in exactly the same way, nor should anyone.

Once the upper portion of the perineal body is reestablished, one or more vertical sutures on either side of the midline should be placed to firmly reconnect the perineal body with the rectovaginal septum (Figure 11-13). The sutures of the fourchette area must not produce a constricting effect but rather should take just enough tissue to allow for an outwardly funneling introitus to favor coital function. As mentioned earlier, one or two interrupted horizontal closure corner sutures, placed before the midline vaginal closure comes too low, can avoid reduction of vaginal entry to nonfunctional levels (see Figure 11-8). The base of the perineal body must be restored by bringing adequate tissue to the midline from relatively wide lateral areas to ensure the return of the insertion of the bulbocavernosus and transverse perineum muscles into their normal central attachments. In cases of severe disintegration, this is best performed by using a widely sweeping anterior-posterior figure-of-eight stitch in a plane 5 mm from the surface. Concomitantly such a maneuver will almost close off the raw subdermal area created at the outset by the triangular excision of perineal skin. The surface closure is then completed by a continuation of the vaginal closure suture in nonlocking fashion in the skin. Most operators use a subcuticular suture placement for skin closure, but I gave that up several years ago. I found that the patients have equivalent discomfort regardless of whether the sutures are buried or on the surface and that I give incredible (or so it seems to the patient) relief by simply cutting the surface sutures at 2 weeks postoperatively. This cannot be done with buried stitches.

COLPOPERINEORRHAPHY: COMMENTARY

Standard admonition, seemingly universal, from time beyond time, has prescribed rectal examinations after posterior repairs to detect errant sutures into the rectal lumen. If any are found, we have been taught, they should be severed at once, and this, of course, sacrifices the continued integrity of the repair because, having been cut after the procedure is completed, they will not be replaced. Such advice is absolute nonsense. During my residency, my colleagues in training and I, in hundreds of cases of correctional repairs and episiotomies, found frequent incidents of suture penetration through bowel mucosa. We said nothing, nothing was done, and nothing unusual happened. No increase in postoperative cellulitis was noted, abscesses did not occur, and not one fistula developed.

My curiosity drove me to continue the postrepair rectal checks for several years wherein, despite the discovery of occasional undesirable bowel intraluminal stitches, about which no action was taken, again no untoward consequences developed. As reported by Poth in 1968,[25] the reason for an undisturbed benign course despite the unwelcome suture intrusion is the forced penetration of the exposed stitch through the mucosa to become buried beneath it by attendant usual and expected postsurgical edema. The intestinal mucosa rapidly heals over the small defect, all of this happening in a matter of hours. The corollary factor to this unruffled course is the natural tissue resistance to the customary areal bacteria. Of added note, for those who live in fear of fistulas from stray stitches, such a development will not occur unless penetration runs through two mucosal surfaces by the same thread.

However, if despite this reassurance one continues to worry, then rectal examinations should be conducted at intervals, arbitrarily after two fascial suture placements, while the operative site is still open and vaginal mucosal edges are still separated. Then, if desired, a suture could easily be severed, withdrawn, and replaced with a more satisfactory one. Because there always seem to be exceptions, and even though I long ago stopped doing postoperative rectal examinations for any reason, when I use nonabsorbable sutures, I follow this regimen of intraoperative rectal examinations assiduously. Nonabsorbable sutures are literally forever, foreign bodies that will not go away, so, on general principles, I feel they must be handled differently.

Vaginal packing after reconstructive procedures performed from below should be an invariable finale to guarantee the best healing. Such packing is usually best in the form of layered gauze in a long roll about 2 inches wide, saturated with an antiseptic or antibiotic solution. Using metal ribbon retractors to hold the repaired vagina open to its depth and to prevent friction from the gauze on the mucosa as it is moved into position, every bit of space should be filled snugly. Then the inevitable postoperative edema will help accomplish the first goal of packing, namely, marked deterrence of serosanguinous fluid collection adjacent to raw surfaces. Secondly, the packing will provide inestimable support for the multitude of delicately placed sutures in resisting the potentially destructive Valsalva force of retching, vomiting, or coughing, not uncommon anesthetic aftermaths. Thirdly, as natural settling of tissues develops in the immediate postsurgical phase, appropriately placed packing promotes subsequent natural adherence of tissues in the earliest stages of healing.

Contrary to most common practice, I leave the packing in place for 2 days, not one. Pragmatically this makes more sense and I certainly feel, coupled with the use of propelled lavage throughout the actual surgery, it has markedly diminished the incidence of postoperative infection as explained in Chapter 16. In the same vein, I think there is little argument about the positive role packing well for 2 days has played in our excellent long-term surgical results.

This chapter would not be complete if it did not briefly review why a small but significant percentage of operations fail despite the best of judgment, technique, material, and circumstances. Pelvic denervation and atrophy have been studied extensively over the past 20 years, and with particular intensity in the past 6 years, in consideration of the roles they play in physiologic and anatomic disruption. It is generally concluded that, in the postreproductive woman, it is difficult, and sometimes impossible, to overcome surgically the problems emanating from long-standing denervation and its consequent destructive effects on muscle and connective tissue. The restorative influence of estrogen on all the pelvic tissues is well established but, although astonishingly remarkable in some instances, it is generally limited. A corollary observation to this fact points out that the longer the absence of estrogen, the more deeply ensconced is the atrophy and the less the positive tissue response to replacement therapy. Obviously this is due, in line with the general loss of tissue substance, to the marked diminution and disappearance of estrogen receptors throughout the pelvis. As discussed in Chapter 1, the presence in the healthy pelvis of estrogen receptors in the bladder, urethra, rectum, and anus and the enveloping supportive muscular, connective, and elastic tissues is today scientifically established.

Definitive evidence of the crucial role of denervation in particular, caused primarily by childbirth many years earlier, and often amplified by other conditions with time, can be found in the extensive recent contributions to the literature of numerous investigators.[13,15,16,18,26–29]

Norton has been engaged in extensive clinical studies on collagen deficiency states. In relation to this work, she gives a comprehensive account of weakness and atrophy of pelvic connective tissue in the cause of genital prolapse.[30]

Along the same line, nerve deterioration is an accepted accompaniment of long-standing diabetes mellitus. In these cases, preoperative promises and expectations must be conservative. The same is true in situations of degenerative neurologic diseases and in circumstances of prior cerebrovascular accidents.

Fecal incontinence unassociated with fistulas or chronic fourth degree lacerations seems to be a steadily increasing problem, thereby demanding discussion relevant to the possibilities for correction during the posterior repair. Because pudendal neuropathy can play a role in both urinary and fecal incontinence, when the former is a principal complaint, the patient must be queried about the latter if she does not volunteer any information about it. It is probably good practice to question the patient anyhow about fecal incontinence in all planned pelvic corrective cases because surgery often can help when anatomic sphincter defects are involved in the cause of involuntary stool loss.

Certainly neuromyographic evaluation, when available, may present helpful information preoperatively, as will the presence or absence of the bulbocavernosus reflex contraction. Intentional subjective squeezing during bidigital examination apprises the general level of perineal muscle tone. Obviously the worse the results of these simple tests, the less you may be able to offer surgically. Nonetheless, especially since precise complete determination of the extent of any anatomic defects of both the internal and external sphincter mechanisms can only be made essentially during the surgery, the operator should search for and repair, if discovered, such imperfections.

Usually, in my experience, if the internal sphincter is torn, almost always are the two upper loops of the external sphincter also markedly thinned out. This is best demonstrated after the dissection of the posterior vaginal wall, in colpoperineorrhaphy, has been completed by placing a double-gloved nondominant index finger in the rectum. In the worst situations, all that remains intact between vaginal mucosa and rectum, above the level of the lowermost circular loop of external sphincter ani, is the rectal mucosa itself with minimal or no submucosa and no muscularis. The intrarectal digit can practically be seen through this thin tissue layer. This linear tear in the musculature of the bowel itself should be repaired by a series of interrupted 3-0 Maxon sutures through its extent. I feel that continuous suture closure, although decreasing the number of knots, bunches this very compliant tissue into a constrictive bundle.

Although the superior loop of the external anal sphincter is recognized as the puborectalis muscle, looping posteriorly around the bowel, sutures placed transversely between its two arms anterior to the anus, into connective tissue adjacent to this muscle, can help to correct the attenuation that is contributing to the defective sphincter action. In these situations of obvious sphincter tears, the intermediate loop, consisting of muscle bundles arising from the levator ani posteriorly to swing anteriorly around the anus, counterbalancing the forward pull of the upper loop, the puborectalis, just above it, must be considered disrupted to a varying extent. This muscular defect can usually easily be corrected with a few side-to-side interrupted 2-0 Maxon sutures placed into the fibromuscular tissue lying just above the lower loop, the circular sphincter ani.

As for the lower, or base circular loop, it should be first exposed by dissecting down to it and simultaneously dissecting tissue off the perineal skin. Considering that the perineal body is usually severely disrupted in these cases, combined with an abnormally short anal-fourchette expanse of skin, this can be accomplished quickly and easily. A few more 2-0 Maxon side-to-side stitches, bringing tissue into the midline, obviously thickening the muscle and correcting attenuation, completes the job.

Finally, although discussed in detail in Chapter 18, prevailing integrity of good surgery depends profoundly on a continued never-ending lifelong regimen of sensible habits. Sound nutrition and reasonable exercise remain foremost. Any condition that might induce increased intra-abdominal pressure, either ongoing or repetitive, must be prevented or eliminated, whether originating from disease or habit. A particularly important point in this regard is lifting, which should be avoided anyhow, particularly if more than 10 pounds, but if done, the patient must exhale when she lifts. Jumping can be especially destructive. Girdles are anathema. Diabetes must remain in perfect control. A commitment to estrogen replacement therapy, whether oral, dermal, or intravaginal, is an everlasting contract. In short, postoperative management never stops.

The last word: despite one's self-confidence as a surgeon and great satisfaction with a seeming particularly fine surgical performance with an apparent immediate great-looking anatomic result, no operator should ever make guaranteed promises to the patient postoperatively, just as you should not have made them preoperatively. Even with circumstances at their best in the very early postoperative course, one cannot predict what adverse events may happen in the future nor can one depend on 100% patient compliance any more than one can predict or rely on the quality of the pelvic tissues or their innervation before surgery is begun. Simply stated, as in any phase of pelvic reconstructive or urogynecologic surgery, even the most competent and qualified surgeons can only promise the patient the best possible effort within their capabilities. The balance is up to her and to chance.

Yet, nonetheless, we remain far removed from the time of Berkeley and Bonney[31] who steadfastly proclaimed the impossibility of correcting prolapsed pelvic lesions without limiting coital capability. Similarly, our much improved understanding of pelvic anatomy and our skillful surgical efforts of today defy the contention of Pratt[32] that a loss of 25% to 45% of vaginal depth, despite a surgeon's best attempts to retain vaginal function, was inevitable in secondary procedures of pelvic reconstruction. Using all currently available management techniques and regimens, we have every reason to expect a high level of long-term comfort and good function.

In conclusion, what should the pelvic configuration appear to be after reconstruction according to the discussions and advice of Chapters 9, 10, and 11? Whether any one of these procedures or any combination of two or more of them are performed, namely excision of enterocele sac, SSF, colporrhaphy, or perineorrhaphy, the goal should be restoration of a normal vaginal axis in a functional vagina. Figure 11-14 illustrates an undesirable result with a short vagina, a straight axis, and a vaginal vault anterior to the front edge of the levator plate. In Figure 11-15, in contrast, correct surgical achievement reveals a long functional vagina the vault of which is far posterior to the anterior limit of the levator plate in association with a restored vaginal axis.

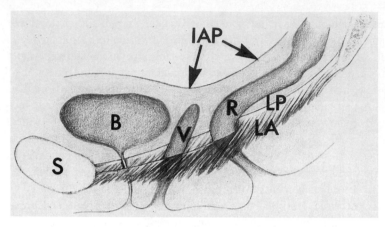

Figure 11-14 Inadequate postoperative result. The vagina is short and vertical. The vaginal vault lies in front of the levator plate. B, bladder; IAP, intra-abdominal pressure; LA, levator ani; LP, levator plate; R, rectum; S, symphysis pubis; V, vagina.

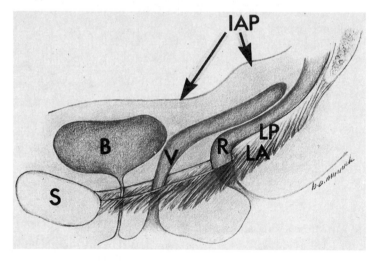

Figure 11-15 Good postoperative anatomic restoration. Normal vaginal axis and deep functional vagina lie with vault well posterior to the anterior edge of the levator plate. B, bladder; IAP, intra-abdominal pressure; LA levator ani; LP, levator plate; R, rectum; S, symphysis pubis; V, vagina.

REFERENCES

1. Nichols DH, Milley PS, Randall CL. Significance of restoration of normal vaginal depth and axis. *Obstet Gynecol.* 1970;36:251–256.

2. Funt M, Thompson JD, Birch H. Normal vaginal axis. *South Med J.* 1978;71:1534–1535.

3. Berglas B, Rubin IC. Study of the supportive structures of the uterus by levator myography. *Surg Gynecol Obstet.* 1953;97:677–692.

4. DeLancey JOL. Anatomic aspects of vaginal eversion after hysterectomy. *Am J Obstet Gynecol.* 1992;166:1717–1728.

5. Tobin CE, Benjamin JA. Anatomical and surgical restudy of Denonvillier's fascia. *Surg Gynecol Obstet.* 1945;80:373–388.

6. Milley PS, Nichols DH. A corrective investigation of the human rectovaginal septum. *Anat Rec.* 1968;163:433–452.

7. Nichols DH. Posterior colporrhaphy and perineorrhaphy: Separate and distinct operations. *Am J Obstet Gynecol.* 1991;164:714–721.

8. Burch JC. Urethrovaginal fixation to Cooper's ligament for correction of stress incontinence, cystocoele, and prolapse. *Am J Obstet Gynecol.* 1961;81:281–290.

9. Burch JC. Cooper's ligament urethrovesical suspension of stress incontinence. *Am J Obstet Gynecol.* 1968;100:764–774.

10. Aldridge A, Watson P. Analysis of end results of labor in primiparas after spontaneous versus prophylactic methods of delivery. *Am J Obstet Gynecol.* 1935;30:554–565.

11. Gainey HL. Post-partum observation of pelvic tissue damage. *Am J Obstet Gynecol.* 1943;45:457–463.

12. Gainey HL. Post-partum observation of pelvic tissue damage: Further studies. *Am J Obstet Gynecol.* 1955;70:800–805.

13. Snooks SJ, Swash M, Mathers SE, Henry MM. Effect of vaginal delivery on the pelvic floor: A five year followup. *Br J Surg.* 1990;77:1258–1260.

14. Peterson I, Franksson C, Danielson GO. Electromyography of the pelvic floor and urethra in normal females. *Acta Obstet Gynecol Scand.* 1955;34:273–285.

15. Snooks SJ, Setchill M, Swash M, Henry MM. Injury to innervation of the pelvic floor sphincter musculature in childbirth. *Lancet.* 1984;2:546–550.

16. Warrell DW. Pelvic floor neuropathy: Partial denervation in pelvic floor prolapse. In: Bensen JT, ed. *Female Pelvic Floor Disorders.* New York and London: WW Norton; 1992:153–156.

17. Anderson RS. A neurogenic element to genuine stress incontinence. *Br J Obstet Gynaecol.* 1984;91:41–45.

18. Smith ARB, Hosker GL, Warrell DW. The role of partial denervation of the pelvic floor in the etiology of genitourinary prolapse and stress incontinence: A neurophysiological study. *Br J Obstet Gynecol.* 1989;96:24–32.

19. Nichols DH, Randall CL. *Vaginal Surgery.* 3rd ed. Baltimore: Williams and Wilkins; 1989:26–30.

20. Dickinson RL. Studies of levator ani muscle. *Am J Obstet Dis Woman.* 1889;22:897–917.

21. Weinstein S. Vault prolapse. *Clin Pract Sexuality.* 1991;7:17–20.

22. Hadra BE. *Lesions of the Vagina and Pelvic Floor. Records.* Philadelphia: McMullin and Co; 1888.

23. Halban J, Tandler J. *Anatomic und Atiologic der Genital prolapse beim Weibe.* Vienna and Leipzig: Wilhelm Braumuller; 1907.

24. Lee RR. *Atlas of Gynecologic Surgery.* Philadelphia: WB Saunders; 1992:88.

25. Poth EJ. Intestinal anastomosis. A unique technic. *Am J Surg.* 1968;116:643–648.

26. Benson JT. In: Benson JT, ed. *Female Pelvic Floor Disorders.* New York and London: WW Norton; 1992:142–152; 380–389.

27. Snooks SJ, Swash M, Henry MM, Setchell M. Risk factors in childbirth causing damage to the pelvic floor innervation. *Int J Colorect Dis.* 1986;1:20–24.

28. Allen RE, Hosker GL, Smith ARB, Warrell DW. Pelvic floor damage and childbirth: A neurophysiological study. *Br J Obstet Gynaecol.* 1990;97:770–779.

29. Gilpin SA, Gosling JA, Smith ARB, Warrell DW. The pathogenesis of genitourinary prolapse and stress incontinence of urine. A histological and histochemical study. *Br J Obstet Gynaecol.* 1989;96:15–23.

30. Norton PA. Histological and biochemical studies. In: Benson JT, ed. *Female Pelvic Floor Disorders.* New York and London: WW Norton; 1992:166–175.

31. Berkeley C, Bonney V. *Textbook of Gynaecological Surgery.* 5th ed. London: Cassel; 1947.

32. Pratt JH. Secondary operations to orrect failures of previous operations for genital prolapse. *Clin Obstet Gynecol.* 1966;9:1084–1099.

Management of Premalignant Lesions of the Vulva, Vagina, and Cervix in the Older Patient

C. William Helm

Premalignant disease of the lower genital tract is dominated by the spectrum of cellular disorders called intraepithelial neoplasia (IN), previously known as dysplasia (Table 12-1). Although these lesions may occur throughout the lower genital tract simultaneously, there are distinct differences related to the exact site of origin, of which three will be discussed. Therefore, they will be discussed by individual location. Because IN in all three sites has the potential to develop into invasive carcinoma, detection and treatment of these conditions plays an important role in maintaining the health of older women.

CERVICAL INTRAEPITHELIAL NEOPLASIA

Cervical intraepithelial neoplasia (CIN) includes a range of abnormality from mild to severe dysplasia of the epithelium (CIN 1, mild dysplasia; CIN 2, moderate dysplasia; and CIN 3, severe dysplasia/carcinoma in situ [CIS]). The details of its pathology are described in depth elsewhere.[1] The significance of CIN is the risk of progression to higher grades of CIN and invasive carcinoma of the cervix.

TABLE 12-1 Classification of Intraepithelial Neoplasia of the Lower Genital Tract

	Vulva	Vagina	Cervix
Squamous intraepithelial neoplasia or dysplasia			
Mild	VIN 1	VAIN 1	CIN 1
Moderate	VIN 2	VAIN 2	CIN 2
Severe/carcinoma in situ	VIN 3	VAIN 3	CIN 3
Glandular intraepithelial neoplasia	Paget's disease		CGIN

CIN, cervical intraepithelial neoplasia; VAIN, vaginal intraepithelial neoplasia; VIN, vulvar intraepithelial neoplasia; CGIN, cervical glandular intraepithelial neoplasia.

Malignant Potential

It is thought that invasive carcinoma is usually preceded by CIN 3[2] and that the risk is related to the degree of abnormality present. CIS and CIN 3 are the most likely to progress to invasive cancer.[2–5] The reported rates of progression to invasive carcinoma over time vary between 1.4% and 66% with the majority of reports indicating a rate in excess of 25%.

The milder forms of CIN can also progress to either higher grades of dysplasia or to invasive carcinoma, and it has been estimated that perhaps 25% of dysplasias overall will progress to invasive carcinoma if left untreated long enough.[2] For ethical reasons, passive observation of development to invasive carcinoma can no longer be taken as an end point in clinical studies and researchers have more recently examined the progression of CIN 1 to higher grades of CIN. Because such studies vary in important details such as the method used to diagnose the cellular and morphological changes, the duration of follow-up without treatment, and the population demographics, comparison of data is difficult.

Stern and Neely estimated that the relative risk of a woman with cervical dysplasia developing CIS in contrast to a woman without dysplasia was 1600:1.[6] They also estimated that the rate of progression of all grades of dysplasia to CIS is 6.4% per year. Koss[7] reported that dysplasia of all types progressed to CIS in 42.3% of cases while Richart and Barron[8] reported progression to higher grade in 28%. As far as CIN 1 alone is concerned, Campion and colleagues[9] reported that 26% of cases of CIN 1 progressed to CIN 3 within 1 year, whereas Richart and Barron[8] and Syrjanen and coworkers[10] reported rates of progression of CIN 1 to higher grades of dysplasia of 14% and 21%, respectively. Syrjanen also reported that CIN 2 progressed to CIN 3 in 21% of cases over 70 months.

Prevalence

The exact prevalence of CIN in older women is unknown. The disease is asymptomatic and detectable only by screening. Not only have older women traditionally

TABLE 12-2 Number of Cases of CIN 3 and Invasive Carcinoma of the
Cervix in Pennsylvania Residents by Age Group in 1990

Age	CIN 3	Invasive Carcinoma
<30	741	35
30–39	665	130
40–49	282	136
50–59	80	108
60–69	41	117
70–79	38	98
≥80	7	42

SOURCE: From Pennsylvania State Health Data Center—1990

been reluctant to take advantage of screening programs, but unfortunately many of these efforts have not been specifically directed at this group.

Figures from the Pennsylvania State Health Data Center (Table 12-2) indicate that 55% of all invasive carcinoma of the cervix in Pennsylvania is occurring in women over the age of 50 years. The incidence of carcinoma of the cervix shows two age peaks, between 40 and 44 years and 60 and 64 years and the Pennsylvania data verifies these age-group concentrations. However, the reported incidence of CIN 3 in Pennsylvania is much lower than the incidence of invasive disease. Because invasive carcinoma is usually preceded by CIN 3, the data underscores the fact that screening is still not being used effectively on this population. Older, urban, lower income women are at particularly high risk for carcinoma of the cervix.[11] Many studies have demonstrated that nonparticipants in screening are at high risk for the development of cervical cancer and, in the United States, previously unscreened elderly women had two to three times more abnormal Pap smears than women under age 65.[12]

Screening

Screening for premalignant conditions of the cervix is based on the exfoliative Papanicolaou smear or "Pap test" that was described by Papanicolaou and Traut[13] and facilitated by Ayre in 1947 after he described his spatula for scraping the cervix.[14] Since its introduction, the widespread use of Pap screening has been thought to help reduce the incidence of invasive carcinoma in screened populations.[15–17] Although the optimum interval between routine cervical Pap smears is unknown in otherwise normal postmenopausal women, the test should ideally be performed as part of an annual checkup whether or not they have had a prior hysterectomy. In recognition of the need for screening in older women, the American Cancer Society now sets no upper age limit for the cessation of screening.

TABLE 12-3 The Bethesda Classification of the Papanicolaou Smear

Epithelial Cell Abnormalities

Atypical squamous cells of undetermined significance

Squamous intraepithelial lesion
Low-grade SIL encompassing either or both:
1. Cellular changes associated with human papilloma virus
2. Mild dysplasia/CIN 1
High-grade SIL encompassing:
1. Moderate dysplasia/CIN 2
2. Severe dysplasia/CIN 3
3. Carcinoma in situ/CIN 3
Squamous cell carcinoma

Glandular cells
1. Presence of endometrial cells in one of the following circumstances:
   a. Out-of-phase in a menstruating woman
   b. In a postmenopausal woman
   c. No menstrual history available
2. Atypical glandular cells of undetermined significance
   a. Endometrial
   b. Endocervical
   c. Not otherwise specified
3. Adenocarcinoma
   a. Endocervical
   b. Endometrial
   c. Extrauterine

Nonepithelial Malignant Neoplasm

CIN, cervical intraepithelial neoplasia; SIL, squamous intraepithelial lesion

Investigation of Abnormal Pap Smears

Abnormalities identified on Pap smears are now classified according to the Bethesda system in the United States (Table 12-3).[18] The management of abnormal Pap smears in the older woman is essentially similar to that for younger patients with colposcopy being the main initial investigation. Those women with moderate or severe squamous dysplasia on cytology and all those with glandular abnormalities require urgent colposcopy. The initial management of mild dysplasia and changes of lesser degree is controversial, but even if colposcopy is not performed in the first instance, all women with persistently mild abnormalities on Pap smear should be further investigated.

The technique of colposcopy has been described elsewhere.[19] The essential elements are (1) examination of the cervix and other areas of the lower genital tract for obvious macroscopic lesions (cancers, condylomata), (2) inspection under magnification for abnormal blood vessels (which might indicate the presence of a microinvasive carcinoma) with the aid of a green filter, (3) application of 3% to 5% acetic acid and inspection for patterns suggestive of CIN: aceto-white staining, mosaicism, and punctuation. For colposcopic examination to be considered complete or satisfactory, the whole cervix and the entire squamocolumnar junction must be visible. The actual diagnosis of CIN is made by biopsy and histologic examination of the suggestive areas.

Colposcopic examination may present difficulties because of the patient's age. Older patients may find it difficult or uncomfortable positioning themselves on the colposcopy bed; it may be necessary to raise the head end and place cushions behind the patient. An assistant may be required to support a patient's leg if she is unable to keep it on the stirrup. Assessment may be made difficult by aging effects on the lower genital tract, i.e., the vaginal epithelium may be atrophic and friable, the introitus and vagina may be narrowed, and the cervical squamocolumnar junction may be invisible or difficult to see.

Provided there is no suspicion of a glandular carcinoma, estrogen treatment for a minimum of 2 weeks may improve the vaginal epithelium. Kishi reports that 1.25 mg oral conjugated equine estrogen (Premarin) orally for 14 days is sufficient.[20] Adequate colposcopic assessment depends on the ability of the clinician to view the whole cervix and adjacent vagina together with the entire squamocolumnar junction. Due to involutional changes secondary to aging, the squamocolumnar junction often comes to lie within the cervical canal. If associated with narrowing of the cervical os, it may be totally obscured. Thus, Toplis and colleagues found that colposcopy was unsatisfactory in 53% of postmenopausal women.[21]

Treatment

The primary aim of treatment is to rid the patient of the dysplastic condition and prevent the development of invasive carcinoma. The principles are essentially the same as for treating younger women except that preservation of fertility is not an issue (Table 12-4).

If a lesion is seen on the cervix and colposcopy is satisfactory then a "punch" biopsy of the lesion should be taken. Sometimes this may be difficult in postmenopausal women where the cervix may be small, firm, and unyielding. In this situation a small "loop" excision biopsy under local anesthetic may be helpful. Biopsies should be kept to a minimum to avoid unnecessary patient discomfort, but diagnostic accuracy must not be sacrificed.

If the biopsy shows CIN 2 or CIN 3, then the lesion should be treated by one of the available techniques discussed below except cryosurgery. Large lesions and those with glandular involvement on biopsy should be excised rather than ablated. If excision is thought to be incomplete because dysplasia extends to the resection

TABLE 12-4   Treatment of Cervical Dysplasia Based on Colposcopic Findings and Biopsy

---

Satisfactory Colposcopy
1. Lesion confined to cervix:
   Biopsy: CIN 2 or 3
       Small lesion (one to two quadrants): ablation or excision/conization
       Large lesion or glandular involvement: excision/conization
   Note: Following excision/conization, if lesion present at endocervical margin or doubts
       about adequacy of excision, then consider hysterectomy
   Biopsy: CIN 1
       Observe, but if persistent, then ablation or excision/conization

2. Lesion extends onto vagina:
   Ablate with either laser or ball electrocoagulation
       or
   Perform hysterectomy to include excision of abnormality

Unsatisfactory Colposcopy
1. Lesion seen but extends upward beyond visibility: conization
2. Abnormal Pap and normal colposcopic view: conization

CIN, cervical intraepithelial neoplasia

margins or is present on the endocervical curettage specimen from the endocervical canal, vaginal hysterectomy should be considered.

If the biopsy shows CIN 1 or evidence of human papilloma virus (HPV) infection, then management is controversial. The lesion can be ablated by one of the available techniques but because in the majority of cases it will probably regress,[10] a good case can be made for regular follow-up only. Synchronous vaginal involvement by dysplasia contiguous with the cervical disease can be treated with laser ablation or ball electrocoagulation. If a hysterectomy is considered appropriate under these circumstances, the abnormal area of the vagina should be excised with the uterus and cervix. It may be easier to ensure complete excision using a vaginal approach.

If colposcopy is unsatisfactory because either the lesion is incompletely seen or the cervix is normal in the presence of an abnormal Pap smear showing dysplasia, then the patient should undergo conization and fractional curettage.

The significance of atypical squamous cells on Pap smear is not fully determined. The cytologic diagnosis is supposed to describe minor reactive changes that do not amount to dysplasia, but colposcopic evidence of dysplasia may be found on the cervix of such women. Older women with this report on a Pap smear should undergo colposcopy. If colposcopy is normal, then the use of estrogen replacement therapy should be considered because in many instances the Pap smear will revert to normal.[22]

Glandular Intraepithelial Neoplasia

Glandular abnormalities on Pap smear suggest the presence of abnormality above the squamocolumnar junction. Colposcopy is usually performed primarily to exclude an associated abnormality on the ectocervix. Further investigation should include exclusion of an endometrial abnormality by fractional curettage, with or without hysteroscopy, together with conization of the cervix. Cytologic suspicion of a glandular abnormality is a contraindication to ablative therapy.[23] Glandular intraepithelial neoplasia of the cervix may be multifocal and conization may not be sufficient treatment. In older women the presence of such an abnormality warrants hysterectomy.

METHODS OF TREATMENT OF PREMALIGNANT CERVICAL DISEASE

Because of proven progression, treatment of premalignant cervical disease must be aimed at its elimination. Either one of two principal methods, excision or ablative destruction, may be chosen. Both are efficient but excision may be more desirable because it provides a specimen for histologic examination and ablation does not. More specifically, microscopic review of an excised lesion reveals whether or not it has been completely removed, especially if invasion, always a possibility, has occurred. Ablation can leave one guessing and may induce wider destruction than is necessary.

Excisional Methods—General

Terminology with regard to excisional techniques or the treatment of CIN has been somewhat cloudy in the past. Such confusion should not exist today. Current categorization includes three methods: cold conization, laser surgery, and diathermy loop incision (LEEP or LLETZ). Each of these methods is capable of accomplishing total removal, which really, in this context, implies severance of both the area of involvement and the associated complete transformation zone. Of these three procedures, the diathermy loop approach seems to be leading in current acceptance. It has proven itself in achieving simultaneous diagnosis and therapy when used in direct conjunction with the colposcope. Knife conization, in use long before the other two techniques, was always intended to be more diagnostic than therapeutic. When used primarily to remove large areas deep in the endocervical canal, though often thereby therapeutic, just as often the volume of tissue removed is much greater than by other means. Laser excision, which enjoyed a remarkably glamorous rise in popularity in the late 1970s and early 1980s, has fallen from

TABLE 12-5 Indications for Conization of the Cervix

---

1. Unsatisfactory colposcopy with HGSIL Pap
2. HGSIL Pap with normal colposcopy
3. Suggestion of invasion (abnormal vessels at colposcopy)
4. Abnormal glandular cells on Pap
5. Recurrent CIN 3

CIN, cervical intraepithelial neoplasia; HGSIL, high-grade
squamous intraepithelial lesion

grace for a number of reasons, not the least of which is cost, but primarily because of overdestruction of margin tissue. Laser use in gynecology today is confined mostly to ablation.

Conization of the Cervix

The indications for conization are shown in Table 12-5. Conization actually can be performed by loop diathermy[24] and laser[25] as well as the more traditional cold knife (scalpel). The loop and laser can be used in the office under local anesthesia because they require less manipulation than does cold knife conization, but they do require good visualization of the cervix in a relaxed patient, not often possible in older women without anesthesia. In addition, when the cervix is small as in the atrophy of menopause, adequate deep cones are difficult to achieve with any of these techniques even under general anesthesia. Yet it is vital in older women to obtain complete cones of adequate length for histologic assessment. Scalpel conization remains the "gold standard" in this respect. Bleeding is kept to a minimum with the injection of lidocaine 1% with 1:100,000 epinephrine, and the residual raw cavity can be electrocauterized at the end of the procedure. Care must be taken not to damage the bladder or rectum in climacteric patients. Because concern with cervical stenosis and subsequent fertility problems is not important in this population but the need to treat effectively and exclude invasive carcinoma is essential, cold knife conization should be preferred. In this age group, conization should always be accompanied by endocervical curettage if not fractional curettage.

Loop Excision

This technique was pioneered by Cartier in Paris during the 1960s using small 7-mm rectangular loops to excise abnormal areas of the cervix in multiple slices.[19] Prendiville and colleagues developed the use of larger loops up to 3 cm in diameter[26] which allowed the entire transformation zone to be removed in one piece in a form of shallow conization. The technique is relatively easy to learn and can be performed more quickly than laser conization. The injection of local anesthetics renders it pain free. Secondary hemorrhage occurs in 4%,[27] and the rate of cervical stenosis is similar to cryosurgery and cold coagulation. When performed correctly, complete excision of CIN may be verified and areas of unsuspected microinvasion identified with more assurance than with the more widely destructive laser conization.

ABLATIVE TECHNIQUES

Cryotherapy

Cryotherapy is a technique of freezing using a special probe applied to the cervix which lowers the temperature to between −65°C and −89°C using either carbon dioxide or nitrous oxide gas. The cryosurgical probe is applied to the cervix with the aim of getting an ice ball extending 5 mm around the circumference of the instrument. The method was first described by Crisp and coworkers.[28] It became popular because it is cheap and easy to use. No local anesthetic is required. The main side effects are a profuse watery discharge lasting approximately 2 weeks. Cryotherapy is effective for the treatment of low-grade lesions but should not be used for large lesions, for CIN 3, or any lesion that has glandular involvement.

Electrocoagulation Diathermy

This approach uses coagulation current applied to the cervix with a needle probe that is progressively inserted into the area of abnormality. A ball electrode is then applied to the surface of the ectocervix. It was first described by Chanen and Hollyock.[29] It can be done quickly and is easy to use but has traditionally necessitated the administration of a general anesthetic. Recently it has been shown that it can be performed under local anesthesia.[30] The main complications are the rare occurrence of primary hemorrhage[23,31,32] and although actual cervical stenosis is reported in only 1% overall,[33] this may be higher in postmenopausal women. The resulting new squamocolumnar junction is invisible, i.e., inside the external os, in 65% of cases.[23,34]

Cold Coagulation

The "cold" coagulator is a machine that allows the abnormal area of the cervix to be heated to 120°C by means of a probe applied to the lesion site much as with cryosurgery. Destruction to a depth of 4 mm occurs with a 20-second application.[35] The technique was invented by Semm.[36] It also is fast, simple, and inexpensive. It causes no bleeding and can be used in the office. Like cryotherapy, it is not suitable for large lesions. It is associated with a 1% incidence of cervical stenosis and a 3.5% incidence of bleeding persisting for 1 to 6 weeks after treatment.

Laser Ablation

The carbon dioxide laser vaporizes cells when directed to the abnormal area of the cervix. This method was first described by Stafl and coworkers[37] and for a time became the most popular method of treating CIN in the United States. The beam is guided via the colposcope, which effects fine control into target areas. The depth of destruction is related to the beam power, size of the beam, and the duration of application. Usually a cylinder of tissue is destroyed extending 3 mm beyond the abnormal area on the ectocervix and 8 mm in depth. The laser can be used under general anesthesia to treat CIN that extends off the cervix. The equipment is expensive, the procedure is relatively difficult to learn, and the risks are considerable. Mild to moderate secondary hemorrhage occurs in 3% to 12% of cases although the rate of severe bleeding is only 1% to 2%.[38–40]

Hysterectomy

The presence of CIN in a postmenopausal woman is not an absolute indication for hysterectomy because local treatment of CIN is so effective. However, hysterectomy may be necessary if constrictive changes associated with aging preclude adequate local treatment. Vaginal hysterectomy when possible can facilitate the removal of adjacent vaginal intraepithelial neoplasia and is systemically less exacting in postreproductive patients than is the abdominal approach.

Results of Treatment

Many studies have reported good success rates with local ablation of CIN by a variety of techniques. However, these investigations have included relatively small numbers of postreproductive women. Problems in accurate assessment include variations in the populations treated, criteria used to rate success, length and methods of follow-up, and systems of data tabulation (Table 12-6).

Under the best conditions, the most suitable method of treatment for each individual patient must be chosen according to size of the lesion, the grade of dysplasia, and the depth of glandular involvement to achieve the best results. The more ominous any of these factors are, the greater the failure rate. When failure occurs via ablation techniques, resort to standard backup treatments of cold knife conization or hysterectomy is necessary. These two directly invasive treatment approaches, used extensively before the introduction of ablative techniques, are associated with a low incidence of subsequent recurrent or invasive disease.[48]

VAGINAL INTRAEPITHELIAL NEOPLASIA

Vaginal intraepithelial neoplasia (VAIN) was first described by Hummer and colleagues in 1933,[49] but the condition went virtually unnoticed until reports

TABLE 12-6 Results of Ablative Treatment of CIN*

Author	Year	Method	Overall CIN n	Failure %	CIN 1/2 n	Failure %	CIN 3 n	Failure %	Criteria for Success
Ostergard[41]	1980	Cryosurgery	274	11	238	6	36	25	Cytology and endocervical curettage 14 mo
Hatch[42]	1981	Cryosurgery	600	12	444	9	156	20	Cytology 6 mo
Townsend[43]	1983	Cryosurgery	100	7	47	5	53	10	Colposcopy/cytology 12 mo
Creasman[44]	1984	Cryosurgery	770	10	511	6	259	18	Cytology (2.5% < 6 mo)
Anderson[38]	1982	Laser	441	24	104	17	337	25	Colposcopy/cytology 4 mo
Baggish[39]	1982	Laser	297	11	170	9	127	13	Colposcopy/cytology 6 mo
Burke[40]	1982	Laser	131	18	91	15	40	23	Colposcopy/cytology 3 mo
Wright[45]	1983	Laser	429	5	229	4	200	6	Colposcopy/cytology 6 mo
Duncan[46]	1983	Cold coagulator	434	2	132	5	302	6	Cytology 12 mo
Smart[47]	1986	Cold coagulator	256	10					Colposcopy/cytology 12 mo
Chanen[33]	1983	Electrocoagulation	1864	3	699		1165		Colposcopy/cytology 12 mo
Woodman[23]	1985	Electrocoagulation	138	8	54	6	84	10	Colposcopy/cytology 10 mo
Giles[32]	1987	Electrocoagulation	232	6	107	5	125	6	Cytology 12 mo
Prendiville[26]	1983	Loop excision	92	2	28		64		Colposcopy/cytology 12 mo
Luesley[27]	1990	Loop excision	403	4	175	5	228	4	Colposcopy/cytology 6 mo

*Only includes patients having a single treatment and who received follow-up. Some figures have been estimated from data given in paper. CIN, cervical intraepithelial neoplasia.

SOURCE: Hatch K, Helm CW. Cancer of the cervix—surgical treatment. In: Blackledge G, Jordan M, Shingleton HM, eds. *Textbook of Gynecologic Oncology*. Philadelphia: WB Saunders; 1991:317. Reprinted with permission.

started appearing in the mid 1970s.[50–53] VAIN is much less common than dysplasia (IN) in other sites of the lower genital tract, representing just 0.4% of preinvasive malignancies,[54] but the disease particularly affects climacteric women. Most studies show a mean age of more than 50 years although the range extends from the late teens into the eighties.[50,54–59]

The histologic features or VAIN are similar to those of CIN. Depending on grade of severity, the categories are VAIN 1 (mild), VAIN 2 (moderate), and VAIN 3 (severe).[60] Atrophic changes occurring in postmenopausal women and radiation effects can lead to difficulty in diagnosis especially if inflammation is present.[60] Vaginal cellular changes of this nature, even in the postmenopausal woman, are commonly associated with HPV infections.[56,59,61] The condition affects the upper part of the vagina in more than two thirds of cases[49,50,52,55–57,59,62] and may be multifocal.[49,56,57,63]

The occurrence of VAIN has been associated with CIN and malignant disease of the genital tract,[50] previous radiation,[64,65] HPV infection,[66] and immunosuppression.[50,67] The majority of cases are found in women previously treated for preinvasive or invasive cancer of the cervix or vulva,[50,56,57,59,68] with the interval from original treatment being up to 24 years.[69] VAIN occurring after a hysterectomy for CIN was considered to be due to disease left behind in the vagina at the time of hysterectomy, but it may also represent multicentric disease of the lower genital tract.[70] It was at one time suggested that VAIN was associated with hysterectomy even for benign disease but this is not so.[71]

Malignant Potential

The major concern with regard to VAIN is the risk of progression to invasive carcinoma. The evidence for progression to invasive cancer is based on the fact that invasive carcinoma can develop from VAIN 3 if left untreated. Areas of VAIN 3 are often associated with unsuspected microinvasive or invasive disease and invasive carcinoma may develop following inadequate treatment for VAIN.

Geelhoed and colleagues reported data on 10 patients with vaginal CIS who were followed for 4 years without treatment, 3 of whom progressed to invasive vaginal carcinoma.[65] Progression to invasive disease has been described by others.[49,52,72–75] Several authors report that, after excisional surgery has been performed for what was thought to be noninvasive VAIN, areas of microinvasion have been found.[76,77]

If invasive carcinoma of the vagina does develop in untreated VAIN, the outlook is poor. Kucera and Vavra reported that the overall 5-year survival rate for 110 patients with vaginal carcinoma was 39.9%.[78] Using International Federation of Gynecology and Obstetrics (FIGO) staging standards, their survival figures revealed 76.7% for stage I, 44.5% for stage II, 31% for stage III, and 18.2% for stage IV. There are no data on the malignant potential of VAIN 1 and 2, but it is probably low. Dysplasias of mild degree can probably be observed only and most will disappear.[79]

Diagnosis

Vaginal intraepithelial neoplasia is a silent disease, essentially asymptomatic, usually detected on Pap smears as part of a screening program or at regular checkups. Until the 1980s, most gynecologists never took routine Pap smears during regular annual checkups in women who had sustained total hysterectomy for benign disease. However, with the progressive recognition of the role of viruses in causing serious dysplastic lesions in the lower genital tract and the associated apparent objective rise in the incidence of these problems, current opinion advises appropriate vaginal vault and vaginal wall smears at least every 2 years in these hysterectomized women. When an abnormal Pap smear is obtained, colposcopy then becomes the main method of further investigation whether the cervix is present or not.

Identification of abnormal areas of the vagina is made primarily by colposcopy. Lesions may be multifocal and thus inspection of the whole vagina is essential as well as cervix, if present, and vulva. The application of 3% to 5% acetic acid reveals aceto-white areas, which may show punctuation similar to that of CIN but mosaicism is rare in VAIN.[59] The application of Lugol's iodine may be useful to delineate more clearly the abnormal areas[50,70,80,81] because it stains normal glycogen-containing epithelium dark brown and leaves dysplastic areas lighter in color. It is best to hold the application of Lugol's solution until after acetic acid has been applied because it interferes with colposcopic visualization.

Colposcopy may be extremely difficult in postmenopausal women, particularly if they are not sexually active and are not on estrogen replacement therapy. Exogenous estrogen therapy by any route, best particularly topically, will facilitate colposcopic examination both mechanically by increasing resiliency and visually by vitalizing the atrophic endometrium.[82] Despite such measures, adequate inspection may not be possible without general or full regional anesthesia in the mechanically compromised older patient. Also, because biopsy of the vagina is particularly painful and difficult without adequate anesthesia, one should not hesitate to use it. One of the great difficulties in assessing the vagina following hysterectomy is the inspection of the so-called dog ears on either side of the vaginal vault, again emphasizing the need for anesthesia in such cases to see these hidden areas that were originally in juxtaposition to the cervix.

Once an abnormal area has been detected by colposcopy, biopsy is essential for diagnosis. This can be either a small punch biopsy or removal by surgical excision. The latter is preferable because it may be at once both diagnostic and curative. The larger specimen permits examination to the borders of the lesion and into the depth of the larger specimen for better assessment of possible invasion.

TABLE 12-7 Treatment Options for Vaginal
Intraepithelial Neoplasia

Surgical
  Ablative
    Cryotherapy
    Laser ablation
    Electrocautery
  Excision
    Local excision by knife, by laser
    Partial vaginectomy
    Total vaginectomy

Medical
  Radiotherapy
  5-Fluorouracil cream

Treatment

Treatment options in postmenopausal women are identical to those in younger
women (Table 12-7). The principle aims of therapy are removal of the premalignant disease, assurance regarding unsuspected invasion, and preservation of a
functioning vagina. Factors that will influence management are the patient's age,
the location and extent of disease, previous treatments, the presence or absence of
a uterus, and the patient's medical condition and immune status.

In general, the disease is better excised surgically because of the need to rule
out invasive disease. Small, unifocal areas of abnormality in the lower and
mid-vagina may be excised and the vagina closed primarily.[63,83] At surgery it is
important to delineate the abnormal area clearly with Lugol's iodine solution and
to take a 3-mm margin of normal tissue. As already implied, surgery is best
performed in older women after several weeks of estrogen treatment. Disease of
the proximal vagina may be best treated by partial vaginectomy in the elderly,
removing the upper part of the vagina containing the abnormal area. The main
concern is to excise disease within the so-called dog ears at the vaginal angles.
Partial vaginectomy can be performed either vaginally,[84] the best route when
feasible, or transabdominally.[85] The vagina can either be closed primarily, ensur-
ing that the edges are everted (pointing into the vagina), or left open to granulate
and reepithelialize. If the uterus and cervix are still present, and disease is present
in the upper vagina, then a hysterectomy should be performed simultaneously to
ensure total excisional continuity of the abnormal area in the upper vagina. This
procedure may be accomplished from above or below. Postoperatively, it is
important to sustain functional and visual capability of the upper vagina by
preventing adhesive occlusion through the use of estrogen and vaginal dilators.
Such a regimen on a regular basis, because of the natural compliancy of the
vagina, will rapidly overcome losses of as much as 4 cm of mucosa, especially if

coital activity is added. A total vaginectomy, rarely performed except when the entire vagina is affected by VAIN,[86–88] requires the use of a split-thickness skin graft if a functional vagina is a goal. Surgery may be extremely difficult following radiation therapy and, under these circumstances, medical treatment may be preferred on a practical basis.

Ablative Techniques

Destructive techniques have been popularized for the treatment of VAIN but have the major disadvantage over excision that invasive disease may be completely treated. Techniques include freezing,[83] electrocautery,[80] and laser application.[55,68,69,89] Because of the lack of glands in the vagina, ablation to a depth of only 3 mm will destroy the entire epithelium containing the VAIN. Either steel wire[75] or lacrimal hooks can be used to evert the vaginal angles. Saline or local anesthetic with a vasoconstrictor agent can be injected under the vaginal epithelium to elevate it and reduce the chance of laser injury to adjacent structures. Extreme care is essential in attacking lesions of the anterior and posterior vaginal walls to prevent the development of fistulae into adjacent hollow organs, particularly in those cases with a previous history of radiotherapy or pelvic surgery.

This approach requires experience and good anesthesia. Local anesthesia may be sufficient for small easily accessible lesions, but a regional or general anesthetic is required for most treatment. The patient should be advised to avoid coitus and the use of tampons temporarily following the procedure and be warned that she may experience a serosanguinous discharge for several days postoperatively.

5-Fluorouracil Cream

5-Fluorouracil (5-FU) is an antimetabolite that interferes with DNA and RNA synthesis and, when applied to the vagina, destroys both normal and abnormal epithelium.[53] Its use was first described in 1975,[67] and since then many studies have suggested variations of dose and time interval.[90–94] The most recent reports advise using either 5 g 5% 5-FU daily for 5 to 10 days repeated at 2-week intervals[94] or 2.5 g 5% at weekly intervals for a total of 10 weeks for either schedule.[93]

Ulceration of the vaginal vestibule can be avoided by the application of a steroid cream and insertion of the medication only at bedtime. Patients should be advised to avoid sexual contact for 24 hours after application. This treatment may present a problem for older patients due to poor compliance. In addition, they may have a problem inserting the cream into the vagina, which will lead to undertreatment and external ulceration. Obviously, the older the patient, the greater must be the involvement of both the physician and the patient's family to ensure appropriate therapy.

Irradiation

Although radiotherapy is a fairly effective treatment for VAIN,[49,73,95] it carries a high risk factor. It may easily produce severe complications, even in expert hands, including fistula, vaginal shortening, and stenosis,[73] and its use should be restricted to a few select patients when all other methods, for whatever reason, are ruled inapplicable.

Results of Treatment

It is difficult to compare adequately the results of different treatment methods for VAIN due to the relatively small numbers of women treated, the paucity of reports to date, and the variable proportions of different grades of disease, techniques, and duration of follow-up. In fact, some papers as recently as 1990 do not even state the duration of follow-up even though this is essential in analysis of success rates.[75] No studies to date have specifically addressed the outcome in older women, but the steadily growing older population and the apparent increase in viral impact on cellular morphology may offer the opportunity for more accurate evaluation in the future. The earliest reports of laser therapy indicated good success rates of around 89%,[89] but two later studies from major centers in England and the United States report high failure rates with laser treatment of 42% and 57%, respectively.[55,96] Even surgical excision of VAIN lesions has a significant failure rate,[50,85] but long-term follow-up seems to show it to be more effective.[97]

VULVAR INTRAEPITHELIAL NEOPLASIA

The principle premalignant conditions affecting the vulva of older women are squamous intraepithelial neoplasia (VIN) and Paget's disease. A variety of benign lesions including the commonly occurring lichen sclerosus and squamous cell hyperplasia affect this age group. Their importance is that their symptoms may mimic those of an invasive or preinvasive malignancy that can develop within areas affected by these conditions. A basic principle of management of vulvar conditions in older women is that preinvasive and invasive disease must invariably be excluded by biopsy.

As with the other intraepithelial neoplasia of the female lower genital tract, VIN is an epithelial abnormality that is divided into grades of severity (see Table 12-1). The histologic features have been well described.[98] The prevalence of VIN is unknown, but severe dysplasia of the vulva (VIN 3) represents 1.8% of all in situ carcinomas of the female genital tract.[54] VIN can affect women of all ages. Before the 1970s it was a disease primarily affecting postmenopausal women, but there has been an increase in incidence in younger women. Factors associated with

VIN are similar to those associated with CIN and not uncommonly include a history of current or previous sexually transmitted diseases, including HPV infection, reduced immunity, and cigarette smoking.[94,99,100]

Diagnosis

This neoplasia is often asymptomatic but, in contrast to CIN and VAIN, symptoms such as pruritus, pain, lumps, and discharge can occur. It can develop anywhere on the vulva but most frequently affects the labia, particularly the posterior part of the labia minora.[101] There are thought to be two clinical variants of VIN, one of which mainly involves older women. In this type, occurring at the mean age group of 60 years, the disease is primarily unifocal, appearing only in the vulva. There is no synchronous involvement of the cervix and vagina and it is usually negative for HPV DNA.[94,99–102] In contrast, the disease type affecting younger women is often multifocal, appearing simultaneously in other sites in the lower genital tract and perianal region.

Vulvar disease has a range of clinical appearances. Lesions may be gray, white, brown, or dull red in color and they may be raised and papular, wartlike, or ulcerative.[103,104] The diagnosis is made only by biopsy and histologic examination. Examination of the vulva using a colposcope (i.e., vulvoscopy) is of particular value in delineating the margin of abnormality and detecting small satellite lesions. Biopsy of any suspicious or overtly abnormal areas should be performed. Although the Keyes punch biopsy may be performed, the only definitive sample is excisional tissue removal to obtain margins and depth.

Malignant Potential

The exact malignant potential of VIN has not been satisfactorily determined but it is thought to be less than that for CIN. The solid evidence for some degree of malignant tendency includes the fact that VIN is found in epithelium adjacent to invasive squamous cell carcinoma, an association not as common as the association of CIN with invasive cervical carcinoma, and areas of "unsuspected" invasion may be found in areas of VIN. Chafe and colleagues reported this occurring in 19% of cases.[105] It has been reported that long-standing, histologically verified VIN progresses to invasion in 90% to 100% of cases[106,107] with transit times of 2 to 10 years, but generally progression rates are thought to be much lower than this, except in those with reduced immunity and the elderly.[99,106–110] Spontaneous regression of VIN has been reported,[99] but it is not possible to predict which lesions will regress. Therefore, one would be hard pressed not to eradicate these "hot spots" when they are uncovered because of patient anxiety and possible later medical-legal entanglements.

TABLE 12-8 Treatment Methods for Vulvar
Intraepithelial Neoplasia

Surgical
Excision
Local excision
Partial vulvectomy
Vulvectomy
Skinning vulvectomy
Ablation
Cryosurgery
CO_2 laser
Cavitronic ultrasonic surgical aspiration
Excision and ablation
Combined local excision and laser vaporization
Medical
Topical 5-FU
Reduction of immunosuppressant dosage

Treatment

The treatment options are listed in Table 12-8. As with CIN and VAIN, the principles involved are exclusion of invasive disease and destruction of all involved epithelium. The precise treatment depends on age, coital aspirations, and medical condition of the patient along with site, extent, and severity of the disease. Most of the data on vaginal intraepithelial neoplasia relate to VIN 3. VIN 1 and VIN 2 (mild and moderate dysplasias) may be treated with observation alone once invasive disease has been excluded, but patient pressure may demand eradication.

Excision

Traditionally VIN has been treated by excisional methods although with the increased incidence of disease in younger women and an increased awareness of sexuality in all ages treatment is becoming much less radical and more tailored to the special needs of each patient. For many older patients unifocal disease can be relatively easily excised with a margin of 3 to 5 mm[111] and the defect closed primarily. Lesions involving the posterior or anterior half of the vulva can be excised by a partial vulvectomy in the shape of a horseshoe. Where there is extensive involvement of both sides of the vulva, simple vulvectomy may be necessary.[112] After excision or simple vulvectomy, healing is usually rapid. The surgery is tolerated well by older women and can be performed under spinal anesthesia. Skinning vulvectomy was introduced to preserve a more normal body image.[105,111,113] In this operation just the skin of the vulva without subcutaneous fat is removed and the area is covered with a split-thickness skin graft usually taken from the inner thigh. The healing time is more protracted, particularly at the skin donor site, but the cosmetic appearance of the vulva is better. Whichever method of excision is used, the margins of resection must be clear to reduce the risk of recurrence.[114–116] It is useful to mark the lines of resection using a colposcope and marking pen at the time of surgery. Excision has been combined with laser ablation[117] in the clitoral and perianal regions to retain more normal anatomic configuration.

Ablation

Although cryosurgery[111] was the first ablative technique to be used for VIN, it was later surpassed in popularity by the CO_2 laser,[118,119] used either alone or in combination with excision.[117] The use of the laser to treat VIN has been excellently described.[120] The vulva contains subepithelial hair follicles and sebaceous glands that may be involved by VIN. Histopathologic study[121] has shown that 99.5% of VIN measured less than 0.77 mm in hairy skin and 0.69 mm in nonhairy skin. It is suggested that removal of VIN to a depth of 1.0 mm in nonhairy and 2.0 mm in hairy skin is all that is required for successful treatment. It is vital not to laser below the third surgical plane, the upper reticular dermis, because this results in prolonged healing and severe scarring.[120]

As with excisional techniques, it is important to ablate with the laser beyond the visibly involved areas to reduce the chance of recurrence. The correct distance is not known and although it is customary to go outside approximately 5 mm, it has been suggested that up to 1.5 cm all around the lesion should be destroyed for the best assurance of total removal.[104] Another technique, cavitronic ultrasonic surgical aspiration, has been reported in the literature, but its role is not yet established.[122]

Ablative techniques should only be used in the climacteric group as an adjunct to primary excisional therapy and to treat recurrent disease if invasion has been excluded on biopsy.

Medical

As in the vagina, the application of 5-FU cream to areas of VIN on the vulva has been reported.[99,109,111,123,124] Response rates have varied from 70%[109,124] to zero.[99,111] 5-FU can cause severe pain and ulceration. It is best reserved for those women in whom all other forms of treatment are felt to be contraindicated or in whom recurrent disease must be controlled.

If VIN occurs in patients already on immunosuppressive therapy, the disease may regress significantly if the dose of the immunosuppressive drug is reduced.

Recurrence after treatment is common in immunosuppressed women and treatment should be conservative once invasive disease is excluded.

Results

It is generally assumed that treatment of VIN will reduce the chance of invasive vulvar carcinoma occurring later. Unfortunately, the recurrence rates of VIN after treatment are high for all methods of treatment. Even after vulvectomy the rate is reported to be between 10% and 25%.[101,105,107,109,111,116] The importance of obtaining clear and wide surgical margins is emphasized by the fact that recurrence rates of 47% occur if margins are not completely negative.[115] Following initial excision, recurrent disease can be treated more conservatively in patients observed closely. Recurrences after laser ablation are reported to be between 12.5% and 30%,[101,125] always higher in cases where destruction is restricted too close to the observable edge of the lesion.

PAGET'S DISEASE OF THE VULVA

Paget's disease is an intraepithelial adenocarcinoma that probably arises from multipotent stem cells in the epidermis and epidermally derived adnexal structures.[98] It was first reported on the mammary areola by Sir James Paget in 1874,[126] but the first case involving the vulva was not described until 1901.[127] It affects mainly postmenopausal Caucasian women[128,129] with a mean age at diagnosis of around 65 years. It is a much rarer disease than squamous cell carcinoma of the vulva. Woodruff in 1955 found only 120 cases in a search of the literature.[130]

The condition presents with pruritus in over 50% of instances[128,129] together with soreness and burning.[131,132] The involved areas may appear as red velvet containing white islands of hyperkeratosis or they may be pinkish and scaly. It often occurs in several different areas of the vulva.[133] The abnormality begins on the hair-bearing portions of the vulva, the genital folds, or the perianal skin, i.e., apocrine gland-bearing regions. The diagnosis can only be made definitively by biopsy which will display a distinctive histologic appearance, always including pathognomonic Paget cells.[98] Treatment must take into account that the histologic abnormality always extends much wider than the visible cellular defect.[134]

Malignant Potential

Although Paget's disease of the vulva is a premalignant condition, progression to invasive disease is rare.[133,135] The main concern is its known potential for association with either an underlying adjacent adenocarcinoma or a malignancy at another site. At one time Paget's disease of the vulva was thought to be commonly aligned with an underlying subjacent glandular apocrine adenocarcinoma,[136] analogous to the situation occurring with Paget's disease of the nipple. In a review of the literature, Chanda found that 24% of 194 patients with extramammary Paget's disease, mainly involving the vulva, were associated with a nearby cutaneous carcinoma.[137] This association may have been overestimated and Helwig and Graham have pointed out the need to differentiate between involvement of adjacent structures by Paget cells within an intact basement membrane and true invasive adenocarcinoma.[138] Some series report no subjacent adenocarcinomas at all.[139,140] Chanda reported that 9% of 109 cases were associated with concurrent malignancy in the cervix, breast, Bartholin's gland, and gallbladder.[137] Other reported sites include the bladder and skin. Perianal Paget's disease has been associated with an underlying rectal carcinoma.

Treatment

The management of Paget's disease of the vulva is defined by the need to exclude an underlying adenocarcinoma and a concurrent carcinoma in the breast and cervix. When discovered perianally, associated rectal or anal canal carcinoma must be excluded.

The possibility of associated underlying adenocarcinoma mandates adequate excision. This may require a total vulvectomy or very wide local excision. Since Paget's disease has been documented histologically in apparently normal vulva skin on the contralateral vulva, some gynecologists favor total vulvectomy.[141] Whatever technique is used, as already noted, wide margins around the visible abnormality are vitally necessary.[134] Frozen section can be helpful in delineating the margin of tumor at the time of surgery but this is not infallible. Inguinal node dissection is unnecessary unless an invasive adnexal adenocarcinoma is found. The clitoris can be preserved by treating that area with laser ablation.

Success of Treatment

Friedrich reported that the recurrence rates for all patients treated surgically, regardless of extent of histologic involvement, was 12.4%.[142] In a review of the world literature, Breen and colleagues revealed a recurrence rate of 11.6% after all forms of surgery.[129]

Recurrence of disease after primary excision can be treated more conservatively if an invasive carcinoma has been excluded originally. Further treatment options include additional local excision and laser ablation. Topical 5-FU cream should be used only in unusual circumstances.[143]

REFERENCES

1. Ferenczy A, Winkler B. Cervical intraepithelial neoplasia and condyloma. In: Kurman RJ, ed. *Blaustein's Pathology of the Female Genital Tract.* New York: Springer-Verlag; 1987:177–217.

2. Buckley CH, Butler EB, Fox H. Cervical intraepithelial neoplasia. *J Clin Pathol.* 1982;35:1–13.

3. Petersen O. Precancerous changes of the cervical epithelium. *Acta Radiol.* 1955;127(suppl):8–163.

4. Fidler HK, Boyes DA, Worth AJ. Cervical cancer detection in British Columbia. *J Obstet Gynaecol Brit Commonw.* 1968;75:392–404.

5. McIndoe WO, McLean MR, Jones RW, Mullins PR. The invasive potential of carcinoma in situ of the cervix. *Obstet Gynecol.* 1984;64:451–458.

6. Stern E, Neeley PM. Dysplasia of the uterine cervix. *Cancer.* 1964;17:508–512.

7. Koss LG. Concept of genesis and development of carcinoma of the cervix. *Obstet Gynecol Surv.* 1969;24:850–860.

8. Richart RM, Barron BA. A followup study of patients with cervical dysplasia. *Am J Obstet Gynecol.* 1969;105:386–393.

9. Campion MJ, Cuzick J, McCance DJ, Singer A. Progressive potential of mild cervical atypia: Prospective cytological colposcopic and virological study. *Lancet.* 1986;ii:237–240.

10. Syrjanen K, Kataja V, Yliskoski M, et al. Natural history of cervical human papillomavirus lesions does not substantiate the biologic relevance of the Bethesda System. *Obstet Gynecol.* 1992;79:675–682.

11. Mandelblatt JS, Hammond DB. Primary care of elderly women: Is Pap smear screening necessary? *Mt Sinai J Med (NY).* 1985;52:284–290.

12. Sieglar EE. Cervical carcinoma in the aged. *Am J Obstet Gynecol.* 1969;103:1093–1097.

13. Papanicolaou G, Traut HF. The diagnostic value of vaginal smears in carcinoma of the uterus. *Am J Obstet Gynecol.* 1941;42:193–206.

14. Ayre JE. Selective cytology smear for diagnosis of cancer. *Am J Obstet Gynecol.* 1947;53:609–617.

15. Fidler HK, Boyes DH, Locke DK. The cytology program in British Columbia. *J Obstet Gynaecol Brit Commonw.* 1968;75:392–404.

16. Guzick DS. Efficacy of screening for cervical cancer: A review. *Am J Pub Health.* 1978;68:125–134.

17. Walton Report. Cervical cancer screening programs. *Can Med Assoc J.* 1976;114:1003–1031.

18. Solomon D. The 1988 Bethesda System for reporting cervical/vaginal cytologic diagnoses. *Acta Cytol.* 1989;33:567–574.

19. Cartier R. *Practical Colposcopy.* Paris: S. Karger; 1977.

20. Kishi Y. Colposcopy for postmenopausal women. *Gynecol Oncol.* 1985;20:62–70.

21. Toplis PJ, Casemore V, Hallam N, et al. Evaluation of colposcopy in the postmenopausal woman. *Br J Obstet Gynecol.* 1986;93:843–851.

22. Kaminski PF, Sorosky JI, Wheelock JB, et al. The significance of atypical cervical cytology in an older population. *Obstet Gynecol.* 1989;73:13–15.

23. Woodman CBJ, Jordan JA, Mylotte MJ, et al. The management of cervical intraepithelial neoplasia by coagulation electrodiathermy. *Br J Obstet Gynaecol.* 1985;92:751–755.

24. Mor-Yosef S, Lopes A, Pearson S, et al. Loop diathermy cone biopsy. *Obstet Gynecol.* 1990;75:884–886.

25. Dorsey JH, Diggs ES. Microsurgical conization of the cervix by carbon dioxide laser. *Obstet Gynecol.* 1979;54:565–570.

26. Prendiville W, Cullimore J, Norman S. Large loop excision of the transformation zone (LLETZ). A new method of management for women with cervical intraepithelial neoplasia. *Br J Obstet Gynaecol.* 1989;96:1054–1060.

27. Luesley DM, Cullimore J, Redman CWE, et al. Loop diathermy excision of the cervical transformation zone in patients with abnormal cervical smears. *Br Med J.* 1990;300:1690–1693.

28. Crisp WE, Smith MS, Asadourian LA, et al. Cryosurgical treatment of premalignant disease of the uterine cervix. *Am J Obstet Gynecol.* 1970;107:737–742.

29. Chanen W, Hollyock VE. Colposcopy and electrocoagulation diathermy for cervical dysplasia and carcinoma in situ. *Obstet Gynecol.* 1971;37:623–628.

30. Chanen W. The efficacy of electrocoagulation diathermy performed under local anesthesia for the eradication of precancerous lesions of the cervix. *Aust NZ J Obstet Gynaecol.* 1989;29:189–192.

31. Hollyock VE, Chanen W. Electrocoagulation diathermy for the treatment of cervical dysplasia and carcinoma in situ. *Obstet Gynecol.* 1976;47:196–199.

32. Giles JA, Walker PG, Chalk PAF. Treatment of cervical intraepithelial neoplasia (CIN) by radical electrocoagulation diathermy: 5 years' experience. *Br J Obstet Gynecol.* 1987;94:1089–1093.

33. Chanen W, Rome RM. Electrocoagulation diathermy for cervical dysplasia and carcinoma in situ: A 15 year survey. *Obstet Gynecol.* 1983;61:673–679.

34. Hollyock VE, Chanen W, Wein R. Cervical function following treatment of intraepithelial neoplasia by electrocoagulation diathermy. *Obstet Gynecol.* 1983;61:79–81.

35. Haddad NB, Hussein I, Blessing K, et al. Tissue destruction following cold coagulation of the cervix. *British Society for Colposcopy and Cervical Pathology.* 1988; Abstracts, p. 6.

36. Semm K. New apparatus for the "cold-coagulation" of benign cervical lesions. *Am J Obstet Gynecol.* 1966;95:963–966.

37. Stafl A, Wilkinson EJ, Mattingly RF. Laser treatment of cervical and vaginal neoplasia. *Am J Obstet Gynecol.* 1977;128:128–136.

38. Anderson MC. Treatment of cervical intraepithelial neoplasia with the carbon dioxide laser: Report of 543 patients. *Obstet Gynecol.* 1982;59:720–725.

39. Baggish MS. Management of cervical intraepithelial neoplasia by carbon dioxide laser. *Obstet Gynecol.* 1982;60:378–384.

40. Burke L. The use of the carbon dioxide laser in the therapy of cervical intraepithelial neoplasia. *Am J Obstet Gynecol.* 1982;144:337–340.

41. Ostergard DR. Cryosurgical treatment of cervical intraepithelial neoplasia. *Obstet Gynecol.* 1980;56:231–233.

42. Hatch KD, Shingleton HM, Austin JM, et al. Cryosurgery of cervical intraepithelial neoplasia. *Obstet Gynecol.* 1981;57:692–698.

43. Townsend DE, Richart RM. Cryotherapy and carbon dioxide laser management of cervical intraepithelial neoplasia: A controlled comparison. *Obstet Gynecol.* 1983;61:75–78.

44. Creasman WT, Hinshaw WM, Clarke-Pearson DL. Cryosurgery in the management of cervical intraepithelial neoplasia. *Obstet Gynecol.* 1984;63:145–149.

45. Wright VC, Davies E, Riopelle MA. Laser surgery for cervical intraepithelial neoplasia: Principles and results. *Am J Obstet Gynecol.* 1983;145:181–184.

46. Duncan ID. The Semm cold coagulator in the management of cervical intraepithelial neoplasia. *Clin Obstet Gynecol.* 1983;26:996–1006.

47. Smart GE. Laser ablation versus cold coagulation for the treatment of cervical intraepithelial neoplasia. *British Congress of Obstetrics and Gynaecology* 1985; Abstract, p. 8.

48. Cavanagh D, Ruffalo EH, Marsden DE. *Gynecologic Oncology: A Clinico-pathologic Approach.* Norwalk, CT: Appleton-Century-Crofts; 1985.

49. Hummer WK, Mussey E, Decker DG, et al. Carcinoma in situ of the vagina. *Am J Obstet Gynecol.* 1970;108:1109–1116.

50. Gallup DG, Morley GW. Carcinoma in situ of the vagina. *Obstet Gynecol.* 1975;46:334–340.

51. Jimerson GK, Merrill JA. Cancer and dysplasia of the posthysterectomy vaginal cuff. *Gynecol Oncol.* 1976;4:328–334.

52. Lee RA, Symmonds RE. Recurrent carcinoma in situ of the vagina in patients previously treated for in-situ carcinoma of the cervix. *Obstet Gynecol.* 1976;48:61–64.

53. Woodruff JD, Parmley TH, Julian CG. Topical 5-fluorouracil in the treatment of vaginal carcinoma in situ. *Gynecol Oncol.* 1975;3:124–132.

54. Cramer D, Cutler S. Incidence and histopathology of malignancy of the female genital organs in the United States. *Am J Obstet Gynecol.* 1974;118:443–460.

55. Woodman CBJ, Jordan JA. The management of vaginal intraepithelial neoplasia after hysterectomy. *Br J Obstet Gynaecol.* 1984;91:707–711.

56. Hernandez-Linares W, Puthawala A, Nolan JF. Carcinoma in-situ of the vagina: Past and present management. *Obstet Gynecol.* 1980;56:356–360.

57. Daly JW, Ellis GF. Treatment of vaginal dysplasia and carcinoma in-situ with topical 5-fluorouracil. *Obstet Gynecol.* 55:350–352.

58. Hoffman MS, Hill DA, Gordy LW, et al. Comparing the yield of the standard Pap and endocervical brush smears. *J Reprod Med.* 1991;36:267–269.

59. Benedet JL, Sanders BH. Carcinoma in situ of the vagina. *Am J Obstet Gynecol.* 1984;148:695–700.

60. Sedlis A, Robboy SJ. Diseases of the vagina. In: Kurman RJ, ed. *Blaustein's Pathology of the Female Genital Tract.* New York: Springer-Verlag; 1987:97–140.

61. Sato S, Okagaki T, Clark B, et al. Sensitivity of koilocytosis, immunocytochemistry and electron microscopy as compared to DNA hybridization in detecting human papillomavirus in cervical and vaginal condyloma and intraepithelial neoplasia. *Int J Gynecol Pathol.* 1986;5:297–307.

62. Sillman FH, Sedlis A, Boyce JG. A review of lower genital intraepithelial neoplasia and the use of topical 5-fluorouracil. *Obstet Gynecol Surv.* 1985;40:190–220.

63. Oliver JA. Severe dysplasia and carcinoma in situ of the vagina. *Am J Obstet Gynecol.* 1979;134:133–137.

64. Muram D, Curry RH, Drouin P. Cytologic followup of patients with invasive cervical carcinoma treated by radiotherapy. *Am J Obstet Gynecol.* 1982;142:350–354.

65. Geelhoed GW, Henson DE. Taylor PT, et al. Carcinoma in-situ of the vagina following treatment for carcinoma of the cervix: A distinctive clinical entity. *Am J Obstet Gynecol.* 1976;124:510–516.

66. Okagaki T, Twiggs LB, Zachow KR, et al. Identification of human papillomavirus in cervical and vaginal intraepithelial neoplasia with molecularly cloned virus-specific DNA probes. *Int J Gynecol Pathol.* 1983;2:153–159.

67. Bowen-Simpkins P, Hull MGR. Intracpithelial vaginal neoplasia following immuno-suppressive therapy treated with topical 5FU. *Obstet Gynecol.* 1975;46:360–362.

68. Capen CV, Masterson BJ, Magrina JF, et al. Laser therapy of vaginal intraepithelial neoplasia. *Am J Obstet Gynecol.* 1982;142:973–976.

69. Petrilli ES, Townsend DE, Morrow CP, et al. Vaginal intraepithelial neoplasia: Biologic aspects and treatment with topical 5-fluorouracil and the carbon dioxide laser. *Am J Obstet Gynecol.* 1980;138:321–328.

70. Marcus SL. Multiple squamous cell carcinoma involving the cervix, vagina and vulva—the theory of multicentric origin. *Am J Obstet Gynecol.* 1961;80:802–812.

71. Herman JM, Homesley HD, Dignan MB. Is hysterectomy a risk factor for vaginal cancer? *JAMA* 1986;256:601–603.

72. Graham JB, Meigs JV. Recurrence of tumor after total hysterectomy for carcinoma in situ. *Am J Obstet Gynecol.* 1962;64:1159–1162.

73. Rutledge F. Cancer of the vagina. *Obstet Gynecol.* 1967;97:635–655.

74. Scokel PW, Collier RC, Jones WN, et al. Relation of carcinoma in situ of the vagina to the early diagnosis of vaginal cancer. *Am J Obstet Gynecol.* 1961;82:397–400.

75. Sherman AI. Laser therapy for vaginal intraepithelial neoplasia after hysterectomy. *J Reprod Med.* 1990;35:941–944.

76. Ireland D, Monaghan JM. The management of the patient with abnormal vaginal cytology following hysterectomy. *Br J Obstet Gynaecol.* 1988;95:973–975.

77. Hoffman MS, DeCesare SL, Roberts WS, et al. Upper vaginectomy for in situ and occult, superficially invasive carcinoma of the vagina. *Am J Obstet Gynecol.* 1992;166:30–33.

78. Kucera H, Vavra N. Radiation management of primary carcinoma of the vagina: Clinical and histopathological variables associated with survival. *Gynecol Oncol.* 1991;40:12–16.

79. Monaghan JM. Vaginal cancer. In Burghardt E, ed. *Surgical Gynecologic Oncology.* New York: Thieme; 1993:171–184.

80. Prangley AG. Premalignant lesions of the vagina. *Clin Obstet Gynecol.* 1962; 5:1119–1126.

81. Gray LA, Christopherson WM. In-situ and early invasive carcinoma of the vagina. *Obstet Gynecol.* 1969;34:226–230.

82. Copenhaver EH, Salzman FA, Wright KA. Carcinoma in situ of the vagina. *Am J Obstet Gynecol.* 1964;89:962–969.

83. Adducci J. Carcinoma in-situ of the vagina. *Geriatrics.* 1972;27:121–123.

84. Monaghan JM. Operations on the vagina. In Monaghan JM, ed. *Bonney's Gynaecological Surgery.* London: Balliere Tindall; 1986:138–142.

85. Curtis P, Shepherd JH, Lowe DG, et al. The role of partial colpectomy in the management of persistent vaginal neoplasia after primary treatment. *Br J Obstet Gynaecol.* 1992;99:587–589.

86. Samuels B, Bradburn DM, Johnson CG. Primary CIS of the vagina. A case report and review of the literature. *Am J Obstet Gynecol.* 1961;82:393–396.

87. Moran JP, Robinson JH. Primary CIS of the vagina, report of laser. *Obstet Gynecol.* 1962;20:405–409.

88. Woodruff JD. Treatment of CIS of the lower genital tract. *Clin Obstet Gynecol.* 1965;8:757–770.

89. Townsend DE, Levine RU, Crum CP, et al. Treatment of vaginal carcinoma in situ with the carbon dioxide laser. *Am J Obstet Gynecol.* 1982;143:565–568.

90. Bleker O, Ketting B, Wayjean-Eecen B. The significance of microscopic involvement of the parametrium and/or pelvic lymph nodes in cervical cancer stages IB and IIA. *Gynecol Oncol.* 1983;16:56–62.

91. Hull MGR, Bowen-Simpkins P. Paintin DB. 5-Fluouracil versus immunotherapy for non-clinical vaginal cancer. *Lancet.* 1976;i:588.

92. Piver MS, Barlow JJ, Tsukada Y, et al. Postirradiation squamous cell carcinoma in situ of the vagina. Treatment by topical 20% 5-fluorouracil cream. *Am J Obstet Gynecol.* 1979;135:377–380

93. Stokes IM, Sworn MJ, Hawthorne JHR. The treatment of vaginal carcinomas in-situ using a new regimen for 5-fluorouracil. *Br J Obstet Gynaecol.* 1980;87:920–921.

94. Caglar H, Hertzog RW, Hreshchyshyn RW. Topical 5-fluorouracil treatment of vaginal intraepithelial neoplasia. *Obstet Gynecol.* 1981;58:580–583.

95. Brown GR, Fletcher GH, Rutledge FN. Irradiation of "in-situ" and invasive squamous cell carcinoma of the vagina. *Cancer.* 1971;28:1278–1283.

96. Hoffman MS, Roberts WS, LaPolla JP, et al. Laser vaporization of grade 3 vaginal intra-epithelial neoplasia. *Am J Obstet Gynecol.* 1991;165:1342–1344.

97. Lenehan PM, Meffe F, Lickrish GM. Vaginal intraepithelial neoplasia: biologic aspects and management. *Obstet Gynecol.* 1986;68:333–337.

98. Wilkinson EJ, Friedrich EG. Diseases of the vulva. In Kurman RJ, ed. *Blaustein's Pathology of the Female Genital Tract.* New York: Springer-Verlag; 1987;36–96.

99. Friedrich EG, Wilkinson EJ, Yao SF. Carcinoma in situ of the vulva: A continuing challenge. *Am J Obstet Gynecol.* 1980;136:830–843.

100. Wilkinson EJ, Friedrich EG, Fu YS. Multicentric nature of vulvar carcinoma in situ. *Obstet Gynecol.* 1981;58:69–74.

101. Bernstein SG, Kovacs BR, Townsend DE, et al. Vulvar carcinoma in situ. *Obstet Gynecol.* 1983;61:304–307.

102. Collins RG, Roman-Lopez JJ, Lee FYL. Intraepithelial carcinoma of the vulva. *Am J Obstet Gynecol.* 1970;108:1187–1191.

103. Shafi MI, Luesley DM, Byrne P, et al. Vulvar intraepithelial neoplasia—management and outcome. *Br J Obstet Gynaecol.* 1989;96:1339–1344.

104. Ferenczy A. Intraepithelial neoplasia of the vulva. In: Coppleson M, ed. *Gynecologic Oncology—Fundamental Principles and Clinical Practice.* Edinburgh: Churchill Livingstone; 1992;443–463.

105. Chafe W, Ferguson K, Wilkinson EJ. Vulvar intraepithelial neoplasia (VIN): Principles of surgical therapy. *Colp Gynecol Laser Surg.* 1988;4:125–132.

106. Japaze H, Garcia-Buneul R, Woodruff JD. Primary vulvar neoplasia. *Obstet Gynecol.* 1977;49:404–411.

107. Jones RW, McClean MR. Carcinoma in situ of the vulva: A review of 31 treated and five untreated cases. *Obstet Gynecol.* 1986;68:499–503.

108. Wilkinson EJ, Rico MJ, Pierson KK. Microinvasive carcinoma of the vulva. *Int J Gynecol Pathol.* 1982;1:29–39.

109. Woodruff JD, Ulian C, Puray T, et al. The contemporary challenge of carcinoma in situ of the vulva. *Am J Obstet Gynecol.* 1973;115:677–686.

110. Buscema J, Woodruff JD, Parmley TH, et al. Carcinoma in situ of the vulva. *Obstet Gynecol.* 1980;55:225–230.

111. Forney JP, Morrow CP, Townsend DE, et al. Management of carcinoma in situ of the vulva. *Am J Obstet Gynecol.* 1977;127:801–806.

112. Parry-Jones E. The management of pre-malignant and malignant conditions of the vulva. *Clin Obstet Gynecol.* 1976;3:217–227.

113. Rutledge F, Sinclair M. Treatment of intraepithelial cancer of the vulva by skin excision and graft. *Am J Obstet Gynecol.* 1988;102:806–818.

114. Benedet JL, Murphy KJ. Squamous carcinoma in situ of the vulva. *Gynecol Oncol.* 1982;14:213–219.

115. Wolcott HD, Gallup DG. Wide local excision in the treatment of vulvar carcinoma in situ. *Am J Obstet Gynecol.* 1984;150:695–698.

116. Iversen T, Abeler V, Kolstad P. Squamous cell carcinoma in situ of the vulva. A clinical and histopathological study. *Gynecol Oncol.* 1981;11;224–229.

117. Bornstein J, Kaufman RH. Combination of surgical excision and CO_2 laser vaporization for multifocal vulvar intraepithelial neoplasia. *Am J Obstet Gynecol.* 1988;158:459–464.

118. Baggish MS, Dorsey JH. CO_2 laser for the treatment of vulvar carcinoma in situ. *Obstet Gynecol.* 1981;57:371–375.

119. Valentine BH. Outpatient laser therapy for vulvar intraepithelial neoplasia: A case report. *J Obstet Gynecol.* 1981;1:260–262.

120. Reid R. Superficial laser vulvectomy. A new surgical technique for appendage-conserving ablation of refractory condylomas and vulvar intraepithelial neoplasia. *Am J Obstet Gynecol.* 1985;152:504–509.

121. Shatz P, Bergeron C, Wilkinson E, et al. Vulvar intraepithelial neoplasia and skin appendage involvement. *Obstet Gynecol.* 1989;74:769–774.

122. Rader JS, Leake JF, Dillon MB, et al. Ultrasonic surgical aspiration in the treatment of vulvar disease. *Obstet Gynecol.* 1991;77:575–576.

123. Carson TE, Hoskins WJ, Wurzel JF. Topical 5-fluorouracil in the treatment of carcinoma in-situ of the vulva. *Obstet Gynecol.* 1976;47(suppl):59–62.

124. Krupp PJ, Bohm JW. 5-Fluorouracil topical treatment of in situ vulvar cancer. A preliminary report. *Obstet Gynecol.* 1978;51:702–706.

125. Ferenczy A. Laser treatment of patients with condylomata and squamous carcinoma precursors of the lower genital tract. *Cancer.* 1987;50:334–347.

126. Paget J. On disease of the mammary areola preceding cancer of the mammary gland. *St. Bartholomew's Hosp Rep.* 1874;10:87–89.

127. Dubreuilh W. Paget's disease of the vulva. *Br J Dermatol.* 1901;13:407–428.

128. Beecham CT. Paget's disease of the vulva. *Obstet Gynecol.* 1976;47(suppl):61–67.

129. Breen JL, Smith CI, Gregori CA. Extramammary Paget's disease. *Clin Obstet Gynecol.* 1978;21:1107–1115.

130. Woodruff JD. Paget's disease of the vulva. *Obstet Gynecol.* 1955;5:175–185.

131. Boehm F, Morris JM. Paget's disease and apocrine gland carcinoma of the vulva. *Obstet Gynecol.* 1971;38:185–192.

132. Creasman WT, Gallagher HS, Rutledge F. Paget's disease of the vulva. *Gynecol Oncol.* 1975;3:133–148.

133. Hart WR, Millman JB. Progression of intraepithelial Paget's disease of the vulva to invasive carcinoma. *Cancer.* 1977;40:2333–2337.

134. Gunn RA, Gallager HS. Vulvar Paget's disease: A topographic study. *Cancer.* 1980;46:590–594.

135. Pierard J, Thiery M, Boddaert J, et al. Maladie de Paget de la vulve avec metastases viscerales. *Arch Belges Dermatol Syph.* 1958;14:87–94.

136. Lee SC, Roth LM, Ehrlich C, et al. Extramammary Paget's disease of the vulva. *Cancer.* 1977;39:2540–2549.

137. Chanda JJ. Extramammary Paget's disease: prognosis and relationship to internal malignancy. *J Am Acad Dermatol.* 1985;13:1009–1014.

138. Helwig EB, Graham JH. Anogenital (extramammary) Paget's disease. *Cancer.* 1963;16:387–403.

139. Fenn ME, Morley GW, Abell MR. Paget's disease of the vulva. *Obstet Gynecol.* 1971;38:660–670.

140. Kaufman RH, Boice EH, Knight WR. Paget's disease of the vulva. *Am J Obstet Gynecol.* 1960;79:451–454.

141. Friedrich EG, Wilkinson EJ, Steingraeber PH, et al. Paget's disease of the vulva and carcinoma of the breast. *Obstet Gynecol.* 1975;46:130–134.

142. Friedrich EG. Intraepithelial neoplasia of the vulva. In: Coppleson M, ed. *Gynecologic Oncology—Fundamental Principles and Clinical Practice.* New York: Churchill Livingstone; 1981:303.

143. Fetherston WC, Friedrich EG. The origin and significance of vulvar Paget's disease. *Obstet Gynecol.* 1972;39:735–744.

Management of Precancerous Lesions of the Endometrium in Postmenopausal Patients

Parviz Hanjani

Management of noninvasive, abnormal proliferations of the endometrium has always been a confusing subject for gynecologists because of the lack of objective criteria for reasonably precise identification of the degree and seriousness of these aberrations. Expressed differently, no uniform classification is supported by the majority of authorities in the field of pathology who, as the leading force, create the guidelines for the general pathologist to follow. As a result, practicing pathologists find themselves mired in a sea of multiple, variant classifications and the reports from them to the gynecologists and physicians treating the patient are, on most occasions, unclear and nondiagnostic. The ambiguity of these reports causes problems for the physician in charge, increasing the potential for mismanagement.

Abnormal endometrial proliferation is divided into noninvasive and invasive forms. This chapter discusses the noninvasive type. Terminologies and available classifications are reviewed, with recommendations for the most helpful identification, using histopathologic features, the natural history of the proliferative abnormality, and the potential for progress to endometrial cancer. Emphasis is placed on management relevant to the particular behavior of each lesion with reference to subsequent invasive potential in older patients.

CLASSIFICATION

A useful classification of abnormal proliferation of the endometrium for clinicians is one that histologically and clinically can be reproducible in multiple patients and will help clinicians decide the course of therapy, from observation only at one end of the spectrum through hormonal manipulation in the middle to hysterectomy at the other end. Such classification should help clinicians understand the difference between an abnormality with low risk of developing into cancer, which can be treated conservatively, and a high-grade lesion with the potential to progress and become malignant, obviously requiring a more aggressive approach. Definitive clarity and simplicity are imperative for clinicians at the front line managing this disease for them to select an appropriate course of therapy that will be adequate even if the final diagnosis shows a more serious lesion than the primary diagnosis. If clinicians understand in the simplest way the degree of potential for the endometrial lesion to develop into carcinoma, it will help them to communicate with the pathologist to receive the kind of report that is most helpful. The pathology report must be evaluated in conjunction with the presence or absence of influencing factors such as use of exogenous estrogen or the possible presence of an estrogen-producing ovarian lesion. Inherent in the analysis of the abnormality must be consideration of its aggressiveness, which may vary significantly from one patient to another. Thus, at times, a benign lesion under the microscope is best treated as though it were an early cancer. Good communication between pathologist and gynecologist is the single most important factor in initiating effective care.

A review of the literature of the past two decades on abnormal proliferation of the endometrium illustrates the confusion encountered by the inquisitive physician who can only be hopelessly frustrated by the endless variations in terminology that defy correlation to a rational approach treating endometrial disturbances. Different authors use the same or similar diagnostic terms but with different histologic criteria.[1,2] Accordingly, a uniform treatment plan cannot be applied to similar diagnostic terms because it will cause over- or undertreatment. Clinicians and pathologists in community hospitals are confused and unable to communicate, to understand, or to be practical in response to a diagnosis with so many different nomenclatures that even the authors do not agree with each other. In this chapter I will try to support a simple classification from a comprehensive review of the literature that will be consistently uniform and will correlate with expected outcomes of particular therapies. For clarification, initially I will discuss briefly some of the terms that have been used in describing premalignant lesions of the endometrium. In the past, Winkler and colleagues established the three benign histologic diagnoses of anovulatory persistent proliferative endometrium, cystic glandular hyperplasia, and adenomatous hyperplasia. Corresponding respectively with these diagnoses, the treatments have been observation only, hormonal therapy, and hysterectomy.[3] Winkler's fourth diagnostic category is cancer, and its therapy and follow-up, naturally, are quite different from the others. Clinicians are currently usually familiar with but not always understanding of nomenclature such as cystic hyperplasia, adenomatous hyperplasia, and adenomatous hyperplasia with atypia. Occasionally terms such as metaplasia and cystic atrophy appear in pathology reports and the nonplussed physician unwittingly and erroneously associates them with premalignancy. Neither has carcinogenic probability.

Cystic Hyperplasia

Cystic hyperplasia is characterized principally by focally dilated glands of varying size. The terms cystic glandular hyperplasia, simple hyperplasia, glandular hyperplasia, and endometrial hyperplasia are used synonymously. The glands in cystic hyperplasia may range from small, round, and regular to focally, cystically dilated ("Swiss cheese"), to moderately crowded and irregular in shape. There is proliferation of both glands and stroma. These glands may be lined by either tall, columnar, or cuboidal epithelium which may show mild stratification or some mitotic activity. This entity should be differentiated from endometrial polyps, chronic endometritis with glandular proliferation, cystic (senile) atrophy, and focal dilatation of glands which, on some occasions, is seen in normal proliferative and secretory endometrium. The cystic adenomatous lining is most commonly characterized by single layers of low cuboidal epithelium. "Swiss cheese hyperplasia" not only describes focal cystic endometrial overgrowth but sometimes refers to inactive flattened epithelium with cystic changes.[4] It has been suggested that this term be used exclusively for patients with totally inactive endometrium because these cystic changes can be seen to a limited extent in almost every endometrium of early menopausal women, where the designation becomes inactive endometrium with cystic changes.[4] Regardless of which term is used, cystic atrophy should be differentiated from hyperplastic endometrium because the former does not have any premalignant potential.

Adenomatous Hyperplasia

The term adenomatous hyperplasia is applied to vastly different patterns of proliferation of the endometrium by different experts to describe a more serious precursor of endometrial carcinoma. It may include at one extreme only minimal adenomatous overgrowth to extensive crowding of the glands with a thin rim of stroma at the other. Although occasionally some out-pouching of the gland can be seen in cystic hyperplasia, extensive crowding and out-pouching at the expense of stroma should be limited to adenomatous hyperplasia. Gusberg used this term to include all categories of hyperplasia of the endometrium beyond cystic hyperplasia.[5,6] He divided this process into mild, moderate, and severe forms. The latter corresponds with a pattern of hyperplasia that others call atypical hyperplasia. When the proliferation or crowding of glands is so great as to minimize intervening stroma, the descriptive term "back-to-back" enters the vernacular of the pathologist. The endometrium may be involved focally or diffusely. Hertig and colleagues describe glandular projections and budding in the surrounding stroma also as adenomatous hyperplasia.[7,8] In contrast, Buehl and coworkers restricted the term to endometrium with little or no cytologic atypia.[9] Adding to the confusion of descriptive terminology are such phrases, often obscure in themselves, as generalized glandular architectural atypia, crowding without cytologic atypia, the so-called finger-in-glove complex, serrated or papillary pattern, with and without cytologic atypia, budding, and confluent glandular formation. Faced with such an array of often intimidating and pseudoscientific jargon, it is no wonder that the conscientious gynecologist frequently is frightened into a path of surgical overtreatment "just to play it safe."

Atypical Hyperplasia

Despite extensive discussion in the scientific literature, uniform agreement as to what precisely constitutes atypical hyperplasia is still lacking. The term was first introduced by Novak and Rutledge, who described abnormal proliferation of the endometrium characterized by a large increase in the number of glands and minimal intervening stroma.[10] Their definition did not include nuclear atypia even though, in their descriptions, they mentioned the presence of large uniform nuclei. To Vellios, atypical hyperplasia meant an abnormal endometrium showing some degree of cellular atypia even though there was no glandular crowding.[11] Campbell and Barter used terminology similar to Novak and Rutledge to describe atypical hyperplasia but divided this abnormality into grades I, II, and III according to the degree of resemblance of the lesion to carcinoma of the endometrium.[12] Creasman and DiSaia defined cellular atypia in their description of adenomatous hyperplasia.[4] Some authors refer to atypical hyperplasia as an abnormally complex architectural pattern regardless of the degree of cytologic atypia.[10,12] Others use this term to describe endometria with cytologic atypia regardless of the extent of the pattern of architectural complexity.[1,13,14] Some authors will require both cytologic atypia and complex architectural pattern to classify hyperplasia as truly atypical.[14,15]

Carcinoma in situ of the Endometrium

Hertig reported on carcinoma in situ as a focal lesion of cytologic alterations without prominent glandular crowding.[15,16] His diagnosis was based on the presence of large glandular eosinophilic cells with abundant cytoplasm the nuclei of which were pale, contained small granular chromatin, and were irregular. This cytologic atypia was confined to the epithelium with no stromal invasion. Buehl and colleagues defined carcinoma in situ of the endometrium, or stage 0, as severe atypical adenomatous hyperplasia approaching cancer but confined to the endometrial glands.[9] The absence of stromal invasion was a key factor in limiting the definition. Welch and Scully used the term carcinoma in situ to describe a small focal lesion involving no more than five or six glands in which the cytologic feature of carcinoma was present and there was no evidence of invasion.[17] If these changes were extensive or the glands were crowded together to the point that stromal invasion could not be ruled out, a diagnosis of invasive carcinoma was made. The cumulative reports of a multitude of investigators lead to one clear conclusion: there is no precise dividing line between severe atypical hyperplasia of the endometrium and the lesion called adenocarcinoma in situ of the endometrium.

Without such distinction between late severe endometrial proliferation and in situ adenocarcinoma of the endometrium, this latter term serves no purpose in guiding the management of patients with severely atypical adenomatous hyperplasia of the endometrium. In fact, it causes confusion in regard to the therapeutic approach to this problem. The important factor is distinguishing between atypical proliferation of the endometrium without stromal invasion and frankly invasive adenocarcinoma that is well differentiated.

Metaplasia of the Endometrium

The replacement of glandular epithelium with a cell type not normally present in the endometrium is called metaplasia. This benign type of epithelial change may involve squamous, ciliary, and eosinophilic cells. Tubal surface syncytial patterns and papillary formations may be seen. Squamous metaplasia is the most frequently seen and may be associated with hyperplastic and carcinomatous endometrium but itself is benign. Sometimes it is found in an otherwise normal endometrium. These lesions by themselves do not share the criteria of atypical hyperplasia, and if present in the absence of hyperplasia or carcinoma, there is no particular clinical significance. Importantly, even though they are associated with hyperplasias and carcinomas, they do not seem to have any effect on the behavior of these lesions. These lesions, if present by themselves, must be differentiated from hyperplasia.

When we more thoroughly delineate terms such as cystic hyperplasia, adenomatous hyperplasia, atypical adenomatous hyperplasia, atypical hyperplasia,

TABLE 13-1 Abnormal Proliferation of Endometrium

Noninvasive
  Simple hyperplasia
  Complex hyperplasia
  Atypical hyperplasia
Invasive

adenocarcinoma in situ, and metaplasia, which have been in the literature for the past 20 to 25 years, we will similarly become enabled to use better directed uniform and appropriate management. A simplified classification corresponding with these entities will enable gynecologists and pathologists to communicate more easily within their own specialties and with each other. Management of patients afflicted with these benign entities can then be carried out universally with reasonably clear understanding of the potential for each of these lesions to develop into adenocarcinoma of the endometrium. At this point, I will now crystallize the discussion by presenting a classification formulated by a large group of prominent investigators in an attempt to achieve these goals of clarity and uniformity. Their conclusions have been endorsed by the Society of Gynecological Pathologists and recommended for communication and planning to the pathologist and the clinician.

Table 13-1 presents the classification proposed by the International Society of Gynecological Pathologists. In this classification, abnormal endometrial proliferations are divided into noninvasive and invasive according to the presence or absence of stromal invasion. Noninvasive proliferation of the endometrium is divided into simple hyperplasia, complex hyperplasia that is adenomatous hyperplasia without atypia, and atypical hyperplasia. Atypical hyperplasia included adenomatous or complex hyperplasia with atypia and any hyperplasia other than adenomatous hyperplasia that has cellular atypia.

The World Health Organization Committee on Endometrial Tumors has proposed a classification of endometrial hyperplasia that corresponds with the International Society of Gynecological Pathologists which is under the auspices of the World Health Organization. This latest classification categorized endometrial hyperplasia into four subtypes (Table 13-2): simple without atypicality, simple with atypicality, complex without atypicality, and complex with atypicality. The

TABLE 13-2 Categories of Endometrial Hyperplasia

Simple hyperplasia without cellular atypia
Simple hyperplasia with cellular atypia
Complex hyperplasia without cellular atypia
Complex hyperplasia with cellular atypia

TABLE 13-3 Classification Based on Presence or Absence of Cellular Atypia

Simple hyperplasia
Complex hyperplasia
Atypical hyperplasia

term complex or complexities refers to a severe architectural atypicality and the term atypicality refers to cellular atypicality with or without a complex architectural atypicality. These two classifications are similar in most respects, and we can create one classification that is simple for the pathologists and the gynecologists to use in deciding the management of patients with this abnormal proliferative process.

Although the classification in Table 13-3 seems similar to that of Table 13-1, the emphasis is placed primarily on the absence or presence of cellular atypia. Thus, the divisions are defined as simple hyperplasia (including cystic) without cellular atypia, complex hyperplasia without cellular atypia, and atypical hyperplasia in which the prominent feature is cytologic atypia. This latter category can be simple hyperplasia with cytologic atypia or complex hyperplasia with cytologic atypia.

Simple Hyperplasia Without Cytologic Atypia

The endometrium is thickened and its volume has increased by proliferation of both glands and stroma, more of gland than stroma. Glands are dilated and increased in number with some out-pouching and invagination causing an irregular outline to the enlarged gland.[1,15,18,19] These glands are scattered and surrounded by a significant amount of dense stroma. The crowding of the glands is minimal and is not back-to-back.[2,15,16,18–21] On gross examination of the endometrium, it appears thick and pale, but no characteristic findings suggest grossly the process of hyperplasia.[4,19] On curettage, even though the endometrium is hyperplastic and occasionally may produce a significant amount of tissue, in an older patient usually the tissue retrieved is scant and the hyperplastic areas are found not be extensive.[4]

Simple hyperplasia may be focal or diffuse and may coexist with metaplasias or any other endometrial proliferation.[2,18,19] Usually the glands are proliferative but small portions may show some secretory changes. In simple hyperplasia, even though the glands can be crowded and irregular in shape, a significant amount of stroma should be present. With minimal intervening stroma and significant irregular glandular out-pouching approaching "finger in glove," a diagnosis of complex hyperplasia should be made and this type should not be categorized as simple hyperplasia.[2,18,19,22]

Simple hyperplasia in an older woman should be distinguished from cystic atrophy or senile atrophy of the endometrium. In cystic atrophy of the endometrium, the epithelium is flattened and inactive and the glands are lined by single layers of low cuboidal cells without any of the features seen in proliferative glands. The stroma is generally inactive and atrophic. Stromal cells are usually without mitosis and little cytoplasm. Fibrosis may be present. This cystic atrophic or cystic dilatation of the glands of the endometrium is a more common feature in the endometrium of some normal menopausal women. Some degree of "Swiss cheese" morphology, more or less, can be seen in simple endometrial hyperplasia, cystic dilatation with hyperplasia, inactive endometrium, or senile endometrial atrophy. The endometrium in these cases is not hyperplastic but thin and atrophic. It appears that it will be better if this term is dropped altogether or used only for atrophic endometrium with cystic changes.[4] Endometrial polyps are distinguished not only by a polypoid configuration but by large, thick-walled blood vessels and the presence of fibrosis in the stroma.[2,18,19,23]

Because this book deals only with postmenopausal patients, distinguishing simple hyperplasia from endometritis and normal proliferative endometrium will not be discussed and the reader is referred to extensive literature written on these subjects.

In summary, then, simple hyperplasia without atypia describes and includes all the terms such as cystic glandular hyperplasia, glandular hyperplasia, and simple glandular hyperplasia when no cytologic atypia is present.

Complex Hyperplasia Without Cytologic Atypia

Complex hyperplasia without cytologic atypia is a term that describes a process of generalized complex glandular crowding and irregular glandular borders, separated from each other only by thin rims of stroma (architectural atypia). No cytologic atypia is present. Silverberg describes this as follows: "Extensive finger-in-glove serrated or papillary appearance justifies a diagnosis of complex hyperplasia as does the finding of glands that are extensively crowding out the intervening stroma."[18,19] Corresponding to Silverberg's description Kurman and colleagues categorize this crowding as "back-to-back" showing architecturally packed complex glands that are separated from each other by narrow bands of stroma.[15,16] Silverberg uses the term "back-to-back" to describe glandular proliferation without intervening stroma corresponding to the description by Kurman and associates of a confluent glandular pattern. There is no cytologic atypicality, but the cells are columnar with elongated nuclei and varying degrees of mitotic activity. Epithelial pseudostratification may range from two to four cell layers in some of the glands. The presence of back-to-back glands, less stroma, and intraluminal papillae distinguishes this complex hyperplasia without cellular atypia from simple hyperplasia with no atypia. Differential diagnosis in younger perimenopausal patients will include late proliferative and disorder proliferative endometrium as well as well-differentiated very early adenocarcinoma. In a postmenopausal patient, well-differentiated adenocarcinoma must be distinguished from very complex hyperplasia with minimal or no intervening stroma. When there is no intervening stroma in association with a confluent type of glandular structure, it may be difficult to separate this very complex hyperplasia from early well-differentiated adenocarcinoma. It should be reported by the pathologist to the clinician as possible well-differentiated adenocarcinoma to prevent any undertreatment.[1,8,15,16,18,19,24,25]

The terms complex hyperplasia without cellular atypia, adenomatous hyperplasia without cellular atypia, and complex glandular hyperplasia without cellular atypia are all used to describe the above lesion and they all should be treated as such. To prevent confusion, this nomenclature should not be used to describe lesser lesions. In summary, this terminology includes all lesions that have architectural atypia of varying degrees of severity lacking any cellular atypia.

Atypical Hyperplasia

All lesions with hyperplastic glandular changes that feature cellular atypia are classified as atypical hyperplasia. The cellular aberrations distinguish this group from simple hyperplasia and complex hyperplasia. The cells are enlarged, polarity is lost, and the nuclear-to-cytoplasmic ratio is increased. Nuclear membranes are thickened and irregular in size and shape, nuclei are prominent and a coarse chromatin texture and clumping is present.[1,15,16,18,19,21,26] Stratification can be significant or negligible, mitotic activity can be conspicuous or insignificant, and the degree of atypia can range from minimal to marked. Severe atypical hyperplasia with extensive architectural and cytologic atypia is not easily distinguishable from carcinoma. When such questions exist, the pathologists's report to the clinician should include the question of malignancy. Atypical hyperplasia usually involves some endometrial glands but not the entire endometrium.[18,19,22] Although multiple endometrial sites may be afflicted, the areas are separated from each other by either normal, atrophic, or sometimes simple or complex hyperplasia without cellular atypia. Foci with cytologic atypia may involve bands of simple or complex hyperplasia or both.[18,19] The stratification of the glands is not artefact and the features seen in these patients are not seen usually in patients with simple or complex hyperplasia without atypia.[23]

Reactive atypia constitutes focal changes in glands after mechanical trauma, such as diagnostic curettage, or after radiation. It should be differentiated from atypical hyperplasia by the rather simple glands lined with single layers of cells without any stratification.[18,19]

In summary, atypical hyperplasia, practically speaking, includes a spectrum of lesions ranging from simple hyperplasia with cellular atypia through minimal complex hyperplasia with cellular atypia to highly complex hyperplasia with extensive architectural and cytologic atypia. Currently carcinoma-in-situ is categorized together with severely atypical hyperplasia. Any attempt to separate the two is purely academic and serves no practical purpose because the treatment is the same for both. The term adenomatous hyperplasia with atypia is superfluous because such a title is just another to cover the same lesions already described. To avoid confusion, it should not be used, even though it is still popular.

FACTORS IN MANAGEMENT DETERMINATION OF ENDOMETRIAL HYPERPLASIA

Correct choices in the treatment of hyperplasia of the endometrium depend on the following two factors: (1) distinction between the severe form of typical endometrial hyperplasia and the least advanced cancer (well-differentiated adenocarcinoma) and understanding the importance of this distinction in regard to the statistical effect on prognosis, and (2) the significance of hyperplasia as a premalignant lesion of the endometrium and the statistical incidence of progression to adenocarcinoma.

Criteria to Distinguish Atypical Hyperplasia from Carcinoma

Responsibility for correct clinical management rests almost entirely on the decisive pathologic distinction of a benign precancerous lesion without significant risk from a lesion with the potential for myometrial invasion and metastasis leading to death. In this diagnostic range, more specifically, the knowledgeable physician must not overtreat the former or undertreat the latter.

Several authors have described their own criteria to differentiate between the most severe type of atypical hyperplasia and well-differentiated adenocarcinoma of the endometrium.[1,15,16,18,19] The standards of Kurman and Norris have more reproducibility and thus, acceptance, than all others. Objectively speaking, if pathologists generally were to use these criteria, with minimal modification, in most cases they will accurately separate that group of patients with the higher risk of invasion and metastasis from precancerous lesions of much lower potential for this grave change.[1,15,16] This information is vitally important because the curettage specimen usually gives no indication of whether or not myometrial extension of the tumor already exists.

Kurman and Norris recommended the use of stromal invasion as the criterion of malignancy. To identify these patients, these investigators, using stromal interaction with invasive carcinoma, came up with four principles, each of which may identify stromal invasion in curetted specimens. They classify them as follows:

1. Desmoplastic response, an irregular infiltration of the gland associated with an altered fibroplastic stroma (fibrose stroma).

2. Cribriform pattern, a confluent complex glandular pattern with each individual gland merging into each other without any intervening stroma, and some bridging of the epithelium from one gland to another. (The cribriform pattern must occupy at least half of a low power field of 4.2 mm in diameter).

3. Excessive complex papillary patterns with branching and fibrose processes involving at least half of the low power field.

4. Masses of squamous epithelium replacing gland and stroma forming a solid sheet at least through half of a low power field.

Silverberg, while agreeing with these criteria for predictable stromal invasion, does not accept benign squamous epithelial masses replacing the stroma as a criterion of carcinoma, but he does believe that any quantity of these four patterns of Kurman and Norris, which correspond with stromal invasion, can predict the likelihood of myometrial invasion.[18] The absence of these standards clearly does not deny the possibility of invasion but certainly makes it much less likely. However, adherence to these criteria as suggestive of stromal invasion will help the pathologist to report to the clinician a presumptive diagnosis that will guide the practitioner toward adequate therapy. Basically, the prognostic value of this information guards against undertreatment. Without the presence of these criteria, when simple hysterectomy was performed, 15% to 17% of the uteri were found to contain carcinoma.[1,16,27] All patients in one of these studies and most of the patients in another revealed carcinoma confined to the endometrium or only superficially involving the myometrium. Simple hysterectomy was adequate treatment. When stromal invasion was predicted, according to the standards of Kurman and Norris, residual carcinoma was found in 50% of the patients. In this group, 24% had moderately to poorly differentiated tumor and 34% had deep myometrial invasion. This suggests that use of these criteria may differentiate between the lesion for which the treatment is limited to preventive measures (i.e., simple hysterectomy) and the lesion that needs to be treated as cancer (i.e., extensive node sampling). Thus, it seems reasonable to use the Kurman criteria in defining stromal invasion to help the clinician plan appropriate management. Interpreting more completely, the general gynecologist can manage the cases of premalignancy, including those formerly called carcinoma in situ, by total hysterectomy, whereas those with more ominous prognosis should be handled by the gynecologic oncologist with extreme extirpative surgery and ancillary measures.

Benign Hyperplasia of the Endometrium as a Premalignant Lesion of the Endometrium

Certain studies have suggested that endometrial tumors are divided into two different types with dissimilar pathogenesis. One type usually associated with endometrial hyperplasia is generally well differentiated with better prognosis. This subset of cases are relatively young women with exogenous or endogenous excess estrogen. The second group includes those who do not show hyperestrogenism and obviously a different unexplained mechanism of carcinogenesis is operating. In this array, the setting is considerably more somber and the prognosis is usually unfavorable.[1,13,28]

The implication of these observations suggests no relationship to hyperplasia in the latter subset. However, the probability of progression from hyperplasia to cancer, initially catalyzed by estrogen, has been a matter of much debate and controversy because the precise degree of premalignant potential of hyperplasia has never been clearly defined. It has been strongly suggested that hyperplasia and carcinoma represents a continuum and that all these carcinomas arise from benign hyperplasia. If a simple hyperplasia progresses to a malignant lesion, it will only happen after passing through the stages of complex and atypical hyperplasia. Evidence supporting hyperplasia as a premalignant lesion comes from the following observations:

1. Presence of endometrial hyperplasia in uteri removed for carcinoma.
2. Presence of hyperplasia in the previous biopsy of the patient later diagnosed to have endometrial carcinoma.
3. Prospective study of following patients with known endometrial hyperplasia later found to have endometrial carcinoma.

The last of these three observations is the most convincing. Gusberg and Kaplan reported 12% of adenomatous hyperplasia progressed to carcinoma between 18 months and 9 years.[6] Wentz reported 27% adenomatous hyperplasia advanced to carcinoma within 2 to 8 years.[29,30] When the diagnosis was atypical adenomatous hyperplasia, 82% evolved into cancer. Chamlin and Taylor reported a 14% progression within 1 to 14 years.[31] Sherman and Brown reported a 10% progression for cystic hyperplasia, 22% for adenomatous hyperplasia, and 57% for atypical adenomatous hyperplasia within 2 to 18 years.[32] Kurman reported a simple hyperplasia continuation rate of 1% within 1 to 26.7 years, whereas complex hyperplasia progressed to malignancy in 3%, simple atypical hyperplasia in 8%, and complex atypical hyperplasia in 29%. From the review of this literature it is apparent that all hyperplasias have some potential to progress to malignancy. Thus, the practitioner is hard put ever to accept observation only as opposed to some form of definitive treatment, principally hysterectomy.

CLINICAL MANAGEMENT OF ENDOMETRIAL HYPERPLASIA

In treating patients with endometrial hyperplasia or noninvasive endometrial proliferation, certain factors must be considered. Not to be forgotten or ignored is the patient herself. Her age and her general medical condition play distinct roles in decision-making. The family history and the patient's own trepidations must be respected. She may fear the potential for cancer, but she may dread surgery even more. A sick husband or parent may demand her attention and move her to opt for observation at least temporarily. The desire to continue estrogen replacement therapy may dictate an immediate recourse to hysterectomy. What may have happened to friends or relatives in similar or seemingly similar circumstances can act as a profound influence on the patient's choice of direction. Whatever the situation, in no other setting will the practitioner ever be called on more to exercise skill in the art of medicine. Thorough discussion and ample explanation with the patient by the doctor, not an aide, is not only considerate and humane, it is mandatory. It is most desirable to have relatives present and most certainly the doctors should document the discussion, using quotes of the patient liberally. The keynote of all such consultation, all things considered, is sound advice in the very best judgment of the practitioner.

In no way can the clinician proceed with consultation with any patient without first having available all necessary pathologic information. Is the diagnosis based only on the finding of endometrial cells, normal or abnormal, coincidental with a Pap smear? Was the patient subjected only to an endometrial biopsy or washings in incidences of abnormal bleeding to satisfy a diagnosis? In essence, in any given case, have adequately reliable diagnostic studies been performed so that the responsible physician, the one who will ultimately prescribe the particular course of treatment, can be as confident as possible that he or she is giving the best advice to the patient and her family? More bluntly stated, underreporting, either from inadequate sampling or careless interpretation, of potentially serious or serious lesions, may lead to disaster.[33]

Most commonly, trouble is initially signaled by abnormal bleeding in the perimenopausal, menopausal, or postmenopausal woman. Occasionally discovery may begin with the inadvertent finding of endometrial cells in the Pap smear taken at a regular checkup. Optimal surveillance is obligatory in the patient who, for one reason or another, is being carried on unopposed estrogen replacement therapy. Although common practice today commands combination of exogenous estrogen with sufficient progesterone in opposition to negate its proven carcinogenic property, a significant number of cases are not so covered. In these instances, some kind of periodic endometrial sampling, to detect hyperplasia in its earliest phase, well before manifest bleeding occurs, is a stringent requirement. Even those patients on adequate combined hormonal replacement therapy, when bleeding occurs at noncyclical or unexpected times, should be given immediate attention via special sampling.

Obtaining an initial specimen when suspicion calls for it may be easily accomplished in an outpatient setting. This can be done by obtaining endometrial aspirations, washings or scrapings using such instruments as the vibra-aspirator, the Novak endometrial curette, or a form of suction pipette (pipelle). However, office procedures which give only cytology evaluation are often not specific enough in identifying the degree of endometrial hyperplasia.[33] When accuracy is in question, especially if the presenting symptom is bleeding, and endometrial sampling reveals anything less than malignancy, a dilatation and curettage (D. and C.), with or without hysteroscopy, *must* be performed.

The threat or underdiagnosis cannot be emphasized enough. The D. and C., when indicated, cannot be ignored on the basis of inconvenience, discomfort, or cost since diagnostic accuracy is so vital. Also, it has been proven that even a D. and C. not infrequently is inadequate for accuracy (see Chapter 15) and that combining it with hysteroscopy increases diagnostic precision.

Although there may be disagreement as to the degree of malignant probability, little controversy exists about premalignant potential of some degree at any level of endometrial hyperplasia. The age of the woman at the time of diagnosis of hyperplasia has a significant effect because, in a woman less than 40 years of age, hyperplasia usually is self-limiting and the incidence of progression to malignancy is lower.[34] Also, the interval from progression of hyperplasia to malignancy is longer. In one typical study in women under age 40, with severe atypical hyperplasia in the curettings, the incidence of true carcinoma was low, involving only 2 of 17 patients. Both had well-differentiated disease confined to the endometrium.[35] The incidence of carcinoma in excised uteri under similar circumstances is much higher in patients older than 40 years and especially higher in women over 50 years of age. Thus, as women grow older, a higher incidence of progression of hyperplasia to malignancy occurs and the interval from the time of diagnosis of hyperplasia to one of malignancy is shorter. Also, there is a much higher coincidence of association of hyperplasia, especially atypical hyperplasia, with endometrial cancer in the hysterectomy specimen.[16]

In the suggested classification using cytologic and architectural abnormalities to describe hyperplasia, the incidence of progression to carcinoma is very low, less than 2%, when hyperplasia is classified as simple. For architecturally complex hyperplasia, this incidence is about 3%. Simple hyperplasia with cytologic atypia will have about an 8% chance of progressing to malignancy, and in complex hyperplasia with cytologic atypia, about 29%. As might be expected, the transition time of hyperplasia to carcinoma is much longer for simple hyperplasia than for atypical or complex atypical hyperplasia, i.e., 10 years and 4 years, respectively.[16]

Several reports have given figures of 17% to 25% presence of carcinoma in excised uteri in patients who were diagnosed to have atypical hyperplasia in curettings.[1,3,6–8,15,22,25,27,28,32,36–46] These procedures were done within a month of curettage and all patients had well-differentiated carcinoma. On the other hand, consider a major series of studies of long-term follow-up showing that only 11% to 23% of women with atypical hyperplasia will develop carcinoma if a hysterectomy is not done.[1,6–8,15,25,28,36–42] This suggests that these lesions usually are slow growing and are stable for a long period. One point that should be kept in mind is the fact that in all these investigations usually a very severe degree of atypical hyperplasia was chosen as the indication for hysterectomy. Cases of lesser degree were followed with conservative management, and the final figure of the incidence of progression is affected by this factor. However, there is no question that carcinoma found in extirpated uteri in which prior curetting revealed atypical hyperplasia is well differentiated and rarely invades the myometrium. Tavasolli and Kraus reported carcinoma in 25%, or 12 of 48 uteri removed after a diagnosis of a typical hyperplasia but only one of these patients had minimal myometrial invasion.[23] Kurman and Norris reported 17%, or 15 of 89 cases of coincidental carcinoma in which the prehysterectomy diagnosis had been atypical hyperplasia.[1,15] Even though 8 of these patients had carcinoma confined to the endometrium and the rest revealed myometrial invasion, it was confined in each case to the inner third of the uterine wall. A study from 1937 reported a 2.4% progression of hyperplasia to carcinoma in premenopausal patients and 11% in postmenopausal patients.[47] In one of the early studies a figure of tenfold risk for postmenopausal women with hyperplasia was discussed.[48] In another study a 3% risk for premenopausal and 25% risk for postmenopausal patients was given.[49] Wentz reported detailed data on patients with all classifications of complex hyperplasia and atypia showing a significant number of patients with adenomatous hyperplasia and atypical hyperplasia progressing to invasive cancer in 2 to 8 years.[29,30] An investigation by Sherman following patients for 2 to 15 years showed a high rate of subsequent carcinoma and very low rate, about 20%, regression to a benign stage without treatment.[32] Kurman's study of 170 patients with all grades of endometrial hyperplasia with a follow-up of 1 to 26.7 years, using new classifications, revealed that simple hyperplasia, previously called cystic hyperplasia, has a very low rate of progression to malignancy.[15] However, as the degree of cellular and architectural atypia increases, the incidence of progression to malignancy increases. From all these data and so much more for which we have no space, it is clear that some patients with atypical hyperplasia will have associated carcinoma that is undiagnosed via endometrial sampling. Regardless of whether these lesions are slow growing or confined, they need to be treated vigorously to prevent death from this disease. Because these lesions generally will be well differentiated and confined to the endometrium only, there is no necessity for advance studies and sophisticated staging. With this type of lesion, total hysterectomy will offer a very good prognosis. The patient will not have been undertreated. Also, in view of all these data, even with the low rate of progression in the more simple types of hyperplasia, all things considered, hysterectomy today cannot be considered overtreatment. Present research continues in the development of more sophisticated methods to help in evaluating the degree of risk of progression to malignancy, such as DNA measurements, roles of estrogen and progesterone receptors, and plasminogen activators as catalysts.

Although this publication centers on the older woman and the elderly, the substance of this chapter must adjunctively include a discussion of endometrial hyperplasia in the premenopausal woman, particularly if she is under 40 years of age. If hysterectomy is the choice of treatment of both patient and doctor, then further discussion is obviated. However, for a variety of reasons, not the least of which may be retention of fertility, the patient may desire a nonsurgical channel of therapy, in which case a uterus of known disease implication may be carried into the postmenopausal state. At that time a new set of problems must be faced, particularly if she will desire estrogen replacement therapy at that stage of life.

If this younger patient presents simple hyperplasia with no atypia and no complex facets, simultaneously ruling out any source of estrogen overstimulation, she has a very low risk of progression to carcinoma. Once a dilatation and curettage has been performed to rule out atypia, depending on the circumstances, timely administration of progesterone can produce a thorough chemical curettage. This can then be followed by a series of estrogen-progesterone cycles similar to a birth control program. In nonsmoking women, a regimen such as this can be carried on safely in continuous or interrupted fashion to the age of 50 years or even beyond. Safety is contingent on periodic checks of the endometrium via simple outpatient sampling techniques such as afforded by the suction pipette (pipelle). When objective evidence of hyperplasia cannot be demonstrated, if the patient is capable of ovulation, conception may be attempted, because this goal is the primary reason for the delay in resorting to more definitive surgical therapy for cure in this preclimacteric age group. Because endometrial overgrowth may only be suppressed but not cured by cyclical combined hormone therapy, once it is stopped, militant vigilance is vital.

In patients aged 40 and younger who demonstrate more complex histologic changes, including atypia, as discovered when abnormal bleeding has occasioned endometrial retrieval for one form or another, nonsurgical management presents a greater challenge. If the desire for childbearing is compelling enough, profound hormonal suppression is advised for at least 3 to 4 months. Then thorough resampling of the endometrium must be performed. If the hyperplastic process has been objectively eliminated, attempts at conception should be made at once. When pregnancy is successful, one should delay minimally after its conclusion before periodic sampling begins anew. At the slightest signal of reversion to abnormality, either cellular or architectural, the patient is well advised to undergo hysterectomy without delay.

If on the other hand the intensive exogenous endocrine suppression proves inadequate in controlling the hyperplasia after 3 to 4 months, especially if there is any other indication that the patient is prone to endometrial cancer, further postponement of uterine extrication is assuredly imprudent.

Because it has been proven that potential for progression to cancer increases significantly with each successive decade regardless of the level of disease at the time of first discovery, the patient in the 40 to 49 age group is in greater jeopardy than one under age 40. Similarly a woman over age 50 is even more susceptible. Thus, the older the patient, the more insistent should be the urge for hysterectomy at the earliest reasonable time after discovery of hyperplasia of any significance.

However, when there exists a profound medical infirmity of cardiovascular, pulmonary, renal, or metabolic origin that poses a greater surgical risk than the consequences of endometrial hyperplasia, if left alone, then certainly a pharmacologic route of therapy would seem propitious. Logically the older the patient or the more advanced the lesion, the more intensively should such a course be pursued, and the earlier, the better. Heavy doses (200 to 400 mg) of depot progesterone administered intramuscularly and repeatedly over a long period of time, to produce an atrophic endometrium, have been effective in suppressing not only endometrial hyperplasia but also extremely early well-differentiated endometrial cancer. With relevance to earlier sections of this chapter, it must be remembered that 50% to 60% of cases of atypical hyperplasia will regress after a curettage or hormonal therapy, but a significant number of these will retain persistent disease, some of which will progress to malignancy eventually. Our major problem in this regard, at the present time, is lack of knowledge and methods of detection to delineate which patients will have the potential toward cancer and which ones will not. Thus, we must treat all patients today as though they have some risk of developing endometrial carcinoma with the understanding that the majority will not become so afflicted. Again, the patient and, when available, her family must be fully informed, especially when severe medical conditions preclude surgery.

Treatment by different methods of irradiation leaves the patient with additional options but that subject is not within the province of this book.

In conclusion, although there remains a margin for conservative therapy in young people when the diagnosis is endometrial hyperplasia, postmenopausal women currently are best served by hysterectomy.

EDITORIAL COMMENTS

Marvin H. Terry Grody

Over many decades, the traditional dilatation and curettage, especially if fractionated by including endocervical scrapings as a separate specimen, has been the "old reliable" standard as the most precise method for diagnosis in the case of abnormal endometrium. Whenever there has been a question of inadequacy, gynecologists automatically have resorted to it, either as in recent years in an out-patient setting under paracervical block, or under more old-fashioned methods of general anesthesia in the hospital when preferred.

Yet the "blind" dilatation and curettage has come under intense criticism in multiple studies as being capable at best of only clearing 30% to 40% of the endometrial surface, even when engineered by expert hands. Because of this shortcoming, foci of hyperplasia can be bypassed in otherwise normal endometrium, or atypical and more ominous centers of endometrial activity can similarly be missed in a bed of hyperplasia far less threatening. The answer to this critical dilemma is the hysteroscope. Authorities today universally agree that the new dimension afforded by hysteroscopy in enabling the trained eye to spot definitively the most atypically active endometrial areas gives us superbly accurate detective capability. Curetting under such visual guidance, thereby retrieving specimens from the most suspicious points, ensures maximum diagnostic dependability, assuming correct microscopic interpretation (see Chapter 15). Thus, the door of confidence is opened to the practitioner who now can choose the best available course of management for that particular patient.

Almost automatically today's gynecologist, in the face of all the material presented thus far, almost certainly, in every case of endometrial hyperplasia of any degree of atypia, be it cellular or architectural, excluding purely cystic hyperplasia, will strongly consider hysterectomy as the best treatment option. The argument behind such a recommendation lies squarely on the accepted potential for malignant development or possible already coexistent early malignancy. Unquestionably the current very low surgical risk of hysterectomy, either abdominal or vaginal, helps to motivate such a decision. Perhaps equally important, by choice of surgery over all other options, one eliminates ongoing uncertainty and fear. Also removed are the tedium and discomfort and expense of periodically repeated tests, some of which will be invasive, all of which are a serious burden to both patient and doctor. Yet however strong or seemingly logical the operative inclination, the gynecologic surgeon should be thoroughly cognizant of all the related facts in the further chronology of this peculiar entity known as endometrial hyperplasia as revealed in a wealth of accumulated authoritative literature. So, without any substantial criticism, hysterectomy, considered aggressive in one light but conservative and thorough in another, is the primary choice of therapy for hyperplasia, a benign disease that can become deadly if left alone. The ultimate evidence in support of such a decision should be firmly etched within the cognizance of the clinical gynecologist who remains abreast of current established standards.

Because hysterectomy is the preferred method of treatment of hyperplasia, a brief digression on the route of hysterectomy is in order. In general, as discussed in Chapter 4, when reasonable, the vaginal route is preferable, particularly in older women who tolerate surgery so much better from below than from above. However, many practitioners will always insist that the abdominal route is best as the only way for absolute assurance of concomitant oophorectomy. Certainly no argument can be presented denying the crucial necessity of simultaneous bilateral ovarian removal, especially if there exists any suspicion of an associated functioning ovarian growth such as granulosa cell tumor.

As already discussed earlier in this book, almost without exception in women other than the very aged, ovarian retrieval accompanying vaginal hysterectomy is no problem for the trained gynecologic surgeon. Unfortunately, almost all younger gynecologic oncologists today have left behind any skills in vaginal hysterectomy and oophorectomy that they may have developed during their primary residency training. As a result, their thinking is channeled only toward the abdominal route from which they can always not only assuredly remove both ovaries but, as they insist, always examine the lymph nodes of uterine drainage and take peritoneal washings. As presented earlier in this chapter, if hyperplasia has unknowingly progressed to true cancer, it is practically always well differentiated and well confined. Thus, hysterectomy in itself, without peritoneal washings and node inspection, is quite satisfactory treatment, an argument favoring the vaginal approach when not mechanically prohibited.

However, suppose an ovarian tumor significantly enlarged beyond the limits of the average normal ovary is palpated on preoperative examination. Here intelligence dictates the suprapubic route. There is also no debate in this matter if manual examination is deemed inadequate and more objective methods of ovarian depiction display an adnexal enlargement sufficient enough to jeopardize mechanical extirpation vaginally. Such visualization can be mediated via ultrasonography, computed tomography scans, or magnetic resonance imaging. These diagnostic methods might also, in cases of extreme cellular and architectural atypia, render clues pertinent to undetected malignant change with early invasion, but these methods are not recommended as a routine, they are not cost effective, and regular usage could hardly even be termed academic.

Another diagnostic method, easily administered, for use as an adjunctive determinant in choice of approach, is laparoscopy. A quick intra-abdominal diagnostic scan immediately after the patient is anesthetized can be most effectively informative in immediate decision-making at the time of the operation itself. An expanded in Chapter 15, consideration of laparoscopy as a diagnostic aid probably is not included often enough in our planning strategy. In the situation under discussion, using intra-abdominal endoscopy initially, in moments one can analyze the peritoneal surface, measure ovarian size, and judge ovarian mobility and availability for vaginal extirpation accessibility. Removal of the ovaries in the realm of treatment of endometrial hyperplasia as a separate procedure through the laparoscope is not a recommendation of any of the authors of this book.

REFERENCES

1. Kurman RJ, Norris HJ. Endometrial neoplasia: Hyperplasia and carcinoma. In Blaustein A, ed. *Pathology of the Female Genital Tract.* 2d ed. New York: Springer-Verlag; 1982;311–351.

2. Silverberg SG, Makowski EL, Roche WD. Endometrial carcinoma in women under 40 years of age. Comparison of cases in oral contraceptive users and non-users. *Cancer.* 1977;39:592–598.

3. Winkler B, Alvarez S, Richart RM, Crum CP. Pitfalls in the diagnosis of endometrial neoplasia. *Obstet Gynecol.* 1984;64:185–194.

4. DiSaia P, Creasman W. *Endometrial Hyperplasia, Clinical Gynecologic Oncology.* 4th ed. St. Louis: Year Book 1993:133.

5. Gusberg SB. The individual at high risk for endometrial carcinoma. *Am J Obstet Gynecol.* 1976;126:535–541.

6. Gusberg SB, Kaplan AL. Precursors of corpus cancer. IV. Adenomatous hyperplasia as stage 0 carcinoma of the endometrium. *Am J Obstet Gynecol.* 1963;87:662–678.

7. Hertig AT, Sommers SC, Bengloff H. Genesis of endometrial carcinoma. III. Carcinoma in-situ. *Cancer.* 1949;2:964–971.

8. Hertig AT, Sommers SC, Bengloff H. Genesis of endometrial carcinoma. I. Study of prior biopsies. *Cancer.* 1949;2:946–956.

9. Buehl IA, Vellios F, Carter JE, Huber CP. Carcinoma in situ of the endometrium. *Am J Clin Pathol.* 1964;42:594–598.

10. Novak E, Rutledge F. Atypical ndometrial hyperplasia simulating adenocarcinoma. *Am J Obstet Gynecol.* 1948;55:46–51.

11. Velios F. Endometrial hyperplasias, precursors of endometrial carcinoma. *Pathol Annu.* 1972;7:201–229.

12. Campbell PE, Barter RA. The significance of atypical endometrial hyperplasia. *J Obstet Gynaecol Br Commw.* 1961;68:668–672.

13. Bokhman JV. Two pathogenic types of endometrial carcinoma. *Gynecol Oncol.* 1983;15:10–14.

14. Kraus FT. High risk and premalignant lesions of the endometrium. *Am J Surg Pathol.* 1985;9(3):(suppl):31–37.

15. Kurman JR, Kaminski PF, Norris HJ. The behavior of endometrial hyperplasia. A long-term study of untreated hyperplasia in 170 patients. *Cancer.* 1985;56:403–412.

16. Kurman RJ, Norris HJ. Evaluation of criteria for distinguishing atypical endometrial hyperplasia from well-differentiated carcinoma. *Cancer.* 1982;49:2547–2559.

17. Welch WR, Scully RE. Precancerous lesions of the endometrium. *Hum Pathol.* 1977;8:503–508.

18. Silverberg SG. Hyperplasia and carcinoma of endometrium. *Semin Diagn Pathol.* 1988;5:135–153.

19. Silverberg SG. New aspects of endometrial carcinoma. *Clin Obstet Gynaecol.* 1984;11:189–208.

20. Kurman RJ, Norris HJ, Hendrickson MR, et al. Endometrial stromal invasion in the diagnosis of well-differentiated carcinoma. *Am J Surg Pathol.* 1984;8:719–720.

21. Norris HJ, Tavasolli FA, Kurman RJ. Endometrial hyperplasia and carcinoma. Diagnostic considerations. *Am J Surg Pathol.* 1983;7:839–847.

22. Fox H. The endometrial hyperplasias. *Obstet Gynecol Annu.* 1984;13:197–209.

23. Tavasolli FA, Kraus FT. Endometrial lesions in uteri resected for atypical endometrial hyperplasia. *Am J Clin Pathol.* 1978;70:770–775.

24. Beutler HK, Dockerty MB, Randall LM. Precancerous lesions of the endometrium. *Am J Obstet Gynecol.* 1963;86:433–443.

25. Kurman RJ. Endometrial hyperplasia and its relationship to certain types of carcinoma. In: *Surgery in the Treatment of Gynecologic Cancer.* Proceedings of the International Symposium. Antwerp: University Press; 1988: Sept 30-Oct 1:11.

26. Norris HJ, Connor MP, Kurman RJ. Preinvasive lesions of the endometrium. *Clin Obstet Gynecol.* 1986;13:725.

27. King A, Seraj IM, Wagner RJ. Stromal invasion in endometrial adenocarcinoma. *Am J Obstet Gynecol.* 1984;149:10–14.

28. Koss LG, Schreiber K, Oberlander SG, et al. Detection of endometrial carcinoma and hyperplasia in asymptomatic women. *Obstet Gynecol.* 1984;64:1–11.

29. Wentz WB. Effect of a progestational agent on endometrial hyperplasia and endometrial cancer. *Obstet Gynecol.* 1964;24:370–376.

30. Wentz WB. Progestin therapy in endometrial hyperplasia. *Gynecol Oncol.* 1974;2:362–368.

31. Chamlian DL, Taylor HB. Endometrial hyperplasia in young women. *Obstet Gynecol.* 1970;36:659–666.

32. Sherman AC, Brown S. The precursors of endometrial carcinoma. *Am J Obstet Gynecol.* 1979;135:947–956.

33. Bonte J. Diagnosis and treatment of precancerous endometrial lesions. In: Schultz B, ed. *Endometrial Cancer.* Internation Symposium. Marburg; 1986:26.

34. Trope C, Lindahl B. Premalignant lesions of the endometrium. Clinical features and management. *Gynecologic Oncology.* 2d ed. New York: Churchill Livingstone, 1992;34–36.

35. Kurman RJ, Norris MJ. Endometrium. In: Henson D, Saavedra A (ed). *The Pathology of Incipient Neoplasia.* Philadelphia: WB Saunders; 1986:265.

36. Hendrickson MR, Kempson RL. Endometrial epithelial metaplasia: proliferations frequently misdiagnosed as adenocarcinoma. *Am J Surg Pathol.* 1980;4:525–542.

37. Hendrickson MR, Ross JC, Kepmson RL. Toward the development of morphologic criteria for well-differentiated adenocarcinoma of the endometrium. *Am J Surg Pathol.* 1983;7:819–838.

38. Jones WM, Kurman RJ. New ways of managing endometrial hyperplasia. *Contemp OB/GYN.* Dec 1990:36.

39. Katayama KP, Jones HW. Chromosomes of atypical (adenomatous) hyperplasia and carcinoma of the endometrium. *Am J Obstet Gynecol.* 1967;97:978–981.

40. Kistner RW. The effects of progestational agents on hyperplasia and carcinoma in situ of the endometrium. *Int J Gynecol Obstet.* 1970;84:561–566.

41. Kistner RW. The treatment of hyperplasia and carcinoma in-situ of the endometrium. *Clin Obstet Gynecol.* 1982;25:63–74.

42. Kjorstad KE, Welander C, Halvorsen T, et al. Progesterones as primary treatment in pre-malignant changes of the endometrium. In: Bush KT, King B, Taylor CR (eds). *Endometrial Cancer.* London: Bailliere Tindall; 1978:188.

43. Wentz WB. Progestin therapy in lesions of the endometrium. *Semin Oncol.* 1985;12:23–26.

44. Wentz WB. Treatment of persistent endometrial hyperplasia with progestins. *Am J Obstet Gynecol.* 1966;96:999–1004.

45. Wolfe SA, Mackles A. Malignant lesions arising from benign endometrial polyps. *Obstet Gynecol.* 1962;20:542.

46. Hertig AT, Sommers SC. Genesis of endometrial carcinoma: study of prior biopsies. *Cancer.* 1949;2:946–952.

47. Payne FL. The clinical significance of endometrial hyperplasia. *Am J Obstet Gynecol.* 1937;34:762–769.

48. Christopherson WM, Alberhaskey RC, Connelly PJ. Carcinoma of endometrium. I. A clinicopathological study of clear cell carcinoma and secretory carcinoma. *Cancer.* 1982;49:1511–1515.

49. Kucera F. The histogenesis of carcinoma of the body of the uterus. *Zentralbl Gynakol.* 1957;79:345–350.

The Pelvic

Mass

Carolyn V. Kirschner
John H. Isaacs

The average life expectancy of a woman in the United States is approximately 78 years. A woman at age 60 is expected to live another 20 years; at age 70 she should live an additional 13 years and at 80 another 7 years.[1] Elderly patients who present with a gynecologic condition, therefore, may benefit for many years from aggressive management of their disease.

Numerous studies have indicated that elderly patients will benefit from gynecologic surgery and that acceptable mortality and morbidity may be achieved in the treatment of gynecologic malignancies.[2,3] With the recent advances regarding ultrasound and laparoscopy in evaluation of pelvic masses, more conservative treatment approaches may be preferable.

SIGNS AND SYMPTOMS OF PELVIC MASSES

Smith and Anderson evaluated characteristics of symptoms and delay in seeking diagnosis of ovarian cancer in 83 women.[4] Contrary to previous impressions, most early stage cancers in their study did produce symptoms and were more likely than late stage cancer to cause fatigue and urinary symptoms. Late stage cases were most often accompanied by abdominal pain and swelling; only pain was likely to convince women to seek care. Their conclusion was that women, particularly those with high-risk factors, should be made aware that apparently benign disease symptoms are characteristic of early ovarian cancer.

Symptoms from ovarian masses are in general related to tumor size or manifestations of associated ascites and expanding ovarian lesions in the pelvis will cause pressure on the bladder or rectum. In addition, ovarian tumors may undergo torsion, which results in infarction or rupture, often leading to acute onset of lower abdominal or pelvic pain. Ascites may cause shortness of breath or increasing abdominal girth. In evaluating a patient with a pelvic mass, physical examination should be directed toward the abdomen to identify the presence of a fluid wave, which would indicate the presence of ascites. Although ascites is usually associated with ovarian cancer, patients with Meigs syndrome classically have an ovarian fibroma and right pleural effusion. Severe cirrhosis or congestive heart failure may also present with the development of ascites. Pelvic examination is usually compatible with a benign neoplasm in the case of a mobile unilateral cystic lesion. Solid fixed bilateral tumors, associated with nodularity in the cul-de-sac on rectovaginal examination, are more consistent with malignant neoplasms.

Another characteristic of ovarian neoplasms which is felt to indicate malignancy is the bilaterality of the mass. Koonings and colleagues reviewed data on 861 patients with ovarian tumors.[5] Among patients with unilateral tumors, 16% had malignant lesions in contrast to 40% of those with bilateral neoplasms. The women with bilateral neoplasms had a 2.6-fold increased risk of malignancy compared with women with unilateral neoplasms. Thus, bilateral ovarian neoplasms are two times more likely to be malignant than are unilateral lesions.

LIMITATIONS OF THE PELVIC EXAMINATION

Another recent review by Koonings and coworkers indicates that the overall risk that an ovarian neoplasm is malignant is 45% in postmenopausal women.[6] In their study, the highest risk for malignancy was in the age group 60 to 69 and declined slightly after age 70. This study did not specifically discuss tumor size or preoperative work-up but instead reviewed data on 861 women with a postoperative diagnosis of an ovarian neoplasm.

Rulin and Preston also found that the proportion of malignancies increased with age.[7] In their study, pelvic examination missed 10% of tumors less than 10 cm in diameter. It is apparent that pelvic examination alone is not optimal in screening for ovarian cancer nor in evaluating a patient with a pelvic mass. It is also apparent that additional studies are often required to adequately screen or evaluate these patients.

ULTRASOUND IN THE EVALUATION OF PELVIC MASSES

Ultrasound has been used extensively in obstetrics. With higher resolution scanners, however, the role of ultrasound in gynecology has greatly expanded. The higher resolution afforded by vaginal probes, which operate at a higher frequency than do standard transducers, has allowed for the detection of much smaller structures that may or may not have clinical significance. In addition, a cystic unilocular adnexal mass on abdominal ultrasonography may in fact display septation on vaginal ultrasonography.[8] Campbell and colleagues used both abdominal and vaginal ultrasonography to screen 5479 postmenopausal women. These patients were screened annually for at least 3 years. Five patients with primary ovarian cancer and 3 with metastatic disease were detected. They had a false positive rate at the time of the initial scan of 3.5%. The additional advantage of transvaginal scanning is that a full urinary bladder is not required. Thus, vaginal ultrasound scanning appears to be more amenable to routine office screening as part of the pelvic examination while the patient remains in the lithotomy position.

Many women currently undergo pelvic ultrasound to investigate vague abdominal or pelvic complaints, either at their own request or at the direction of their attending physician. Pelvic ultrasound is often done despite a negative pelvic examination result, either at the patient's request or due to patient obesity or inability to cooperate with optimal pelvic examination. It is, therefore, likely that many masses which may otherwise have gone undetected are being recognized.

Transabdominal Ultrasound

Much has been written recently regarding the role of ultrasound in the evaluation of the postmenopausal patient with a pelvic mass. Luxman and coworkers reported data on 102 postmenopausal women who underwent ultrasonographic evaluation of adnexal masses before surgery.[10] Previous studies have used sonographic size, morphology, and echogenicity of the adnexal masses to predict the likelihood of malignancies.[7,11–13] According to these studies, ovarian cysts smaller than 5 cm in diameter and those that are unilateral, unilocular, simple cysts would have a low risk for malignancy and could, therefore, be managed conservatively. In the Luxman study, abdominal ultrasonography had a positive predictive value of 39% and a negative predictive value of 94%. Two of 33 patients who had a simple cyst on abdominal ultrasound eventually proved to have ovarian carcinoma, both of which were smaller than 5 cm. Thus, abdominal ultrasonography is a sensitive method for predicting the malignancy of adnexal masses in postmenopausal women, but it is not specific. Goldstein and colleagues had no malignancies in their series of 48 postmenopausal patients with a unilateral simple cyst.[14] Nineteen were neoplastic. The authors concluded that these lesions can be followed with serial ultrasound without surgical intervention.

Herrmann and coworkers studied 404 women with suspected pelvic masses in a prospective study designed to assess the accuracy of sonography in confirming or excluding the presence of ovarian cancer; 312 of these patients underwent surgical exploration.[12] The ultrasound scan predicted malignancy in 38 of the 52 patients who eventually were found to have a malignancy, whereas benign tumors were predicted correctly in 177 of 185 (96%) of patients.

Transvaginal Ultrasound

Transvaginal ultrasound has been advocated as a way of optimizing ultrasound evaluation of pelvic masses. Transvaginal scanning may provide a clearer picture of the ovary in patients in whom abdominal ultrasound may be technically compromised, specifically obese patients or those unable to tolerate the full bladder required for transabdominal scanning.

Sassone and colleagues studied 143 patients specifically with ovarian lesions. They developed a scoring system for the objective description of ovarian masses based on the transvaginal sonographic appearance of the lesions. Variables included inner wall structure, wall thickness, septa, and echogenicity. In their study, size of the mass was not significant. Thirteen patients had malignant lesions. Of these, ascites was present in only two instances. In all patients, the inner wall structure was not smooth and the echogenicity was other than sonolucent in 13 of 14 tumors. The wall was thin in only 1 of the 14 and of 29 simple cysts there were no carcinomas.

The role of color flow Dopplers is currently being explored as a method of determining benign from malignant neoplasms.[16,17]

Ultrasound as a Screening Test for Ovarian Cancer

Several studies have examined the role of ultrasound as a screening test for ovarian cancer. Andolf and coworkers performed ultrasound scanning as an adjunct to pelvic examination in 800 women between 40 and 70 years of age presenting for a variety of gynecologic complaints.[18] Among 167 patients with abnormal ultrasound scans, one case of ovarian carcinoma of low malignant potential was detected, and this patient had both an abnormal pelvic examination and pelvic pain.

Bhan and coworkers have also evaluated the use of pelvic ultrasound as a screening test.[19] A total of 15,977 scans was performed on 5479 self-selected, asymptomatic women. Five women (0.1%) were found to have a primary ovarian malignancy, all diagnosed as stage IA or IB. In their series, 10% of women had a positive initial ultrasound screen which became negative with successive scans. Two hundred seventy-one women underwent surgical exploration. Twenty-five percent of these patients had benign epithelial tumors and 35% were classified as "tumor-like conditions." Five primary ovarian cancers were detected as well as four metastatic carcinomas. Abdominal ultrasound, then, appears to have a low yield for ovarian cancer, with a high rate of operation for benign ovarian tumors.

Van Nagell and colleagues used transvaginal sonography to examine 1300 postmenopausal women.[20] Ovarian abnormalities were detected in 33 women (2.5%), and 27 patients underwent exploratory laparotomy. Ovarian tumors were found in all patients who were explored, including two primary ovarian cancers and 14 serous cystadenomas. The 2 patients with cancer had normal pelvic examination and normal serum CA-125 levels. Both had stage I disease. In another study, Higgins and coworkers performed ultrasound screening on 1000 asymptomatic women aged 40 or older.[21] Twenty-four of those patients were explored for adnexal masses which were detected by the study. One of these patients proved to have cancer, but this was not a primary ovarian carcinoma and was metastatic from a primary adenocarcinoma of the colon.

Finkler and coworkers have shown that the combination of ultrasound and CA-125 levels provides a high positive and negative predictive value in postmenopausal women.[22] Using ultrasound and a CA-125 level greater than 35 U/mL, they correctly predicted 19 malignancies in a series of 74 postmenopausal women with adnexal masses. With the advent of transvaginal color flow imaging, ultrasound screening may be helpful in even earlier detection of neovascularization, which is associated with invasive disease.

It is not appropriate at present to advocate ultrasound as a screening test for ovarian cancer, because of its low yield. The role of combined ultrasound and CA-125 is promising but remains to be established.

Serum CA-125

Zurawski and colleagues screened 950 nonhospitalized Roman Catholic nuns with a median age of 55 years to determine the utility of serum CA-125 levels as a screening test for ovarian cancer.[23] Thirty-six women (4%) had serum levels greater than 35 U/mL and only 7 (1%) had serum CA-125 levels above 65 U/mL. Among the 7 women with values above 65 U/mL, 5 were found to have benign or malignant neoplasms at the time of entry. No studies to date have addressed the false negative rate of CA-125 screening. It is well known that CA-125 levels may be elevated in benign gynecologic as well as benign nongynecologic conditions. Nongynecologic malignancies may also be associated with elevated CA-125 levels. Classically, 80% of serous ovarian carcinomas are associated with elevated CA-125 values. Elevations with other ovarian malignancies are variable.

Magnetic Resonance Imaging

The role of magnetic resonance spectroscopy (MRI) in the evaluation of pelvic tumors remains in question. Mountford and colleagues studied 51 biopsy specimens from patients with cancer of the ovary or colon to determine whether it was possible to identify tumor subtypes with metastatic potential.[24] Primary carcinomas with metastasis gave T2 values greater than those carcinomas not associated with known metastasis.

Laparoscopy for Cystic Ovarian Masses

Although well established as a diagnostic tool in the field of gynecology, laparoscopy is not without risk. Complications of laparoscopy may include:

1. Complications referable to the creation of pneumoperitoneum (7.4/1000 cases), including cardiac arrest, hypercarbia, gas embolism, and pneumothorax

2. Electrical complications (2.2/1000 cases), including abdominal wall and bowel burns

3. Hemorrhage (6.4/1000 cases)

4. Penetration complications (2.7/1000 cases), including injuries to the gastrointestinal tract and blood vessels as well as perforation of the uterus

5. Infection (1.4/1000 cases)

Other rare complications include herniation of omentum or small bowel through the trocar and postoperative adhesions requiring laparotomy.[25]

Parker and Berek studied 25 patients with cystic adnexal masses by operative laparoscopy.[26] Candidates for laparoscopic management included patients with a negative serum CA-125 tumor marker plus ultrasound criteria of tumor size less than 10 cm cystic, distinct borders, no irregular solid parts or thick septa, no evidence of ascites, and no matted bowel. Operative findings were benign in all 25 patients. Mean operative time was 73 minutes and mean hospital stay was 12 hours. Two patients sustained complications of surgery. The first patient had a perforation of the bladder with a 5-mm trocar which was managed with indwelling catheter drainage at home. The second patient sustained injury to the sigmoid colon during enterolysis, and this required laparotomy. Another patient had a frozen section diagnosis that was inconclusive, requiring laparotomy to accomplish removal of the mass. Final pathologic diagnosis was a benign serous cystadenofibroma. A third patient required laparotomy despite laparoscopic confirmation of a benign paratubal cyst. At laparoscopy incidental papillary excrescences were noted on the contralateral ovary and omentum. Biopsy revealed metastatic breast carcinoma.

Obviously patients selected for conservative management of adnexal lesions must be chosen carefully. It is important that correct preoperative evaluation be performed before any surgical intervention. Maiman and coworkers reported on a total of 42 women who had laparoscopic management of ovarian neoplasms that were subsequently found to be malignant.[27] Thirty-one percent of these patients had unilateral, unilocular cystic lesions less than 8 cm in diameter, all of which normally would have suggested a benign lesion. The role of cyst aspiration at the time of laparoscopy remains controversial. Theoretically, a malignancy that would otherwise be confined to an ovary would be upstaged as the result of cyst puncture with subsequent spillage into the abdominal cavity. A technique has recently been developed in which the cyst is aspirated under negative pressure without spillage. The mass is then placed in a plastic bag and withdrawn through the scope or through a colpotomy incision.

PREOPERATIVE MANAGEMENT OF THE ELDERLY SURGICAL PATIENT

Once the decision for surgery has been made, both patient and physician must be appropriately "tuned" and prepared for the operation. Watters and McClaran enumerate seven critical factors to obtain the best outcome in the preoperative management of the elderly surgical patient.[28] These include:

1. Careful preoperative preparation of the patient and optimization of medical and physiological status
2. Appropriate anesthesia and physiologic monitoring
3. Recognition of alterations in clinical pharmacology
4. Minimization of the postoperative stresses of hyperthermia, hypoxemia, and pain
5. Prevention of alterations in blood pressure and heart rate
6. Avoidance of disturbances of fluid, electrolyte, and acid-base status
7. Careful surgical techniques

Relative inactivity may limit the symptoms of cardiac, pulmonary, or peripheral vascular disease. In addition, symptoms may be attributed to changes of advancing age rather than to significant physiologic impairment. Memory or hearing deficits may make it difficult to obtain a reliable history, and in addition, elderly patients may have a higher pain threshold than younger patients. Febrile responses may be less marked in elderly patients and hypothermia is more common in elderly patients with serious illness.

History is extremely important and may aid in the management of the postmenopausal patient with an equivocal finding of pelvic examination or ultrasound. Epidemiologic factors associated with an increased risk for ovarian malignancy include Caucasian race, positive family history in two or more first degree relatives, infertility, nulligravidity, previous breast or colon carcinoma, concurrent endometrial or cervical adenocarcinoma, and Peutz-Jegher syndrome.[29] Genetic syndromes associated with ovarian cancer include Peutz-Jegher syndrome, multiple basal cell carcinoma, and gonadal dysgenesis.[30]

It is important to assess the preoperative medical status of the patient. In particular, the cardiovascular and pulmonary systems should be thoroughly evaluated to avoid a potentially preventable preoperative mortality or morbidity. A thorough preoperative history, physical examination, electrocardiogram, and chest x-ray are essential. If any abnormality is detected in these screening tests, medical evaluation by an internist or cardiologist is indicated. Further testing may include a treadmill test or echocardiography scan. Abnormalities detected in these tests may require cardiac angiography. Mild essential hypertension of itself is not a contraindication to surgery; however, the possibility of end-organ manifestations, such as renal, cerebral, or cardiac impairment must be evaluated. Preoperative serum, creatinine, and liver function tests would be helpful as a further screening test to rule out renal or hepatic disease. (See Chapter 3 for further amplification.)

Preoperative evaluation of the elderly patient with a pelvic mass should include lower gastrointestinal radiologic studies. It is the opinion of many gastrointestinal specialists, however, that colonoscopic examination is more accurate. Barium enema studies range in accuracy from 90% in cooperative and well-prepared patients to as low as 50% in uncooperative or improperly prepared patients.[31] It is important that the gynecologic surgeon ensure that the patient is properly prepared for the x-ray studies of the colon and to ensure that the studies are of the air contrast type. Without air contrast the colonic mucosa cannot be adequately outlined and colon lesions may be mistaken for fecal material or be hidden by stool collection.

Prior to laparotomy, an intravenous pyelogram is also indicated in the patient with a pelvic mass. If a computed tomography scan (CT) has been performed with contrast, then this step may be eliminated. Intravenous pyelogram or CT establishes the function of the kidneys and determines the presence of a pelvic kidney or a partially obstructed ureter.

The ovary is a common site of metastasis from other primary sites. From 10% to 25% of all ovarian malignancies are actually metastatic in origin.[32] The most common sources of metastasis to the ovary are the gastrointestinal tract, the breast, and the uterus. When the ovarian metastasis is from the gastrointestinal tract, it is almost always bilateral. If metastatic disease is a consideration, then upper gastrointestinal x-ray, careful breast examination, and mammography are important components of the preoperative evaluation.

Laboratory studies preoperatively should include liver function tests and a serum CA-125 tumor marker. The latter is positive in approximately 80% of women with a serous cystadenocarcinoma, but also may be elevated in benign ovarian neoplasms. The main value of CA-125 before laparotomy is not in diagnosis but rather as a baseline before treatment. If the level is elevated preoperatively, the physician may follow levels serially during treatment and for subsequent follow-up. A prompt return to normal during treatment is associated with a more favorable prognosis, and an elevation of CA-125 may precede clinical evidence of recurrence by 1 to 6 months.

Advanced age and pelvic surgery are two well-known risk factors for the development of postoperative deep vein thrombosis. Liberal use of sequential compression devices on the lower extremities is prudent and is essential for any elderly patient undergoing laparotomy. The use of sequential compression devices in the setting of laparoscopy has not been studied, but at worst would not be a detriment. (See Chapter 18 for complete details.)

Preparation of the Patient for Surgery

Preparation of the patient for surgery for a pelvic mass begins with the establishment of as accurate a diagnosis as possible. This allows for planning for the appropriate extent of surgery and perioperative patient care. It is imperative that the patient and her family be informed as well as is possible. The patient should understand that bowel or bladder resection may be required and that a colostomy is a possibility.

If there is any possibility that surgery might involve a bowel resection, bowel preparation should always be performed preoperatively. Even if bowel resection is not performed, the bowel preparation allows for complete collapse of the intestine and greater ease of surgery, even perhaps allowing for a smaller incision than otherwise might be required.

The most important component of the bowel preparation is the mechanical cleansing. Although a 3-day mechanical preparation including oral antibiotics has been advocated, a single-day preparation with Go-Lytely (a solution of balanced electrolytes) allows a simple and effective means of cleaning the bowel without a prolonged time in which the patient is not allowed to eat. The day before surgery, the patient should be allowed only a clear liquid diet and Go-Lytely should begin at approximately noon, with the patient drinking 8 ounces every 10 to 15 minutes until the rectal discharge is clear. This usually requires 2 to 4 quarts Go-Lytely, which may be mixed or "chased" with a clear liquid juice or soda, thus limiting the salty taste for which the fluid is known. The role of oral antibiotics has recently been questioned. Erythromycin 1 g and neomycin 1 g have traditionally been given four times a day on varied schedules the day before surgery. These antibiotics, however, do add a significant amount of gastrointestinal upset, with limited therapeutic value. Parenteral antibiotics, however, have been well established to aid in prophylaxis for wound infection and also in the event of bowel surgery.

SURGICAL EXPLORATION

Often in the evaluation in a postmenopausal woman with a pelvic mass an exploratory laparotomy is necessary. The volume of any abdominal fluid should be recorded, and the fluid should be aspirated and submitted for cytologic examination. If no ascites is found, washings for cytology should be taken from the right diaphragm, right and left gutters, and pelvis. The right diaphragm washing is facilitated by insertion of a Robnell catheter above the liver to which is attached an Asepto syringe with 50 mL saline. The saline is injected and aspirated for cytology. Similarly, installation of fluid and aspiration should be performed in the areas of the right and left colonic gutters and finally of the pelvis. Saline is the preferred fluid for cytologic examination because water will lyse these cells and result in a false negative examination.

Careful abdominal and pelvic exploration should then be performed of all serosal surfaces. The surgeon should develop a personal method of exploration so that no area is missed. For example, a methodical examination would include the right and left lobes of the liver, gallbladder, right kidney, omentum, transverse colon, stomach, spleen, left kidney, para-aortic area, cecum and appendix, ascending colon, descending colon, sigmoid, small intestine, running the small bowel from the ileocecal valve to the ligament of Treitz, and finally, attention directed to the pelvis. A standard order of exploration is also helpful for later dictation of operative findings.

Careful examination of all surfaces should be made to assess for tumor nodularity and any suspicious area should be biopsied. The mass should then be excised, sent for frozen section, and if malignant, full staging and debulking should be performed. Standard staging for malignant ovarian tumor would include bilateral salpingo-oophorectomy with total abdominal hysterectomy and biopsies of peritoneal surfaces, including right diaphragm, right and left gutters and pelvis, as well as omentectomy and washings for cytology. Pelvic and para-aortic lymph node sampling is also desirable.

If at the time of frozen section the histology of a mass is in question, it is best to proceed with a limited staging surgery so that if the final pathology report is malignant, then as much information as possible is gained without subjecting the patient to another operation. It has been our policy in the case of large mucinous tumors or in cases with papillary excrescences not clearly malignant that the patient undergo abdominal hysterectomy, bilateral salpingo-oophorectomy, pelvic and upper abdominal biopsies, an omental biopsy and washings for cytology. Lymph node dissection should not be performed because of the added morbidity, unless malignancy is clearly identified.

CLINICAL CASES

The following are some clinical scenarios with recommendation for management.

Postmenopausal Palpable Ovary Revisited

The classic paper on the postmenopausal palpable ovary syndrome, written in 1971, described the indications for surgical exploration of a postmenopausal woman as any patient with a palpable ovary in the postmenopausal period.[33] After Barber's editorial in 1971, surgical exploration became the standard of care for managing any patient with palpable ovaries in the postmenopausal period. More recently, however, Barber has commented that this practice should not be extended to the asymptomatic, nonpalpable ovarian cyst.[34] Barber would advocate repeat ultrasound examinations and continued follow-up as long as the cyst size remains stable. Three dimensional ultrasonography is currently being developed in western Europe and may prove invaluable in this regard.

Familial Ovarian Cancer Syndrome

B.G. is a 65-year-old woman who presents for routine annual examination. She states that her sister died at age 64 with ovarian cancer and that her daughter was recently diagnosed with ovarian cancer. She is concerned with her own chances for developing the disease. *Answer:* Patients with two first degree relatives with ovarian cancer are at particularly high risk for developing ovarian cancer. Familial ovarian cancer is thought to be inherited as an autosomal dominant pattern with variable penetrants and, as such, women and families with a history of familial ovarian cancer may have as high as a 50% chance of developing ovarian cancer.[35] This patient's risk for ovarian cancer may be as high as 50%. She is clearly beyond childbearing age and a prophylactic oophorectomy should be strongly recommended. Alternatively, the patient could be followed with CA-125 tumor markers and ultrasound scanning every 6 months, but unless the patient is medically inoperable, she should undergo oophorectomy.

Adnexal Mass with Low Suspicion of Malignancy

P.C. is a 67-year-old woman who sees her internist because she has lower abdominal discomfort. She is eventually found to have a diverticular disease, but the work-up includes a pelvic ultrasound, which shows a 2-cm cystic mass on her right ovary. The internist consults you for recommendation for management of the abdominal ultrasound. *Answer:* New technology and high-resolution ultrasound scanning have resulted in the detection of many lesions that have probably been present in the past but have not been detected. With a normal physical examination and no evidence of ascites on the ultrasound scan, I would suggest that a CA-125 serum tumor marker be drawn. If this is normal, then both should be repeated in 2 to 3 months. If the patient's symptoms resolve and the mass does not increase in size and the CA-125 level remains normal, the patient can be followed conservatively with serial ultrasounds and tumor markers. If there is any change in any of the above, then immediate oophorectomy is indicated.

Abdominal Ascites of Uncertain Origin

V.T. is a 72-year-old woman who presents with ascites of unknown etiology. You are consulted to rule out ovarian cancer. *Answer:* Work-up should include a pelvic examination and CT scan as well as electrocardiogram, chest x-ray, and CA-125 tumor marker. If the examination and CT scan do not show a mass, then paracentesis should be performed. If cytology is negative, and the CA-125 tumor marker is low, then a diligent search should be made for a medical etiology of the ascites, such as congestive heart failure, renal disease, or hepatic failure. Remember that CA-125 may be modestly elevated in ascites caused by diseases other than ovarian cancer. A primary peritoneal neoplasia needs to be ruled out, but if the CT scan and paracentesis are negative, this is unlikely. If the paracentesis reveals adenocarcinoma or if the CA-125 level continues to rise despite optimization of the patient's medical status, then consideration should be given to surgical exploration.

Pelvic Mass and Multiple Medical Problems

T.A. is an 84-year-old woman with a complaint of left leg pain and swelling. Her internist has performed CT scanning which revealed a multiloculated cystic mass in the pelvis. She has multiple medical problems and her internist is reluctant to clear her for surgery. *Answer:* This may be one indication for a pelvic examination under anesthesia with transvaginal needle biopsy of the lesion. Although disruption of a pelvic mass in general is contraindicated because of the potential of seeding the peritoneum if the integrity of the capsule of the presumed carcinoma is altered, in this case it may be helpful for the patient to have as much information as possible before the final decision for surgery is made. If the needle biopsy is positive for carcinoma, then chemotherapy or surgery (or both) can be more intelligently discussed with the patient.

Pelvic Mass and a Previous History of Cancer

B.S. is a 73-year-old woman with a history of colon carcinoma. A follow-up CT scan shows a 3-cm mass on the left ovary. The patient is asymptomatic. *Answer:* CA-125 and carcinoembryonic antigen levels should be drawn. With the history of previous malignancy, one should be more aggressive in evaluating this mass. Bilateral oophorectomy should be performed, either via laparotomy or laparoscope.

SUMMARY

The elderly patient with a pelvic mass must be thoroughly examined and evaluated before decisions are made. Improved ultrasound and laparoscopic techniques may allow for conservative management of many ovarian abnormalities. The ideal care for suspected ovarian carcinoma, however, remains exploratory laparotomy with bilateral salpingo-oophorectomy, hysterectomy, and staging or cytoreduction.

REFERENCES

1. Capen VC, Capen JB. Aging and disease in the geriatric gynecology patient. *Curr Prob Obstet Gynecol.* 1983;6:4–44.

2. Kirschner CV, DeSerto TM, Isaacs JH. Surgical treatment of the elderly patient with gynecologic cancer. *Surg Gynecol Obstet.* 1990;170:379–384.

3. Lawton FG, Hacker NF. Surgery for invasive gynecologic cancer in the elderly female population. *Obstet Gynecol.* 1990;76:287–289.

4. Smith EM, Anderson B. The effects of symptoms and delay in seeking diagnosis on stage of disease at diagnosis among women with cancers of the ovary. *Cancer.* 1985;56:2727–2732.

5. Koonings PP, Grimes DA, Campbell K, Sommerville M. Bilateral ovarian neoplasms and the risk of malignancy. *Am J Obstet Gynecol.* 1990;162:167–169.

6. Koonings PP, Campbell K, Mishell DR, Grimes DA. Relative frequency of primary ovarian neoplasms: A ten-year review. *Obstet Gynecol.* 1989;74:921–926.

7. Rulin MC, Preston AL. Adnexal masses in postmenopausal women. *Obstet Gynecol.* 1987;70:578–581.

8. Goldstein SR. Ultrasound for the postmenopausal patient. *Female Patient.* 1990;15:61–65.

9. Campbell S, Bhan V, Whitehead MI, Collins WP, Royston P. Transabdominal ultrasound screening for early ovarian cancer. *Br Med J.* 1989;229:1363.

10. Luxman D, Bergman A, Sagi J, David MP. The postmenopausal adnexal mass: Correlation between ultrasonic and pathologic findings. *Obstet Gynecol.* 1991; 77:726–728.

11. Moyle JW, Rochester D, Sider L, Shrock K, Krause P. Sonography of ovarian tumors: Predictability of tumor type. *Am J Radiol.* 1983;141:985–991.

12. Herrmann UJ, Guttfried W, Locher GW, Goldhirch A. Sonographic patterns of ovarian tumors: Prediction of malignancy. *Obstet Gynecol.* 1987;69:777–781.

13. Andolf E, Jorgensen C. Simple adnexal cysts diagnosed by ultrasound in postmenopausal women. *J Clin Ultrasound.* 1988;16:301–303.

14. Goldstein SR, Subramanyam B, Snyder JR, Beller U, Raghavendra BN, Beckman EM. The postmenopausal cystic adnexal mass: The potential role of ultrasound in conservative management. *Obstet Gynecol.* 1989;73:8–10.

15. Sassone AM, Timor-Tritsch IE, Artner A, Westhoff C, Warren WB. Transvaginal sonographic characterization of ovarian disease: Evaluation of a new scoring system to predict ovarian malignancy. *Obstet Gynecol.* 1991;78:70–76.

16. Bourne T, Campbell S, Steer C, Whitehead MI, Collins P. Transvaginal colour flow imaging: A possible new screening technique for ovarian cancer. *Br Med J.* 1989;299:1367–1370.

17. Weiner Z, Thaler I, Beck D, Sharaz R, Deutsch M, Brandes JM. Differentiating malignant from benign ovarian tumors with transvaginal color flow imaging. *Obstet Gynecol.* 1992;79:159–162.

18. Andolf S, Svalenius E, Astedt B. Ultrasonography for early detection of ovarian carcinoma. *Br J Obstet Gynecol.* 1986;93:1286–1289.

19. Bhan V, Amso N, Whitehead MI, Campbell S, Royston P, Collins WP. Characteristics of persistent ovarian masses in asymptomatic women. *Br J Obstet Gynecol.* 1989;96:1384–1391.

20. Van Nagell JR, DePriest MD, Puls LE, et al. Ovarian cancer screening in asymptomatic postmenopausal women by transvaginal sonography. *Cancer.* 1991;68:458–462.

21. Higgins RV, van Nagell JR Jr, Donaldson ES, et al. Transvaginal sonography as a screening method for ovarian cancer. *Gynecol Oncol.* 1989;34:402–406.

22. Finkler NJ, Benacerraf B, Levin P, Wojciechowski C, Knapp RC. Comparison of serum CA-125, clinical impression, and ultrasound in the preoperative evaluation of ovarian masses. *Obstet Gynecol.* 1988;72:659–664.

23. Zurawski VR Jr, Broderick SF, Pickens P, Knapp RC, Bast RC Jr. Serum CA-125 levels in a group of nonhospitalized women: relevance for the early detection of ovarian cancer. *Obstet Gynecol.* 1987;69:606–611.

24. Mountford G, Saunders JK, May GL, et al. Classification of human tumours by high-resolution magnetic resonance spectroscopy. *Lancet* 1986;1:651–653.

25. Loffer FD, Pent D. Indications, contraindications and complications of laparoscopy. *Obstet Gynecol Surv.* 1975;30:407–426.

26. Parker WH, Berek JS. Management of selected cystic adnexal masses in postmenopausal women by operative laparoscopy: A pilot study. *Am J Obstet Gynecol.* 1990;163:1574.

27. Maiman V, Seltzer V, Boyce J. Laparoscopic excision of ovarian neoplasms subsequently found to be malignant. *Obstet Gynecol.* 1991;77:563–565.

28. Watters JM, McClaren JC. The elderly surgical patient. In: Wilmore, ed. *Care of the Surgical Patient.* New York: Scientific American; 1990.

29. McGowan L. Epidemiology of ovarian cancer. *Oncology.* 1989;3:51–62.

30. Heintz APM, Hacker NF, Lagasse LD. Epidemiology and etiology of ovarian cancer: A review. *Obstet Gynecol.* 1985;66:127–135.

31. Miller RE. Detection of colon carcinoma and the barium enema. *JAMA.* 1974;230:1195.

32. Knaus JV, Barber HR. Metastatic lesions presenting as pelvic mass. In: Isaacs JH, Byrne MP, eds. *Pelvic Surgery—A Multidisciplinary Approach.* Mount Kisco, NY: Futura Publishing Co.; 1987:69–88.

33. Barber HRK, Graber EA. The PMPO Syndrome (postmenopausal palpable ovary syndrome). *Obstet Gynecol.* 1971;38:921–923.

34. Barber H. A second look at the postmenopausal palpable ovary. *Female Patient.* 1988;13:13–14.

35. Piver SM, Baker TR, Mettlin C, et al. *The Gilda Radner Familial Ovarian Cancer Registry Newsletter,* 1990.

Endoscopy in the Postmenopause: Diagnosis and Treatment

Ashwin J. Chatwani

In the current environment of gynecologic surgery, endoscopy undeniably occupies a predominant position. No book centering on general gynecologic surgery is complete without a discussion of endoscopy. Even though this volume is limited to the postreproductive woman, it is no exception. The two principal branches of endoscopy in gynecologic usage, laparoscopy and hysteroscopy, despite initial negative predictions regarding their value in the older female population, now play major diagnostic and therapeutic roles. Adept practitioners in these two sophisticated instrumentally based fields are regarded as essential to the vitality of a geriatric gynecologic service.

A brief historical review on how telescopic principles and mechanics came to exert such a powerful influence as they do today not only in gynecology but in a wide diversity of fields can only enhance the appreciation of the distinctive merits of the laparoscope and the hysteroscope. The birth of visualization of body cavities through reflected light is generally credited to the innovative genius of Bozzini who disclosed the first such capable instrument in 1807.[1] However, it took another 58 years of slow acceptance and refinement until the development of the first truly practical endoscope, considerably more advanced than the original hollow tube. It was put into use by Desormeaux in 1865.[2] The first known specific gynecologic involvement came in 1869 when Pantaleoni, through a hysteroscope, described an endometrial polyp as a source of bleeding in a 60-year-old woman.[3]

Exciting developments followed, leading to Kelling's description in 1902 of laparoscopy in laboratory animals after filling the peritoneal cavity with air.[4] Ten years later Jacobaeus reported the first successful laparoscopy usage in 17 patients.[5] Sporadic slowly increasing numbers of laparoscopic procedures continued to be done until the major breakthrough for all endoscopic surgery occurred in 1965 when a cold fiberoptic light source became a practical reality. The leap forward began and, by 1973, enough work in this new modality had been accomplished and documented to occasion Lindemann's extensive historical review.[6]

Technological improvements followed rapidly with the perfection of an insufflator for pneumoperitoneum, the development of high-flow control of insufflation, the creation of superior intrauterine distending media, the steady refinement of more efficient tools for both laparoscopy and hysteroscopy, and the invention of a succession of sophisticated video cameras that facilitated operative maneuverability beyond anyone's dreams.

Because endoscopic methods seem to be replacing some of the standard gynecologic surgical approaches even in menopausal and elderly patients, awareness of potential hazards is essential. Such emphasis is vital because the margin of safety is so much narrower than in younger women. By the same token, the sphere of vulnerability is so much larger in older people because of the compromises aging has placed on major body systems:

A. Cardiovascular
    1. Reduced tissue perfusion
    2. Reduced cardiac reserve

B. Pulmonary
    1. Decreased vital capacity
    2. Increased functional residual capacity
    3. Greater pulmonary resistance

C. Renal
    1. Slower kidney blood flow
    2. Decreased glomerular filtration rate
    3. Lowered diuretic capability
    4. Decreased concentration capacity

Because of these negative physiologic alterations, the large amounts of fluid, either liquid or gaseous, discharged into the body in gynecologic endoscopy can become dangerously burdensome under anesthesia during surgery of any magnitude. Yet with stringent monitoring, coupled with good sense, experience, and caution, both laparoscopy and hysteroscopy can be successfully applied in the older female patient in avoiding more stressful procedures involving laparotomy and hysterectomy.

At the time of the publication of this book, enthusiasm throughout the world is being generated for "gasless laparoscopy," as reported verbally by several investigators at the annual meeting of the American Association of Gynecological Endoscopists in October, 1993, in San Francisco. This is accomplished by the use of a hydraulic lifter attached to a forked fontlike instrument which, when inserted into the abdomen and opened, can elevate the abdominal wall substantially enough to allow for all the usual laparoscopic endeavors except when extensive adhesions are present. By employing passive entry of atmospheric air, the complications of and contraindications to gas instilled under pressure are eliminated.

LAPAROSCOPY

Originally designed primarily as a diagnostic instrument, over a 25-year span the laparoscope has progressed to become a major operative tool as well. Furthermore, the short hospital stay after diagnostic usage is today almost equalled after major forms of surgery performed through the scope. Additionally, in the postmenopausal woman, the avoidance of the trauma of laparotomy by using laparoscopy instead, even while recognizing its limitations in this age group, make it a reasonable choice in many situations.

In cases of pelvic mass, the diagnostic value of direct visualization through the scope can be immeasurable. Not so long ago, answers could only be found via laparotomy. Today we enjoy all the ancillary benefits of ultrasonography, magnetic resonance imaging (MRI), Doppler interpretations, and tumor markers in providing information before the ultimate diagnostic effort afforded by the laparoscope. Not only can a mass or tumor be seen without incisional opening into the peritoneal cavity, but appropriate biopsies can be taken when deemed feasible, all without a linear abdominal wound and its associated trauma and also without the associated discomfort and expense of a longer hospital stay.

Probably the single most noncontroversial use of laparoscopy, including the postmenopausal age group as well as premenopausal women, is its use in the evaluation of pelvic pain. The only arguments of difference center on whether it should be resorted to sooner or later in the work-up. In other words, some use all the available noninvasive diagnostic methods (ie, barium enema, upper gastrointestinal series, intravenous pyelogram, ultrasonography, MRI, computed tomography [CT] scan) before finally turning to laparoscopy. Proponents of the latter as the most definitive tool often use the scope after only one or two of the above procedures has been effected to find an answer earlier. Also, such an approach in most cases will cut down the expense and time involvement for the patient, not to mention the elimination of the discomfort and x-ray exposure associated with these other tests.

Obviously any discussion of diagnostic evaluation of a pelvic mass by laparoscopy leads directly to the question of judgment and practicality for removal of any pelvic mass by laparoscopic surgery in the postmenopausal woman. This introduces another aspect of argument—that perhaps no laparoscopic investigative venture in both young and old patients—should be undertaken without preparation for simultaneous removal of any discovered mass. Referring back to the complete discussion of Chapter 14, we are cautioned by the reminder that the risk of malignancy in an ovarian mass premenopausally is only 13%,[7] whereas it is 45% in the postmenopausal woman.[7,8] Thus, we have the basis for those who propose full use of all other diagnostic means before laparoscopic intrusion. The key warning message points out that any intraoperative rupture of an adnexal mass that turns out to be malignant immediately creates a more ominous situation than that existing before the operation.

Opponents of the preliminary full work-up point out the false positive aspects of ultrasonography, MRI, tumor markers, and CT scans. They argue that laparoscopy in experienced hands can ever so quickly, in one combined effort, both diagnose and remove or correct an old residual pedunculated fibromyoma, a previously undiscovered dermoid, or an adhesive adnexal mass left over from an inflammation or infection of premenopausal years. They further reason that if a mass is truly malignant, considering the sophistication of current instruments, a direct look into the abdomen by endoscopy can immediately give information about the extent of any malignancy, particularly when the lesion is thought to be early, that can only be presumed in many cases by preoperative testing. Thus, more definitive therapeutic planning results.

The conclusions remain unsettled; the guiding principles, as always, are good judgment and appropriate caution, catalyzed by skill and experience.

Postmenopausal operative laparoscopy can be most useful in a significant percentage of cases of vaginal hysterectomy where accompanying bilateral salphingoophorectomy (BSO) is deemed desirable. All authorities agree that the indications for accompanying oophorectomy are the same regardless of the route chosen for hysterectomy. Yet it is well established that the percentage of bilateral oophorectomy associated with uterine extirpation abdominally in the perimenopausal and postmenopausal woman is overwhelmingly higher than the miniscule incidence occurring with vaginal hysterectomy. Much of this difference occurs because of lack of skill in adnexal removal from below. Additionally a considerable number of cases are planned for extensive reconstruction to accompany the vaginal hysterectomy, and bilateral oophorectomy is skipped for reasons of time involvement. Not infrequently pragmatic reasoning that inadvertent complications of incidental oophorectomy might cancel the job of reconstruction, the major justifying determinant for the operation to begin with, explains why oophorectomy is so often omitted. It is also well known that commonly in women over 60 years of age, the ovaries have retracted far out toward the pelvic sidewalls, thereby presenting mechanical difficulties for removal that are extremely challenging even to the most competent vaginal surgeon.

In all such cases, BSO by laparoscopy can be accomplished in the same coincident time frame of the continuing vaginal procedure by another surgeon working from above. Considering that cancer of the ovary, a devastating disease in itself, is no longer regarded as uncommon, especially in a patient with a threatening relevant family history, this perspective of concomitant laparoscopic BSO is unquestionably not only acceptable but in many instances indicated.

HYSTEROSCOPY

Background

Intrauterine endoscopic invasion began its steady road to acceptance as a major gynecologic technique some 20 to 25 years before the publication of this book. Originally it was greeted disdainfully by the average practitioner as an implement that, beyond its use for retrieval of a contraceptive intrauterine device (IUD) that could not be extracted by other means, it was only just another instrument "out looking for a job." Its place currently in gynecologic practice at all levels is well established, especially as accelerated over the past few years by major technological advances. These include improved lens systems, the introduction and refinement of cold light fiberoptics, more practicable distention media, an expanding variety of progressively more efficient ancillary tools, and the introduction and perfection of videocameras.

The steadily growing list of indications for diagnostic and therapeutic hysteroscopy include uterine ablation for disabling and intractable menometrorrhagia, treatment of Müllerian fusion defects, infertility evaluation, transuterine tubal sterilization, tubal canalization techniques, removal of submucous leiomyomata, endometrial polyps and foreign bodies, and the most important of all in the perimenopausal and climacteric woman, investigation and analysis of abnormal uterine bleeding.

Inadequacy of Dilatation and Curettage

Diagnostic dilatation and curettage (D and C) of the uterus has been and remains one of the most frequently performed surgical procedures in the United States. The most common reason for any exploration of the uterine cavity, traditionally done by D and C, is abnormal uterine bleeding at any age level. Because of the ominous potential for premalignant or malignant endometrial lesions as a cause of aberrant bleeding in the perimenopausal and postreproductive woman, accuracy in diagnosis is at a premium. Because D and C is a blind procedure and serious endometrial abnormalities often begin focally, using this diagnostic method can easily miss the lesion. This is emphasized by the stark realization that, after a century of experience with D and C, tissue yield and accuracy continue to be poor. Obviously this can lead to a false sense of

TABLE 15-1 Inadequacy of Dilatation and Curettage

Author	No. of Patients	Comment
Englund et al.[14]	124	Adequent in only 35%
Word et al.[13]	512	Missed 9.5% of lesions
Gribb[15]	80	Provided diagnosis in 14% and incorrect information in 35%
Smith and Schulman[11]	1383	Missed diagnosis of abnormalities in 60%
Stock and Kanbour[12]	50	Less than 75% surface curetted in 84% of cases
Brooks and Serden[16]	29	Lacked accuracy in 82%
Loffer[17]	187	Sensitivity rate of only 65%
Valle[18]	550	Missed 31% of lesions

security and postponement of diagnosis. The gravity of such a situation becomes readily apparent in the reality of the following sets of statistics. The incidence of focal symptomatic (i.e., gross bleeding) lesions has been reported to vary from 19% to 65%.[9,10] Smith and Schulman, on reviewing the record of 1383 consecutive cases involving diagnostic D and C, found that 60% were deficient in significant diagnosis later discovered by additional investigative means.[11] A study by Stock and Kanbour verified the long-established inefficiency of D and C in revealing that, in 84% of such procedures, less than three fourths of the uterine cavity is scraped.[12] In the other 16%, less than one fourth of the endometrial surface had been sampled. Word and colleagues found that, in a series of 512 consecutive cases, 49 serious lesions revealed via hysterectomy were missed by preceding D and C.[13] A more complete summary of reports illustrating the inadequacy of D and C is listed in Table 15-1. All such evidence has led Grimes to condemn the continued dependence on D and C as a sole diagnostic method, if to be used at all.[19]

As a corollary to this discussion, it must be mentioned that, contrary to anecdotal claims, no scientific evidence exists to show D and C to be therapeutic, whether the problem is dysfunctional or anatomic. Even if the successive sequential blind thrusts of the curette fortuitously gather the atypical tissue of a focal lesion, it is extremely unlikely that it will be completely removed. False presumption of possible cure could lead to unnecessary delay of definitive therapy. On the other hand, with particular attention to the perimenopausal woman, missing a benign bleeding polyp or finding no abnormal cells after an isolated instance of ovulatory bleeding often leads to an unnecessary hysterectomy simply from fear of the unknown.

TABLE 15-2 Hysteroscopic Findings in Postmenopausal Women

	Focal Lesions, %	Endometrial Hyperplasia, %	Normal Cavity, %	Atrophy, %	Malignancy, %	Other, %
Siegler[21]	36	0	36	28	0	0
Lin et al.[9]	19	0	42	12	11	16
Sciarra[22]	36	3	33	22	6	0
Motashan[23]	57	17	12	5	9	0
Valle[10]	65	8	0	23	4	0
Loffer[17]	26	28	32	0	12	2
Raju[24]	20	14	20	12	25	9
LaSala et al.[25]	22	13	9	39	12	5
Barbot et al.[26]	34	9	13	10	19	15

Usage of Hysteroscopy

Panoramic hysteroscopy provides a valid alternative to traditional D and C and should be used routinely as a primary procedure in the work-up of the bleeding postreproductive woman. Because of the capability of the qualified hysteroscopist to search into every recess of the uterine cavity, thereby allowing for directed biopsies, it is suggested that, perhaps, the gynecologic practitioner should abandon D and C forever. However, although hysteroscopy is making steady inroads, the prevalence of the D and C continues. This seeming stubborn unwillingness to change can be attributed to "comfortable habit," ignorance, sloth, or lack of instruments, all nonacceptable excuses today.

A number of comparative studies emphatically indicate the superiority of hysteroscopy over D and C. Englund and colleagues found that the uterine cavity was sampled satisfactorily in only 44 of 124 patients undergoing D and C followed by hysteroscopy.[14] Loffer reported hysteroscopy to be 98% sensitive as compared to the 65% of D and C.[17] In a similar study, Gimpelson and Rappold showed D and C to be significantly less revealing in 24% of the subjects.[20]

Numerous investigators have described their hysteroscopic findings in symptomatic (bleeding) postmenopausal women (Table 15-2). Endometrial malignancy was noted in approximately 12% of patients. Otherwise the lesions were benign, that is, normal endometrium, atrophy, polyps, and benign hyperplasia. According to established rates, it is estimated that simple D and C would have resulted in a 52% incidence of inadequate or missed diagnosis in these same women.

A description of the common menopausal endometrial findings under hysteroscopic view is appropriate. Hysteroscopic examination permits accurate location and gross diagnosis of endometrial polyps, a not uncommon cause of early postmenopausal bleeding and a lesion particularly unreliably detected by earlier standard diagnostic tests. In the older woman, polyps are covered by a layer of white, atrophic endometrium. They are usually broad-based, occasionally with an uneven surface secondary to underlying small bluish translucent cysts.[27] Under visual hysteroscopic control, the ability to recover the entire polyp results in more dependable histologic examination.

Submucous fibromyomata, although not generally a problem for the climacteric woman, can produce nonphysiologic bleeding in the perimenopause and early menopause. If pedunculated or submucous, they can be extricated cleanly and atraumatically by experienced operative hysteroscopic manipulation. The characteristic appearances, beside the alteration of contour, is a smoother paler surface than that of the balance of the endometrium.

Benign endometrial hyperplasia, a common menopausal atypia, can be accurately mapped and classified, before any instrumental trauma, through the magnified vision of current hysteroscopes. Focal hyperplasia, often missed by both hysterogram and D and C, can be spotted and diagnosed easily by hysteroscopy, which also becomes invaluable in follow-up assessment of efficacy of therapy of hyperplasia. The diagnostic accuracy of hysteroscopic examination without biopsy for low-risk hyperplasia has been reported to be 65.2% with false positives at 34.8% and no false negatives.[27]

The hysteroscopic parameters of low-risk hyperplasia are abnormal and nonhomogeneous growth of the endometrium, dilatation of the glandular openings, and increased vascularization. Adenomatous or atypical hyperplasia under hysteroscopy is characterized by severe morphologic modification of the uterine cavity. Often one sees polypoid or irregular growth accompanied by both increased and abnormal vascularization.[27] Visually there may be difficulty in distinction from adenocarcinoma, but at least the scope provides accurate pinpointing for biopsy from the most suspicious areas.

Postmenopausal bleeding secondary to endometrial atrophy is common. As part of the differential diagnosis of bleeding in this age group, the best diagnostic approach must be used to rule out carcinoma. Even when negative for malignant cells, cytologic and endometrial biopsy findings are inadequate to exclude its presence. The standard resort to D and C yields no tissue at all, thereby rendering either a false sense of security or raising a quandary regarding a possible missed lesion. All doubt can be rapidly and simply averted through hysteroscopy by which the diagnosis of endometrial atrophy is straightforward. The mucous membrane is reduced to a transparent film that reveals the underlying muscles. A multitude of petechiae accounts for the predilection to bleeding. The panoramic view asserting the atrophic status throughout the cavity negates any need for biopsy.

Occasionally in the postmenopausal woman there is need to locate a lost or neglected IUD. Hysteroscopic examination solves the issue at once, bypassing the standard methods of ultrasonography, hysterography, and blind instrumental search. The success, safety, and effectiveness of IUD retrieval by hysteroscopy has been established.[22,28] The same positive features apply to the recovery of other infrequently involved intrauterine foreign bodies, such as Heyman capsules and broken instrument tips.

Contraindications

The contraindications to hysteroscopy in the postreproductive woman are few. The principal one is cervical malignancy. In the presence of such lesions, theoretically it is possible to spread cancer cells into the upper genital tract. More pragmatically, the trauma of hysteroscopic passage and manipulation may incite hemorrhage that will be difficult to control.

Infections of the genital area should be cleared before any hysteroscopic invasion because the condition could be spread or exacerbated.

INSTRUMENTATION

In the performance of any endoscopic procedure, hysteroscopy included, selection of the most appropriate, reliable, and accurate instruments is of primary importance. Currently the market is flooded by a profusion of competitive instruments and accessories manufactured by a wide range of domestic and foreign companies and offered at varying price levels. The resulting confusion at times confounds even the experts. To aid the practitioner make practical decisions, the following discussion should serve as a basis for fundamental comprehension of the mechanics of hysteroscopy, divided into six categories: (1) telescopes, (2) external sheaths, (3) bridges, (4) fiberoptic bundles, (5) light sources, and (6) operative instruments.

Telescopes

At present, hysteroscopy can be accomplished by panoramic or contact methods. The *panoramic hysteroscope* is a modified cystoscope incorporating a telescope and an outer sheath of stainless steel. Distention of the uterine cavity by some sort of medium is essential for use. Panoramic hysteroscopes are either rigid or flexible. The resolution of the rigid scope is far superior to that of the flexible one. Most rigid telescopes have an outer diameter of 4 to 6 mm although models with smaller diameters are available. The smaller ones suffer from the shortcomings of suboptimal optics. The viewing angles most commonly available are either 0 or 30 degrees. The 30-degree hysteroscope allows more rapid and dexterous evaluation of all the walls and tubal ostia.

In contrast, the *contact hysteroscope,* first developed by Marleschki,[29] does not require uterine distention and consists of an optical glass stem that serves both as a conductor of light to the object being examined and as the conduit for the returning image. In actual performance, the objective lens of the telescope is placed directly in contact with the surface under observation.

The technique of contact hysteroscopy, as popularized by Baggish in the United States,[30] is relatively simple. It does not require any fiberoptic light source; instead it uses ambient light. The important advantage of the contact hysteroscope is its application in the presence of intrauterine bleeding. The main disadvantage is its restricted field of view, but that is precisely and specifically its limited assignment anyhow.

A new instrument, the *microhysteroscope* of Hamou,[30] provides observation both in panoramic and contact modes. Also, it permits visualization of the endocervical canal as well as the endometrial cavity. It uses a 4-mm telescope and a 5.2-mm outer sheath. Its lens system provides observation at 1×, 30×, 60×, and 150× magnifications. The first two of these settings apply to the panoramic view and the latter pair to the contact microscopic analysis.

The light source for the microhysteroscope is the same as that used in conventional hysteroscopy and the distention medium is carbon dioxide. The diagnostic applications of the microhysteroscope are broad including not only those of conventional hysteroscopy but also the special capacity to evaluate the endocervical canal and the transformation zone when it is retracted high in the canal. The high magnifications available for these latter investigations make this instrument particularly desirable.

External Sheaths

Varying from 5 to 8 mm in diameter, external stainless steel sheaths permit the insertion and free movement of the telescopes. Sheaths come equipped with stopcock-controlled channels for the introduction and flow of distention media. The smallest diagnostic sheath (5 mm) is best suited for outpatient hysteroscopy. Some of the available larger sheaths for operative use have attached bridges to permit expanded instrument manipulation.

Bridges

These are attached at one end of the sheath and, when guided by a knob at the other end, provide a distal deflecting mechanism for laser quartz fibers and flexible instruments.

Fiberoptic Bundles and Light Sources

The development and perfection of cold bright light rising from a flexible fiber bundle revolutionized capability in every medical area using endoscopy. Hys-

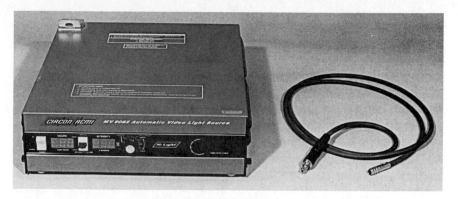

Figure 15-1 Light source *(left)* and fiberoptic light cord *(right)*.

teroscopy is no exception; both panoramic and microscopic views have become refined because of it. The standard models used with different instruments for a variety of hysteroscopic procedures, including the light sources themselves, are shown in Figure 15-1.

Operative Instruments

A progressively increasing armamentarium of rigid, semirigid, and flexible operative instruments has been developed in answer to the steadily widening range of demands and improving skills in hysteroscopic surgery. These instruments range from simple biopsy forceps through scissors and electroresectors to laser tips and roller-ball cauterizers. Most of them are applicable to procedures performed in perimenopausal and climacteric women. Several of the instruments are shown in Figure 15-2.

DISTENTION MEDIA

The cavity of the uterus is potential rather than real. To achieve a panoramic view, that is, maximum exploration of the entire endometrial surface area, distention of the cavity is essential. The ideal distending medium should pose no local or systemic problems. More specifically, it should be isotonic, nontoxic, nonconductive, and rapidly excreted. Additionally, visual clarity and minimal plasma volume expansion are ideals. Also desirable requisites are substances that are easy to handle (watery, not heavy and sticky) and are immiscible with blood. At present the ideal distention medium is nonexistent. Three types of media are currently available and in use:

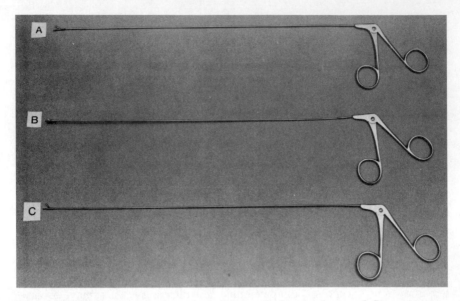

Figure 15-2 Hysteroscopic instruments. A, Scissors. B, Grasping forceps. C, Biopsy forceps.

1. Low-viscosity liquids
   a. 5% dextrose in water
   b. normal saline
   c. 1.5% glycine
   d. 3% sorbitol
2. High-viscosity liquids
   a. Dextran—32% (Hyskon)
3. Nontoxic gas
   a. Carbon dioxide

Distention media are instilled through instrument channels under appropriate pressure by pumps, passive gravity, blood pressure cuff, or syringe.

Carbon Dioxide

Carbon dioxide, the only gaseous medium currently in use, provides a clear view of the endometrium. It is inexpensive, easy to infuse, and the least messy of the common distention fluids. Its use requires a hysteroinsufflator, an instrument devised especially for hysteroscopy. A flow rate of 30 to 50 mL/min. is recommended for visualization inside the endometrial cavity. Occasionally the flow rate must be raised to 100 mL/min., a level that should not generally be exceeded. Pressure of the flow should not surpass 150 mm Hg.

The problems in controlled usage of CO_2 are minimal. If the view is inadequate, coincident with a very low pressure, despite a high flow rate, either a leak in the system or a uterine perforation must be suspected and checked at once, especially in the latter event. Occasionally visualization of the cavity becomes impossible because of bubbles of mucus. Suction often helps to overcome such problems. Although CO_2 is usually ideal for outpatient diagnosis, other than biopsy it is not recommended as a practical medium in association with operative procedures.

With the usage of current hysteroinsufflators, complications from CO_2 are unlikely. Earlier a few cases of cardiac arrest simultaneous with CO_2 hysteroscopy were reported, but this problem potential has been well resolved. The common factor in each of these cases was a distribution of CO_2 greater than 300 mL/min with accompanying alarming pressure levels. Corson and colleagues[32] have recently demonstrated the safety of CO_2 as an intrauterine distending agent when used sensibly. However, they caution against its use in the very high-risk patients with right-to-left intracardiac shunt (septal defect) or pulmonary hypertension. In such cases, other agents should be considered.

Hyskon (Dextran)

The average molecular weight of Hyskon is 70,000. It is thick and heavy, with a sticky consistency, and this makes handling difficult. It is free of electrolytes and slow in absorption. Major advantages are high optical clarity and low miscibility with blood.

Despite the maximum safety level warning of 500 mL Hyskon at one setting noted in the Hyskon package insert, complications have been reported with less than this amount. Most surgeons today abstain from using more than 300 mL.

The complications of Hyskon are pulmonary edema, bleeding time prolongation, disseminated intravascular coagulation, anaphylaxis, and, rarely, pseudo-Meigs' syndrome.

Watery Solutions

Today, 5% dextrose in water or saline, both well tolerated, are used with steadily increasing frequency. They are readily available in all operating rooms. Various mechanical pumps have been introduced recently for delivery of these media into the uterine cavity under constant pressure. More simply, flow can be instituted and maintained by an ordinary syringe, by a pneumatically inflated pressure bag, or by gravity alone.

A cautionary note of extreme importance, however, is relevant to the use of all watery media. Because these liquids flow readily through the tubal ostia into the peritoneal cavity, large quantities may be absorbed during prolonged operative procedures. When careless overflow is permitted, water intoxication and pulmonary edema, even death, can occur. Careful monitoring of flow in and flow out, supplemented by the judicious use of diuretics intraoperatively, can avert dreadful disasters.

OPERATION SETTING

Hysteroscopy can be performed either in an outpatient setting or in the hospital surgical suite. Determinant conditions for the choice of the most practical site for performing this procedure include the patient's medical status, the possibility for concomitant surgery requiring major anesthesia, the level of office or clinic physical operating facility, the quality and quantity of outpatient instruments, and the surgeon's experience. Equally important option factors concern the anticipated procedural goals, that is, purely diagnostic, diagnostic-therapeutic, or therapeutic only. If the latter, will it be minimal (polyps) or extensive (ablation)?

Simplistically, diagnostic procedures lend themselves more readily to a clinic or office setting. Operative ventures, in consideration of more intense and prolonged manipulation than in pure observational identification, should be directed to the hospital operating room where higher levels of anesthesia can be more safely regulated.

Not to be ignored in the choice of operating theater are the particular patient's psyche, her pain threshold, and her own desires. Additionally the postmenopausal patient often presents special or more delicate problems that influence where hysteroscopy may be best performed. For example, an arthritic or orthopedically abnormal condition might render an outpatient approach impractical. Such would also be the case with a constricted introitus, an atrophic narrowed vagina, or a contracted cervical canal. A postmenopausal nulliparous pelvis presents a mechanical problem in itself, best handled under hospital anesthesia. It certainly would compound the conditions already mentioned.

COMPLICATIONS

Significant problems in association with hysteroscopy are uncommon. As with any surgery, the risks in the climacteric group are greater than those in younger women with particular reference to anesthesia and decreased cardiopulmonary reserve. Such physiologic alteration can be compounded by absorption of fluid distention beyond reasonable limits, which are certainly much more restrictive in older women than in young.

Perforation of the uterus is a more likely mishap in older women because of the atrophy and constriction already cited, but ironically the same conditions might markedly restrict any associated bleeding which would certainly be greater in younger women. Dilatation of a stenotic cervix might produce a problematic tear.

Infection is always a possibility but it is not frequently seen. The complications associated with distending media have been discussed in the coverage of the individual substances. Finally potential bleeding problems from any endoscopic surgical site, as is usual in any operation, are omnipresent, especially when sharp and cutting instruments are used. The surgeon must be capable of stopping the bleeding.

CONCLUSIONS

Both laparoscopy and hysteroscopy are currently firmly established modalities for both diagnosis and therapy in the climacteric. Unquestionably both telescopic methods have broadened our capacities to offer the older patient significantly better care in selected areas of diagnosis and therapy. In the postmenopausal woman, laparoscopic importance lies in the realm of adnexal problems, and hysteroscopy is first choice in the solution of uterine bleeding dilemmas. In view of the progress already made, one cannot deny a potential for further positive development. Overall prospects for a continued growth in general usage by practitioners seems bright, especially with apparent increasing learning opportunities available almost universally. The low rate of risks and complications when a careful and conservative approach is followed lend a stimulating appeal to the special role played by endoscopy in the field of geriatric gynecology.

REFERENCES

1. Bozzini P. *Der Lichtleiter oder Beschreitbung einer Einfachen Vorrichtung und Ihrer Anwendung zur Erleuchtung Innerer Hohlen und Zwischenraume des Lebenden Aminalischen Korpers.* Weimer: Landes-Industrie-Comptoir; 1807.

2. Desormeaux AJ. *De l'endoscope et de ses Applications Au Diagnostic et Au Traitement Des Affections De l'urethre et de la Verrie.* Paris: Balliere; 1865.

3. Pantaleoni D. On endoscopic examination of the womb. *Med Press Circ.* 1869;8:26.

4. Kelling G. Uber Oesophagoskopie, Gastroskopie und Colioskopie. *Munch Med Wochenschr.* 1901;49:21–24.

5. Jacobaeus HC. Uber Die Moglichkeit, die Zystoskopie bei Untersuchung Seroser Hohlungen Anzuwenden. *Munch Med Wochenschr.* 1910;57:2090–2092.

6. Lindemann HJ. Historical aspects of hysterectomy. *Fertil Steril.* 1973;24:230–232.

7. Koonings PP, Campbell K, Mischell DR, Grimes DA. Relative frequency of primary ovarian neoplasms: A 10-year review. *Obstet Gynecol.* 1989;74:921–925.

8. Bennington JL, Ferguson BR, Harber SL. Incidence and relative frequency of benign and malignant ovarian neoplasms. *Obstet Gynecol.* 1968;32:627–632.

9. Lin B, Iwata Y, Liu KH, Valle RF. The Fujinon diagnostic fiberoptic hysteroscope. Experience with 1503 patients. *J Reprod Med.* 1990;35:685–689.

10. Valle RF. Hysteroscopic evaluation of patients with abnormal uterine bleeding. *Surg Gynecol Obstet.* 1989;153:521–526.

11. Smith JJ, Schulman H. Current dilatation and curettage practice: A need for revision. *Obstet Gynecol.* 1985;65:516–520.

12. Stock RJ, Kanbour A. Prehysterectomy curettage. *Obstet Gynecol.* 1975;45:537–541.

13. Word B, Gravlee C, Wideman GL. The fallacy of simple uterine curettage. *Obstet Gynecol.* 1958;12:642–648.

14. Englund SE, Ingleman-Sundberg A, Westin B. Hysteroscopy in diagnosis and treatment of uterine bleeding. *Gynakologue.* 1957;143:217–219.

15. Gribb JJ. Hysteroscopy: An aid in gynecologic diagnosis. *Obstet Gynecol.* 1960;15:593–601.

16. Brooks PG, Serden SP. Hysteroscopic findings after unsuccessful dilatation and curettage for abnormal uterine bleeding. *Am J Obstet Gynecol.* 1988;158:1354–1357.

17. Loffer RD. Hysteroscopy with selective endometrial sampling compared with D&C for abnormal uterine bleeding: The value of a negative hysteroscopic view. *Obstet Gynecol.* 1989;73:16–20.

18. Valle RF. Hysteroscopic evaluation of patients with abnormal uterine bleeding. *Surg Gynecol Obstet.* 1981;153:521–527.

19. Grimes DA. Diagnostic dilatation and curettage: A reapprisal. *Am J Obstet Gynecol.* 1982;142:1–6.

20. Gimpelson RJ, Rappold HO. A comparative study between panoramic hysteroscopy with directed biopsies and dilatation and curettage. A review of 276 cases. *Am J Obstet Gynecol.* 1988;158:489–492.

21. Siegler AM, Kemmann E, Gentile GP. Hysteroscopic procedures in 257 patients. *Fertil Steril.* 1976;27:1267–1273.

22. Sciarra JJ, Valle RF. Hysteroscopy: A clinical experience with 320 patients. *Am J Obstet Gynecol.* 1977;127:340.

23. Motashaw ND, Dave S. Diagnostic and therapeutic hysteroscopy in the management of abnormal uterine bleeding. *J Reprod Med.* 1990;35:616–620.

24. Raju KS, Taylor RW. Routine hysteroscopy for patients with a high risk of uterine malignancy. *Br J Obstet Gynaecol.* 1986;93:1259–1261.

25. LaSala GB, Sacchett F, Dessanti L. Panoramic diagnostic microhysteroscopy analysis of results obtained from 976 outpatients. *Acta Obstet Gynecol Scand.* 1987;suppl 141:43–45.

26. Barbot J, Parent B, Dubuisson JB. Contact hysteroscopy: Another method of endoscopic examination of the uterine cavity. *Am J Obstet Gynecol.* 1980;136:721–730.

27. Barbot J. Hysteroscopy for abnormal bleeding in diagnostic and operative hystero-scopy. In: Baggish MS, Barbot J, Valle RF, eds., *Yearbook of Obstetrics and Gynecology.* Chicago: Year Book Medical Publishers 1989;147–155.

28. Taylor PJ, Cumming DC. Hysteroscopy in 100 patients. *Fertil Steril.* 1979;31:301–305.

29. Marleschki V. Die Moderne Zervikoskopie Und Hysteroscopie. *Zentralbl Gynakol.* 1966;20:637.

30. Baggish MS. Contact hysteroscopy: A new technique to explore the uterine cavity. *Obstet Gynecol.* 1979;54:350.

31. Hamou J. Microhysteroscopy: A new procedure and its original applications in gynecology. *J Reprod Med.* 1981;26:375.

32. Corson SL, Hoffman JL, Jackowski J, et al. Cardiopulmonary effects of direct venous CO_2 insufflation in ewes. A model for CO_2 hysteroscopy. *J Reprod Med.* 1988;33:440–444.

Wound Healing and

Suture Selection

in Reconstructive

Surgery

Marvin H. Terry Grody

WOUND HEALING

The capacity for healing after trauma, including surgical invasion, is of much greater concern in the geriatric population than in the younger generations. As middle age wanes, metabolic processes and tissue reproduction slacken, the digestive tract becomes less efficient, the cardiovascular network narrows and diminishes, pulmonary exchange rates recede, the neurologic system atrophies, endocrine glands are less responsive, and the musculoskeletal mass decreases. Of vital importance is the dwindling capacity for immune response. Add to these specific regressions the negative effects of the wear and tear of time on all the body tissues. As if this were not enough, although not so apparent or important at an earlier time, increasingly wider individual variations in overall health and vitality become starkly apparent. These differences among patients, arising from dissimilar genetic inheritance, dietary habits, activity, disease incidence, and general life-style, including drug and alcohol usage and smoking, can create wide gaps in healing potential in older people. The doctor who ignores these danger signals and makes no effort at timely compensatory measures preoperatively courts disaster in the recovery phase, not the least of which is wound dissolution and operative failure.

For the operating gynecologist performing benign procedures in the post-menopausal woman, almost always involving reconstruction, directly or indirectly, two adjunctive factors play a strong role in healing. Firstly, the menopause invokes estrogen depletion and this loss accelerates the aging process, most particularly in the area where the gynecologist works. Pelvic tissues deprived of the positive effects of estrogen are thinner, weaker, drier, and more poorly vascularized than are those under full hormonal stimulation. Hence, a greater incidence of longer and poorer healing and operative failure is apparent.

Secondly, this type of surgery, in contrast to the wide variety of procedures performed in other surgical specialties in this same age group, is totally dependent on the quality of the connective tissue. For starters, the connective tissue of the pelvis is weaker than that elsewhere in the woman because of the trauma endured earlier in life through childbirth. Its function of supporting the weight and pressure of the torso has been so much more demanding than that of connective tissue in the rest of the body that it generally exists in a significantly greater state of attenuation by the time the postmenopause is entered. Thus, the resultant herniations and prolapses requiring repair are more vulnerable for recurrence unless all the negative facets are vigorously dealt with in advance of any scheduled operation. As discussed in Chapter 3, this includes elimination of all elements that cause continuous or repetitive abnormally increased intra-abdominal pressure.

In brief, wound healing begins preoperatively weeks, and often months, before any surgery is performed. An intensive presurgical anabolic corrective pathway is the best insurance for the fast track on the road to recovery after the operation. Our responsibility today, particularly since 60% of the surgery performed on geriatric women is reconstructive and restorative,[1,2] especially in view of increasing life expectancy, is greater than ever to produce good lasting results. It is incumbent on us to pay strict and continuous attention to any and all factors involved in the healing process of the singular surgical wounds we create. Such emphasis becomes particularly vital because we perform our work in the neighborhood of hostile bacteria, the distal end of the alimentary canal, thereby posing the constant specter of infection, the principal threat to good healing anywhere.

The Status of the Patient

Primary consideration must first center on the patient's general constitutional state in preparation for surgery. Deficiencies are more apt to exist in older patients than younger ones and, since evidence as far back as DuNouy's work in 1916[3] suggests slower healing in the former than the latter, measures for compensation must be exercised. The surgical conditions covered by this book are benign, implying no need to rush to the operating room. Time for investigation and preparation, especially because the lesions presenting for correction have usually taken years to reach the point of need for surgery, should be used to create the maximum environment to achieve the maximum long-term outcomes. More and more we will be approached by women in their 60s and 70s and even in their 80s, with projected potential to live several years longer. Many of these women already will have endured one or more operative failures. We must give them their best chance for success.

For decades the hypoestrogenism of the postmenopause has been widely proclaimed as a key factor in the deterioration of pelvic tissues in the parous woman.[4,5] The gross recognition of the frailty of the tissues in the postreproductive woman never subjected to estrogen replacement therapy (ERT) can be observed and palpated in the outpatient examining room. The vaginal mucosa has thinned and dried, the rugae and moisture are gone, and the slightest contact may produce abrasion. The previously rich circulation progressively atrophies and connective tissue strength, texture, and elasticity starkly diminish as the patient ages. Yet as widely accepted as this knowledge has become, how astonishing it is to see one menopausal patient after another either previously having undergone reparative surgery, or having now had it proposed to her, with absolutely no estrogen fortification. No matter how proficient technically, the gynecologic surgeon foolish enough to attempt to operate on such poor tissue condemns the patient to a significantly worse result than that had she been on ERT, often more profound than the presenting lesion before surgery.

Good healing relies on adequate perfusion of oxygen, amino acids, minerals, vitamins, and other catalysts, and this cannot happen in the absence of adequate transporting blood vessels. Although it may take 12 to 14 months for maximum total tissue restoration under the influence of estrogen, in only 4 to 6 weeks mucosal surfaces and underlying circulation can be reclaimed sufficiently to permit effective and lasting good results providing ERT continues postoperatively. As mentioned in Chapter 1, I have been astonished to find absolutely no documentation, not even a declaration, of the need for continued ERT after postmenopausal reconstructive surgery anywhere in the gynecologic literature. My experience of more than 40 years, including thousands of reparative cases of my own and others, augmented by the experience and similar sentiment of seasoned gynecologists I know, dictates stringent adherence to lifelong ERT commitment for maintenance of effective surgery. Logically, if estrogen deficiency is a key player in the scenario leading to symptomatic pelvic structural imperfections, the continuation of replacement is incumbent on continued success.

Two practical notes are important. Preoperatively, oral administration of estrogen is the most practical route because the protrusions existent in most cases render vaginal applications ridiculous. However, postoperatively either method is acceptable, as is the dermal route via the patch. Finally, in low dosage levels regularly used, there is no evidence to support preclusion of ERT at any time, even to the very day of operation, on the basis of possible enhancement of intravascular coagulation (see Chapters 1 and 3).

Older women are often prone to poor nutrition, especially if they live alone or are widowed. Without incentive to eat regular meals or to follow sensible dietary precepts, aggravated by despair, depression, or melancholy, in a setting of more sluggish digestive function than that of her youth, nutrition may fall below levels necessary for sustenance of good health. On a chronic basis, measurable deficiencies can develop that are not directly threatening but which, in critical situations such as impending major surgery, should be and must be identified and corrected to obviate possible dire complications in wound healing.

Hypoproteinemia is the most serious of the likely problems to be addressed. Major surgical research studies have revealed significant tissue edema and marked retardation in gastrointestinal emptying times in association with hypoproteinemia.[6,7] Experimentally, wound disruption after laparotomy was found to be frequent[7] in hypoproteinemic animals, and later marked impairment in wound healing resulting from marked retardation in fibroplasia was revealed in similar subjects.[8] Subsequent investigations of hypoproteinemic states delineated decreased resistance to infection,[9] delayed antibody production,[10] and strong correlation with infectious complications, including wound infections and postoperative disruptions.[11–13] Sandblom and Lindstedt, in a classic study in Switzerland, showed that patients with low serum albumin or low serum total protein levels had distinctly weaker wounds than did patients who had normal levels.[14] They also revealed poorer wound healing in older patients.

Although nutritional states uncommonly drop so low that vigorous efforts must be expended preoperatively to attain more normal levels in the usual cases presenting for pelvic reconstruction, one must be prepared for the geriatric patient who needs such help. Dudrick showed that, on average, 5 days of correction time was the minimum to show significant presurgical change.[15] He also concluded that 5 days of preoperative nutritional management was much better than 2 weeks of a postsurgical program with the same goals. Basically one must strive to revert a catabolic state to one of positive nitrogen balance before surgery.

Ascorbic acid deficiency has been identified as a cause of decreased tensile strength.[16] Others have emphasized the importance of zinc in good wound healing.[17] Studies of localized applications of specific amino acids such as cystine have shown improved wound healing in human beings.[18] Proline and lysine are known progenitors of collagen formation initiated by the early action of fibroblasts in healing. Methionine and arginine are apparently of equal importance. Vitamin A has been shown to accelerate wound healing.

Most of all, wound healing depends on perfusion and oxygenation. Perfusion demands a rich blood supply, including an effective capillary network in the region of the operative wound. Without ample perfusion, none of the vital nutrients can be transported sufficiently, including oxygen, the overall determinant in the varied healing processes.[19] Oxygenation requires an adequately functioning respiratory system as well as a dependable cardiovascular tree.

Iron and zinc are important in the local healing of wounds. The value of iron in the correction of anemia both preoperatively and postoperatively is obvious. Curiously, although nonanemic patients overall recover somewhat more rapidly than do those with anemia, low hemoglobin is not an impediment to good healing or to infection control so long as perfusion is adequate.[19] Again we must emphasize the vascularizing effects of estrogen.

In summary, initial advance warning signs that might presage poor healing in any patient preparatory to surgery, but particularly in the postmenopausal woman, can be categorized as follows:

1. Poor physical appearance
2. Recent unintended weight loss
3. Indolent life-style
4. Poor eating habits
5. Evidence of fluid retention
6. Manifest protein tissue loss
7. Smoking habit
8. Respiratory impairment
9. Cardiovascular disease

Laboratory danger signals amplify the list:

1. Low serum protein (especially the albumin fraction—less than 3.4 g)
2. Low lymphocyte count (very important, according to many observers)
3. Low hematocrit
4. Low oxygen levels
5. Zinc deficiency
6. Imbalanced electrolytes

Although applicable to all cases of major surgery in either sex at any age, I think certain special complicating circumstances affect wound healing in the older woman undergoing pelvic surgery, especially if reconstructive, more than all other patients. *Uncontrolled diabetes* is an obviously demanding situation, known to all surgeons, and requires no discussion here. Certainly preoperative evaluation and stabilization in all cases, with continued close postoperative management by a qualified diabetologist or internist, is obligatory toward maximum wound healing and infection prophylaxis. *Morbid obesity* speaks for itself. Perhaps more than all other factors, obesity, not even in excess, sets the stage for multiple possible postoperative complications, not the least of which is poor wound healing or wound breakdown. At Temple University Hospital (TUH), for anything less than cancer or lifesaving necessity, we will perform no gynecologic surgery in the presence of overt obesity, especially in the elderly, until substantial objective weight loss, with a pledge from patient and family for postoperative perpetuation of weight control, has been demonstrated. *Continuous steroid therapy,* being administered for sound medical reasons, creates a difficult problem in wound healing. All that can be said in this regard is that everyone involved must understand the increased risk, each case must be tailored to specific management, and the responsible internist must be intimately involved in all care. *Distant active infection* is a constant threat for bacteremia. A healing surgical wound provides a first class culture site for wandering blood-borne bacteria. The fragile older woman with a dental abscess or a parenechia, for example, no matter how slight, supplies an excellent target in a fresh operative wound. If such a source is found, even on the morning of surgery, the procedure should be canceled until infection is obliterated, no matter where in the body it is located. *Immunologic impairments* perhaps present the greatest difficulties of all in wound healing. Risks of healing must be well articulated to all concerned. Close and continued consultation with both internist and infectious disease specialist is crucial in correct management.

A special notation about *cigarette smoking* must be made. This repugnant habit seems to be increasing steadily universally among women, particularly older women, by my own perception and that of my colleagues. This may be explained as a sociologic accompaniment of loneliness and inactivity. Smoking presents a major obstacle to good healing in general but especially so in the pelvis, where tissues are relatively fragile and where any chronic increase in intra-abdominal pressure, even intermittently, threatens operative integrity. A recent report indicates significantly poorer healing capacity in women who have ever smoked versus those who have never smoked.[20] This analysis of 606 patients centers primarily on the incidence of incontinence as affected by smoking, but other studies substantiate the direct negative effects of smoking on collagen synthesis, vital in the healing process.[21] This subject is discussed in Chapter 3. All smokers cough, no matter what they profess, and considering the long time necessary for healing of pelvic fascial tissue, only one coughing attack per day can wreck a technically fine operation. An additional note warns that ascorbic acid (vitamin C) should probably be given in doses of 1000 mg/d to current smokers because of nicotine-induced oxidation of ascorbic acid. At TUH we do not face this problem because we will not perform corrective surgery on those avowed to continued smoking. Smoking or not, it is a good idea to give 500 mg/d of vitamin C.

Infection as a Deterrent to Good Healing

A vast array of readily available literature verifies infection as the single greatest detriment to surgical healing.[22-27] Before the mid-nineteenth century and the introduction of antisepsis, infection, pus formation, and secondary hemorrhage posed enormous problems in sutured surgical wounds. In Austria, Semmelweiss emphasized simply the necessity of washing one's hands between patient visitations. Lister, in England, introduced specific antiseptic routines, the rationale for which was being proven by the documentation of the germ theory of disease by Pasteur in France. Hutchinson introduced the steam sterilizer, Lister promoted chromic catgut sutures, Halsted advanced aseptic techniques, and finally Claudius, in 1902, introduced potassium iodide sterilization of suture materials. The war against infection had begun. We have won many battles since then, through better techniques, superior materials, and all manner of antibiotics, but the war will never end. What can we do to stay ahead and to protect our patients, particularly the older ones? The gravity of the problem is statistically borne out in the revelation that patients older than 66 years are six times more prone to infection than those 1 to 14 years of age.[28] Put more precisely, people over 65 are twice as likely to develop operative wound infections as those between 21 and 50.

The Operating Gynecologist

The physician can be a principal purveyor of infection. Simple hand care must be a constant. The skin should be kept hydrated and not allowed to crack in the winter, when protective gloves should be worn at all times outdoors. Frequent applications of nondehydrating substances, such as Silicon Glove (Avon), which is nongreasy, are dependably protective. The fingernails should be kept short and uncovered hands should not be exposed to infected areas.

The human nose is the principal source of *Staphylococcus aureus* infections in operative wounds. This mandates the use of properly affixed operating room masks. Additionally, physicians should keep their hands away from the nose at all times. Washing the hands after nose-blowing is a good idea.

Except for examination, the doctor should not touch the patient at the bedside or in the operating room preoperatively. An estimated 1000 bacteria are transferred each time. Similarly, as Semmelweiss demonstrated, bacteria can be spread by the doctor from one patient to another. These newly transferred bacteria on a doctor's hands can live for 20 to 150 minutes. Hands should be cleaned before and after seeing or examining a patient. Waterless agents (Alcare, Cal-Stat, Hibistat, Septisol) should be used. Finally, the caring surgeon, before going home from the office or the hospital, should habitually cleanse the hands with a waterless alcohol emollient solution for 10 to 15 seconds.

The anus is an obvious major source of contamination. A significant percentage of people, surgeons not exempted, harbor *S. aureus* in the anorectal area. Studies involving cultures from ordinary seats have proven this. Hands should be washed after using the toilet. When public toilets are used, one should flush with the foot. Toilet door handles should not be touched directly. Observation of doctors' disregard for simple toilet hygiene is sometimes appalling.

Scrubbing the hands in the operating room preoperatively today is fairly simple.[29–31] Three currently used agents are equally effective in killing 99.7% or better of all bacteria:

1. Chlorhexidine gluconate—4% (Pre-op II—Davis and Geck; Hibiclens-Stuart)

2. Povidone—1% (Iodophor—Davis and Geck; Betadine-Purdue-Frederick)

3. 70% isopropyl alcohol (ironically, 95% alcohol is inferior)

A 2-minute scrub or contact rids the skin of well over 99% of its bacteria, both transient and resident types. Bar soaps are essentially worthless. The scrubbing action should favor those areas harboring the greatest bacterial concentrations, i.e., under the fingernails (prescrub nail-pick helps), at the cuticles, and in the finger webs. Before vaginal surgery, extra scrubbing on the nondominant index finger is indicated because almost invariably the glove is inadvertently pierced in that area during the operation. In scrubbing, many feel that the more vigorous the agitation, the better the efficacy.

Surgical gloves unquestionably help. They protect the patient from the surgeon's residual bacteria especially if the surgeon relies more on the glove than the scrub; the surgeon also needs protection from the patient's body fluids. Bacteria can and do grow inside gloves, proportionate to the time they are worn, especially as perspiration accumulates inside. When gloves are penetrated, appropriate changes of glove and offending needle are in order. However, appropriate preoperative scrubbing with either povidone or chlorhexidine seems to preclude propagation of infection from glove punctures during surgery. Presumably organisms escape into the wound but in insufficient numbers to act as a serious menace in an otherwise clean wound in the presence of normal host resistance. Double gloving has been considered as increased protection for the doctor but many surgeons complain of resulting decreased tactile sensitivity. In consideration of protection of the surgeon from the patient's fluids, eye shields are suggested either as large plastic glasses or a clear visor.

The Patient

Preoperative bathing is a hygienic consideration for the patient. It is good for her and good for those who attend her, especially because she may not have a chance to bathe well again for a few days. Ask her to concentrate on the area of intended surgery, i.e., the vulva and the lower abdomen. If possible, chlorhexidine should be used in those areas as well as those of the anus, umbilicus, and skin creases. In a monumental study, the infection rate was 2.3% in consecutive major surgical cases of varied nature when the patient did not shower before surgery.[28] If a preoperative shower was taken, using ordinary soap, the rate was 2.1%, but if directed scrubbing with hexachlorophene was used, the infection incidence dropped to 1.3%.

Preoperative shaving of hair at the intended operative sites the night before surgery can raise the infection rate markedly and is not advisable.[32] If the surgeon insists on shaving the operative site, it should be done just before the operation is to start, thereby reducing the infection rate sharply but not nearly as much as when the hair is simply clipped at that time. With clipping, the infection rate is 1.8%, and this can be reduced to 0.9% when no hair is removed at all.[28] Our routine at TUH is restricted to clipping, performed just before the start of laparotomy cases only, not vaginal cases. In my own travels across the United States, I am chagrined at the number of facilities that still shave the patient's pubic and perineal areas before operating room arrival for both abdominal and vaginal cases. At TUH, we neither shave nor clip prior to any vulvar or vaginal approach.

Few physicians are truly cognizant of the effect of length of hospital stay on infection incidence. According to Cruse and Foord, from their prospective 10-year study of 62,939 operative wounds, the longer the preoperative hospitalization, the greater the incidence of postoperative wound infection.[28] They conclude unreservedly that all nosocomial (hospital-acquired) wound infections occur entirely as a result of the preoperative hospital stay and the intraoperative events. No matter what the postoperative management, it does not alter the rate of wound infection.

Preoperative douching, regardless of whether the surgical approach is vaginal or the vagina is opened during abdominal laparotomy, is of questionable value in the prevention of postoperative infection anywhere within the operative field. Common knowledge accepts the impossibility of sterilizing the vagina presurgically by any practical means. It is also known that bacterial population reduction in the vagina is equivalent regardless of the agent used, whether it be a strong sterilizing solution, saline, or just water. Thus, the real value of douching is its bacterial dilution capacity. The prevailing prophylactic balance lies with host tissue resistance and the delicacy in tissue handling and suturing during the operation itself. However, as repeated throughout this text, the value of a positive patient psyche can never be underestimated. So, with this in mind, at TUH we ask each relevant patient to douche the night before surgery with a povidone (1%) solution. Saline or water will not be acceptable to the patient because too many of them know that their friends and relatives all received "a special sterilizing douche" preparation before their operations. Because there is basically no real harm, we have made no effort to alter this routine.

Recently at TUH, as at a few other institutions, we have considered the wisdom of giving a short-term intravaginal treatment preoperatively to all patients showing an alkaline pH in their vaginal secretions. Consider that bacterial vaginosis is extremely widespread, both symptomatic and asymptomatic, reckoned today by most observers to be the leading vaginal contaminant, and that one or more of its principal constituents are in the anaerobic bacteroides family. The virulent bacterial composition almost always responsible for pelvic cellulitis when it occurs after pelvic surgery includes both aerobes and anaerobes, the latter principally of the bacteroides group. The cost of treatment for postoperative pelvic cellulitis, with special reference to medication and probable prolonged hospitalization, can amount to several hundred dollars, not to mention the threat to the integrity of a presumed fine operation. Vaginal secretions always reveal an alkaline pH in the presence of bacterial vaginosis. The vaginal pH test is painless, quickly done, and inexpensive. To be even more certain, the simple "whiff test," easily accomplished in a few seconds, can offer further verification of bacterial vaginosis. It is done by placing a single drop of KOH (10%) solution on a Q-tip containing vaginal secretions. A fishy odor is a positive result. The medication to be used would be a recently developed Food and Drug Administration approved vaginally inserted cream or gel of low allergic potential to be used once or twice a day for 5 or 7 days before surgery. Use of metronidazole vaginal gel—0.75% (MetroGel Vaginal) —or clindamycin phosphate vaginal cream—2% (Cleocin Vaginal Cream— 2%)—is a relatively inexpensive and minimally involved method of eradicating anaerobic bacteria before surgery. When one weighs the generally accepted probability of at least a 15% to 20% incidence of cellulitis after 2 or more hours of vaginal reconstruction, especially with significant resident participation, even after standard preoperative antibiotics, this option for presurgical antibacteroides vaginal prophylaxis seems reasonable. At TUH during the 2 years prior to this publication we have pondered running a clinical series to prove the efficacy of this preventive measure but have found it to be impractical in view of our mounting highly favorable statistics using other methods.

During the 2 years referred to above, and encompassing in that time only those cases performed through the vaginal approach that have required more than 150 minutes of open operative wound exposure, we have noted an astonishing progressively decreasing rate of postoperative infection. We classify these cases as pelvic reconstructive, vaginal, and urogynecologic procedures, and almost all have required at least three different components, some as many as six, in the total operation as performed by our special gynecologic surgical service. As a referral center, we operate primarily on postmenopausal women, sent to us by other gynecologists; the patients present complicated structural and urogynecologic problems, almost always including both pelvic prolapse of one sort or another and severe anterior compartment deficiency. Most have experienced at least one previous pelvic operative failure and many more than two. The age range of this group of patients has been 45 to 89, averaging about 69, and the surgical times have varied from 150 to 260 minutes. The prolonged operating times are a direct result of the complex nature of the surgery, secondary to distortions from previous operations and the multiplicity of procedural components, and significant resident participation as a part of a teaching program. Unquestionably such situations present enormous potential for a high rate of postoperative wound infection, principally pelvic cellulitis, despite accepted standard preoperative and intraoperative antibiotic prophylaxis. This series of almost 200 consecutive operations will have been presented in three separate manuscripts for journal publication by the time this book is completed. One of the most astounding features of these studies will be a postoperative infection rate that has averaged about 4% but which, since July 1, 1992, has dropped close to 3%. The criteria for infection are listed in Chapter 18. The major benefit of this low infection incidence has been excellent wound healing, not to mention rapid recovery and short hospital stay.

What have we deduced as the reasons for this remarkable phenomenon? The major change in our management has been almost constant jet-propelled saline lavage from the beginning to the end of each operation. The value of lavage in helping to reduce infection in abdominal laparotomy has long been recognized. It is standard procedure in operating rooms everywhere to wash the abdominal cavity lavishly with saline before closure to clear out, as much as possible, blood clots, cellular debris, and incidental bacteria, all elements that could promote postoperative infection. Such lavage has been impractical in vaginal cases, especially those of extensive reconstruction, because different areas are opened and closed sequentially. In essence, repair and closure are synonymous vaginally, and to duplicate the abdominal type of lavage, bowls full of saline would have to be tossed into the vaginal site repetitively, soaking the operators and flooding the operating room floor. So vaginal surgeons have depended entirely on suction and sponging to clean the often wide raw areas, not nearly as efficient as a liquid wash.

Since January 1991, our second assistant has been commissioned to use one hand to lavage and suction simultaneously almost constantly through every vaginal case by using a newly developed instrument called Vital Vue (Davis and Geck). This cleverly contrived multipurpose slightly curved tool (Figure 16-1), which also has a light bulb at its end and can retract tissue for better exposure in narrow areas if necessary, can project a narrow stream of fluid under measured pressure into an operative site by finger application on a button, while simultaneous suction prevents any dripping and wetting outside the surgical margins. Blood is collected before clots can form, surgical debris is removed instantaneously, and bacteria have no chance to gain a foothold before being washed clear and sucked out of the area. The Vital Vue device has allowed us to defy a guiding precept of Cruse and Foord that states that the potential for infection doubles with every hour of exposure of an operative

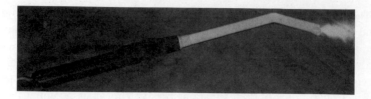

Figure 16-1 Vital Vue handle provides suction, lavage, and light simultaneously and additionally retracts and dissects in narrow places.

wound. We have found no reason to add antibiotics to the saline. It has been suggested that water might be even more effective than saline because of its hemolytic effect on red blood cells, but we feel this also is unnecessary in view of our superb results with saline, obviously more physiologic than water. Studies have shown that 0.9% saline is nontoxic to tissues.[33]

Several adjunctive measures incorporated into our vaginal surgical regimen have also helped substantially in combating infection. All patients are well primed with estrogen and are well nourished at the time of surgery. Where necessary, obesity has been eliminated or curtailed and sensible eating and exercise habits have hopefully been installed as a permanent routine. When indicated, diabetes and other metabolic problems are under control. Standard preoperative bowel clearance has been ensured. All patients, with extremely rare exception, are admitted to a preparation area between 6:30 and 8:00 AM on the same day as scheduled surgery; 80% of all cases are started by 9 AM and 95% by 1 PM.

As noted in Chapter 3, appropriate antibiotic medication is administered intravenously on entry into the operating room. No further attempt at antibiotic prophylaxis is made once the patient leaves the operating suite.

Surgical preparatory scrubbing by medical students and junior residents is strictly supervised. The operative field is thoroughly and widely painted with povidone solution and the anal area is done last. A single-opening preshaped coverall paper drape is carefully applied in vaginal as well as abdominal cases, and the contamination that often occurs in separate leg draping (see Chapter 3) is avoided. Specific attention is given to perianal coverage.

Other than constantly repetitive lavage, perhaps the most important preventive factor is meticulously gentle handling of tissues during the surgery, particularly avoiding unnecessary crushing action. Cautery is used judiciously and precisely so as to prevent excessive necrosis. Bleeding is quite thoroughly controlled, often by pressure alone. Synthetic sutures only are used; natural sutures, like catgut, are totally avoided, even for hysterectomy. Finally, as vaginal reconstructive operations are completed, vaginal packing (see Chapter 18) is snugly placed and kept in position for 2 days, not 1, to prevent serosanguinous pooling and to avoid any threat to surgically approximated tissue from inadvertent increased intra-abdominal pressure.

With reference to abdominal entries, incisions are best made by a sharp cold scalpel blade in a single clean stroke to produce the least tissue trauma. Although many young surgeons today love to use "fancier" seemingly more sophisticated methods for skin incision, like electrocautery or the laser beam, explicitly for "immediate hemostasis," the resultant tissue damage and necrosis, well beyond the wound edge, is extensive and provocative for infection and wound breakdown.[34,35] These techniques should be avoided. Of incidental note is the time-honored ubiquitous but ridiculous custom of changing knife blades once the outer skin has been penetrated. The use of two scalpels has no effect on the infection rate.[36] Closure of abdominal skin incisions, including fascial layers, will be covered as part of the discussion on suture selection.

The use of drains should be discouraged. When deemed absolutely necessary because of continuously seeping raw areas, only closed system "active" suction tubes should be used, always through a separate incision, never through the original operative entry. Static Penrose drains are archaic and must be forbidden; they provide a free ride for bacteria into an operative site, thereby promoting infection and wound breakdown. Even active drains (Hemovac or Jackson-Pratt), when used, should be removed as soon as the suction becomes empty.

THE PHYSIOLOGY OF WOUND HEALING

To bridge the gap between the discussion up to this point of both mitigating and interfering background factors in wound healing and the upcoming presentation featuring sutures and closure, a brief discussion of the details in the physiology of wound healing is appropriate. Although the wound healing process is well documented throughout the general surgical literature, no operating gynecologist can expect to enjoy the best results without a working knowledge of how the surgical wounds heal and, what's more, heal best. Since reparative phenomena are essentially the same throughout the body, with slight differences from one tissue to another, primarily in the face, as the "glue" called scar forms, a general description of the involved physiology is applicable.

Certain dicta that earmark best results must first be presented. Perpendicular wound edges that are also sutured to be perpendicular, not slanted, present smaller uniting surfaces, thus stronger and more rapid healing. Edges well approximated and free of tension provide superior scars. For this to happen in the already heavily scarred and distorted tissues of so many of the older women we approach vaginally in the operating room, wide and thorough dissection aided by the pliancy afforded through estrogen is crucial. Careless negligence involving vitamin and mineral deficiency, malnutrition, and inadequate control of diabetes, plus such negative influences as coincident chemotherapy, steroid medication, and renal deficiency, can interfere significantly with the normal physiologic process of good wound healing. One must never forget that general constitutional anabolic promotion through early mobilization postoperatively overrides the catabolism of the patient who remains in bed. Strangely, as long as sufficient blood volume maintains normal circulation, anemia, apparently for the same reason that it does not encourage infection, will not impair wound healing as long as circulation and perfusion are adequate.

Although some lining surfaces (bladder and peritoneum) may seal in a matter of hours, fascia, ligaments, other connective tissue, and skin require many days to attain reliable strength. A series of orchestrated biologic events occur through which scar tissue evolves, beginning with the *inflammatory phase*.[37,38] In this immediate postinjury period, "cleanup" of debris occurs with the associated appearance of concentrations of leukocytes, platelets, a variety of body chemicals, including prostaglandins, prostacyclins, and histamine, erythrocytes, and blood vessel endothelial cells, thereby starting up the well-ordered sequence.

The *migratory phase* then takes over, during which mesenchymal cells and more inflammatory cells move into the injured area followed by concentrations of macrophages which replace neutrophils. Studies have revealed that macrophages are integral to healing, whereas neutrophils play no such major role.[39,40] Fibroblasts, attracted by growth factor and fibronectin, join the parade.[41,42] Many other factors develop in the wound site that both bind mesenchymal cells to the wounded tissues and cause these cells to proliferate.[43–46] Platelets and macrophages contribute vital mitogenic factors. Angiogenesis starts within the first 2 to 3 days after an incisional wound is made, stimulated also by derivations from platelets and macrophages.[47,48] Capillaries develop from older vessels and progress through fibrin clot away from the edges of the wound toward areas of deprived perfusion at the wound center. As they advance and begin functioning, capillary consolidation occurs to form larger blood vessels.

While this is going on, surface epithelialization begins and progresses as cells migrate from the basal layers on either side of the wound until they meet within the first 4 days after creation of the wound.[49]

Five days into the healing process the *proliferative phase* begins, the hallmark of which is collagen synthesis.[50] The fibroblasts that now have migrated into the wound have begun to predominate and progressively synthesize glycosaminoglycans and collagen. For the first time strength comes to the wound and increases steadily concomitant with remarkable augmentation of collagen synthesis. Myofibroblasts appear and simultaneously wound contraction, not afforded heretofore by collagen, begins and progresses,[51] strength improving substantially as the tensile strength of support sutures wanes.

The period of wound contraction averages about 12 to 15 days, ending when the wound edges are totally united, and the *late phase of scar remodeling* begins 3 weeks after initial wound infliction. This stage in healing is characterized by rapid breakdown of old collagen with simultaneous reformation of new collagen.[52] This new realigned, highly cross-linked collagen continues to extend its tensile strength over days and weeks until it attains a maximum, never quite to the level of the adjacent unharmed tissue.[53]

A pragmatic addendum is appropriate at this point as a finale to the discussion of the physiology of wound healing. Conspicuous unattractive scars that will interfere with function almost invariably result from elective incisions made in the direction of dynamic skin tension.[54] Such unaesthetic healing can be avoided by incision placement perpendicular to the dynamic tensions of the skin, leading to an inconspicuous scar. This is why, at TUH, we encourage transverse lower abdominal incisions whenever reasonable rather than vertical ones. A good example occurs in our choice of a Cherney incision over a long midline vertical one when we combine an abdominal sacralcolpopexy with a bilateral Burch procedure. Similarly, in younger women with large fibromyomata uteri, when for one reason or other we are committed to an abdominal hysterectomy, we start the procedure vaginally until we have cleanly interrupted the cardinal-uterosacral attachments bilaterally. Then, through a wide Pfannenstiel opening abdominally, using a large uterine corkscrew to lift the very large, now unattached, uterine mass gently through the dilatable aperture, an ugly long vertical scar is avoided in favor of an ultimate rather obscure low transverse scar.

WOUND DISRUPTION

Abdominal superficial wound dehiscence down to the fascia occasionally occurs despite all precautions. Although remedies are thoroughly covered in many major surgical texts and in many other published monographs, this chapter would be incomplete without at least some brief direction on current advice on management.

Until relatively recent times, most treatment of such wounds followed the lines of healing by secondary intention. The basic principles involved have always centered on keeping the wound clean and moist with debridement as necessary, covering the wound between dressings, and allowing healing to occur only from inside out. Surgeons have quite some time ago learned that our natural "first-aid" intentions of placing solutions in this wound "to help it heal," i.e., 1% povidone-iodine, 0.25% acetic acid, 3% hydrogen peroxide, and 0.5% sodium hypochlorite, are cytotoxic and destructive, thereby acting to delay healing.[55] Because open moist wounds develop their own immune capabilities as they heal, it is doubtful if any added antibiotic media help. To dissipate further any fear we might have to any role to be played by infection in these subdermal areas, I interject the results of an unusual experiment that illustrates the high degree of contamination required to produce infection in and

under skin. In 1957, Elek and Conen had to inject at least 6 million staphylococci intradermally to overcome host resistance to infection and produce a
pustule in the healthy tissue of volunteer medical students.[56] However, contrast-
ingly, an infected lesion can be caused by a silk suture hiding as few as a
hundred staphylococci.[57] The greater the foreign body present in a wound, i.e.,
suture, especially silk, the greater the bacterial proliferation.[58]

The time-honored clinical axiom, "Never put anything into a wound that you
would not put inside your own eyelid," is best obeyed.

Passing mention, stimulated by two recent articles in the literature,[59,60] and
by intermittent proposals of doctors who have practiced at times in primitive
areas, of the ameliorating and healing properties of natural honey, should arouse
curious interest in the reader. Reports reveal that honey, poured into and onto
open wounds, including open superficial dehiscences, because of its complex
polysaccharide composition, discourages bacterial growth and accelerates healing by secondary intention to as little as 2 weeks.

At present, secondary closure of superficially dehisced wounds seems to be
growing rapidly in popularity. As success in this healing venture has grown, the
cost-saving and time-saving benefits have become joyfully obvious, not to
mention the remarkably decreased aggravation of the patient. A recent significant study, which highlights the need to consider secondary closure in preference to closure by secondary intention, compared the healing times in a sizeable
group of successive patients randomized to either method. Those subjected to
secondary closure required a mean of 18 days from dehiscence to full healing,
whereas those in the secondary intention contingent needed 61 days to achieve
the same objective.[61]

Initially secondary closure must be approached by sharp debridement, including excision, under local anesthesia, until only healthy tissue appears and
blood oozes subcutaneously. Following thorough saline irrigation, the wound is
gently packed with saline-soaked gauze, covered then by a dry dressing. After
changing such a wet-dry dressing three times per day for an average of 4 days, a
healthy bed of granulation tissue usually has formed. The appearance in the
incision becomes beefy red with obvious neovascularity and absence of infected
or necrotic elements. Then, under local anesthesia, depending on the depth of
the wound, interrupted full en bloc or vertical figure-of-eight sutures are placed,
down to the fascia, uniting the wound surfaces on tying, closing the wound
space. Steristrips may be used to augment skin approximation. Patients can
be discharged to home on the day following this secondary closure to return
on an outpatient basis in a week. The sutures are usually removed within a
short time after that visit when objectively the wound seems healed and fully
epithelialized.

Dehiscence of abdominal wounds below the level of the fascia, with or
without evisceration, with or without sepsis, is beyond the scope of this book. A
wealth of information on this subject can be garnered from any number of

surgical textbooks and manuscripts in the literature.[62–75] However, brief mention must be made that obesity is the most commonly occurring risk factor for this most feared complication of surgery, particularly with midline incisions. In such cases, in premenopausal or perimenopausal women, who are obese, who require hysterectomy for benign reasons, and with whom for one reason or another the operator is genuinely committed to an abdominal midline approach, a combined entry can drastically cut the odds on occurrence of dehiscence. The case should be started vaginally with dissection of both the bladder and the cul-de-sac well off the cervix and isthmus uteri. Then the cardinal-uterosacral complex should be clamped, cut, ligated, and tagged, clearing up to the uterine vessels. Now a transverse entry can be made into the abdomen rather than a vertical one and, by using a corkscrew and ample lubricating jelly, the uterus, unattached at its bottom, can be eased up through the incision. If it is still too large, a wedge taken from the center section with a large vascular limiting suture on each side will permit its elevation. Two to three clamps, at the most, on each side then allow for the hysterectomy to be completed quickly with negligible blood loss.

Rodeheaver and colleagues have conducted major studies on polybutester, manufactured as Novafil (Davis and Geck), and shown it to be the suture of choice in patients with high risk for dehiscence in the event of postoperative distention.[76] These investigators have shown Novafil to tolerate a much greater increase in abdominal volume than all other commonly used sutures, including nylon, before it will cut through the tissues. This event was proven for both interrupted and running mass closures, greater for the latter because of the high degree of elastic stretch inherent in polybutester. A running suture is best also because, besides spreading the strain of intestinal distention throughout the entire length of the heavy bore thread, the knots limited to the two ends decrease the possibility for sinus tracts to those two sites only.

SUTURE SELECTION

In essence, all of my basic discussion on choice of suture is applicable to wide varieties of surgery. However, any latitude in choices significantly diminishes in contemplation of operative correction in older versus younger people. Options narrow even further in consideration of the peculiar types of procedures constituting the major subject matter of this volume. Thus, this section both updates concepts on suture materials and usage in general and then specifies choices and methods thought to be preferable for surgery in geriatric women.

Bad habits in suture choice and usage inured from days gone by must be discarded in favor of modern trends toward remarkable newer materials and methods of suture application currently proven and recommended. During the two decades preceding this publication, clinical research on quality and capability of suture, paralleled by the manufacture of exciting innovative materials, has opened up wide opportunities to us for improvement in technique and outcome. Yet amazingly I see almost everywhere in my travels and observations an inexplicably stubborn and illogical resistance to change from outmoded and inferior practices and preferences to newer and better ones. The best example I can offer of such irrational reluctance is the persistent use by many of our top-rated surgeons and gynecologists of natural substances, principally catgut and silk, both of which should be deemed obsolete.

Perhaps the best method for awakening the intellect and conscience of the operating gynecologist is to present initially a series of factual statements and admonitions as interpreted primarily from the teaching of B. J. Masterson of the University of Florida, currently the leading gynecologic clinician in the research of suture material and wound healing.[77]

1. The basic goal of reconstructive healing and wound closure is optimal connective tissue formation. This can be strongly encouraged by the most favorable suture selection and placement.

2. The condition of the operative wound itself influences choices of sutures and outcome. This is determined not only by the status of the tissues as presented to the surgeon but also by the extent of the operation's alteration of the tissues both in making the incision and in further handling technique.

3. The healing properties of the particular type of tissue play a strong role in options.

4. Major factors in selection include the biologic and mechanical characteristics of the different sutures available.

5. Sutures are foreign bodies and, as such, all elicit some element of inflammation, even though much less in some of the newer ones than in older so-called traditional materials, like catgut and silk.

6. Tissue infection potential is invariably enhanced in the presence of any suture.

7. The larger the quantity of suture material (caliber, number of stitches, size of knots), the greater may be the damage to host resistance.

8. Similarly, potential for bacterial proliferation is directly related to the diameter and length of each suture and knot size.

9. Use of large traumatic needles or a multitude of unnecessary needle punctures erases considerably the benefits of careful choices of fine suture substances.

10. Choosing absorbable sutures where nonabsorbable material is required, and vice versa, is detrimental to good healing.

11. Pragmatic surgical judgment perceives when persistent strength during healing, as with fasciae and ligaments, is required to attain a preferable outcome.

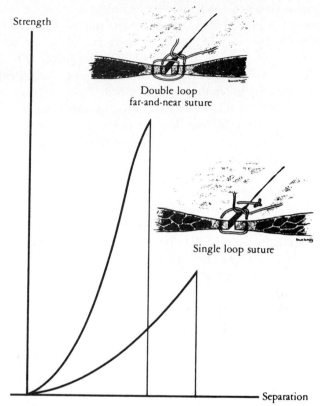

Figure 16-2 Comparison of Smead-Jones (far-near–near-far) single suture versus two single-loop stitches.

12. In abdominal surgical incisions, mass closures with large bites of tissues result in stronger wounds. Generally stitches should be placed as far apart, one from the next, as they are from the wound edge.

13. The efficacy of any stitch depends on the potential for the suture to break, the possibility for it to cut through the tissue, and knot security.

14. Two-loop (Smead-Jones type) far-and-near type stitches lead to greater strength and less wound separation than two single-loop sutures (Figure 16-2).

Definitions

There are three generally accepted categorical arrangements of suture materials:

1. Absorbable or nonabsorbable
2. Natural or synthetic
3. Polyfilament or monofilament

Absorbable sutures all undergo relatively rapid degradation in tissues, losing tensile strength within 60 days. Nonabsorbable sutures maintain tensile strength longer than 60 days after implantation. Essentially there are no "permanent" sutures, a descriptive term used commonly interchangeably with nonabsorbable sutures. All materials, even stainless steel, deteriorate, admittedly at varying rates, under the constant eroding effects of body fluids and chemicals.

Absorbable sutures are further classified as either rapidly absorbable or delayed absorbable, roughly paralleling duration of tensile strength, respectively shorter or longer lasting. One must not be confused, however, by the continued gross visible presence of the newer absorbable sutures in wounds as indicative of continued significant tensile strength. Physically recognized dissolution in some of the rapidly absorbable synthetic sutures may not take place for 90 to 100 days, yet any effective tensile strength may have disappeared within 25 to 32 days. With synthetic delayed absorbables, although dependent tensile strength essentially is lost in 50 to 60 days, the seemingly intact suture may still be found 200 to 250 days after placement. Thus, the term "absorbable" within the 60-day cutoff, in current perception, refers to the time of loss of tensile strength, not physical disappearance, as with traditional catgut, which is fully absorbed generally long before the 60-day limit.

For decade upon decade, natural substances were the only ones from which sutures were fashioned. These materials come not from fabricated chemical formulations but rather from preexisting fundamental matter furnished by nature, such as animal intestine (gut), agriculturally grown products (cotton), or the yield of insect larvae (silk). Because no other choices were available until recent years, except for metal (stainless steel), also to be considered in the "natural" category, but of very limited use, all surgery was conducted using these natural materials. The major problem with natural substances, recognized very early, is tremendous tissue reaction and inflammation, laying the groundwork for possible infection and less successful operative outcome.

Synthetic sutures are manufactured fibers consisting of polymolecular compounds of a steadily growing variety. They vary in property, one from the other, but the distinguishing feature of all, as compared to natural sutures, is the markedly reduced tissue reaction to them. This single quality of relative inertness alone, although there are many other positive characteristics, should have long ago eliminated forever further use of natural materials. Yet custom prevails and persistence of significant natural suture usage can be observed in almost every operating room across the nation. Most annoying is the surgeon's choice of natural materials in situations where they are strictly contraindicated, exemplary of the general ignorance in this area of surgical responsibility, namely, suture selection, despite otherwise good judgment and fine technique.

Polyfilament sutures, including braided substances, whether natural or synthetic, consist of multiple intertwined strands as opposed to monofilaments, which are composed of only one solid fiber. Generally speaking, polyfilament sutures are easier to handle and, if absorbable, dissolve at a faster rate than do their monofilament equivalents, probably because of greater surface exposure to body fluids. In the synthetic category, practically speaking, both types, polyfilament and monofilament, exhibit low tissue reactivity with differences small enough to be unworthy of discussion. However, although in clean wounds the potential for infection with either is very low, if there is high potential, as with diabetes, steroids, immune depression, or the wound is known to be contaminated, monofilaments are indeed preferable. The reason for this is that the hiding place for bacteria provided within the interstices of the filaments, which are large enough to permit bacterial invasion, is inaccessible to granulocytes, lymphocytes, and monocytes in chase of the microbes because they are too large for penetration. Abscess formation may be a sequel in such a situation. No such impenetrable haven is tendered by a single-fibered suture; the bacteria have no place to hide.

Properties of Sutures

In every kind of operative endeavor, it is the surgeon's obligation not just to choose in his or her judgment the best technique for the procedure at hand but to select the most efficacious sutures for each of the different tissues involved. These aims cannot be achieved unless the individual is thoroughly acquainted with the full array of characteristics peculiar to available sutures. Certainly one does not have to be an expert to understand that suture requirements for closure of bladder mucosa ought to be worlds apart from those demanded by sacrospinous ligament fixation. The challenge arises not just with knowing that different tissues in the same or different places, and that the same tissues in different places demand different suture, but in being confidently decisive in making optimal choices to do the best job in each specific circumstance. The delicate nature of tissues in the older woman force the most exacting discrimination.

What constitutes the ideal suture? More pragmatically, what are the desirable qualities that sutures should provide? Various studies[78–96] list the following properties, some of which overlap, that must be assessed in evaluating a suture in selection toward the ideal for each situation.

1. Tensile strength
2. Inflammatory response
3. Ease in handling
4. Conformity and flexibility
5. Memory
6. Knot security

7. Thickness

8. Low tissue drag

9. Elasticity

10. Allergenic potential

11. Maintenance of tensile strength in the presence of infection

12. Predictable rate of absorption

13. Breakdown products

14. Coating

Tensile strength refers to the capacity for sutures to hold sewn edges together, whether it be rectovaginal fascia, abdominal rectus fascia, skin, or vaginal mucosa. Required tensile strength varies widely from one wound or reparative procedure to another, and from one circumstance to another, and it must be carefully assessed in each instance. To use the vernacular, one should not send a boy to do a man's job, nor should a thumbtack be driven with a sledgehammer. Mathematically tensile strength is defined as strength per unit area. It is calculated by dividing the force needed to break a suture by its cross-sectional area. Simple tensiometers can test the relative out-of-package strength of different sutures but do not necessarily reflect comparative changes over time in vivo.

As has already been mentioned, sutures are foreign bodies and, as such, all will stir up some *inflammatory response.* Accordingly, the more inert the suture, i.e., current popular synthetics, the less the inflammation, as opposed to the severe reaction to natural substances. Erroneous thinking from the past, unfortunately still widely prevalent, claims that the more the reaction, the tougher the scar. Nothing could be further from the truth; inflammation only destroys and weakens, particularly undesirable in the already significantly compromised tissue of the geriatric population.

Ease in handling usually refers to facility in tying the suture. The more pliant the suture and the smoother the surface, the greater the comfort in manipulating the suture. Generally, braided sutures are much easier to tie down than single filaments. Ironically, coated catgut and silk seem to tie best of all but yet, as natural substances, disadvantages far outweigh this benefit.

Conformity and flexibility reflect the stiffness of a suture. Obviously a metal suture, like stainless steel, is least apt to conform to tissue contours and is the least flexible in adapting to shifts in tissue position. The thicker sutures, especially if synthetic and monofilamental, are also poorer conformers with decreased pliability as compared to thinner or polyfilamented threads.

Memory refers to the tendency of a suture to return to its original packaged configuration. This can be most annoying in the operating room during a procedure. Almost invariably the scrub nurse, when this happens, will tug hard at each end to straighten out the suture before handing it to the surgeon. Such a maneuver weakens the suture. A suture with strong memory is also more difficult to tie and may threaten knot integrity.

Knot security refers to the snugness of the knot as it is tied down and to its capacity to remain tight. The more flexible the suture, usually the more secure the knot. Coated sutures tie better than plain sutures but some may slip if the coating is slick, thus requiring an extra throw or two. Stiffer sutures give less knot security than more flexible ones and require extra throws to the knot, thereby creating a greater inflammatory source and a larger nidus for bacterial invasion. However, although they tie snugly, knots in natural substances quickly become insecure secondary to the influence of tissue fluids. Popular synthetic polyfilaments, not so affected, sustain good knot security.

Thickness refers to caliber or bore. Although there are thinner and heavier sutures, generally ordinary gross (nonmicroscopic) gynecologic surgery embraces a limited range of suture caliber, within a standardized system, from size 4-0 at the thinnest extreme to size 1 at the thickest limit. The thicker the suture, usually the greater and longer lasting the tensile strength, but the larger the foreign body and its associated deficits. The thinnest sutures should be directed at mucosal and peritoneal surfaces and at subcuticular skin closures. The heavier threads are called for in tissues under the greatest strain during healing, such as fasciae and ligaments, some of which, i.e., rectovaginal fascia, will remain under great perpetual continuous pressure due to the downward force of the erect torso. Although one must always be admonished never to use more or heavier suture than necessary to do a particular job, by the same token heavy tissues that act to support or suspend require tougher and thicker threads that will not only hold better and last longer but are less apt to cut through tissues as will thinner strands that, though strong, may do so under tension.

Tissue drag refers to the friction created between the surface of the suture and the tissue itself as the stitch is pulled through a particular tissue. The smoother the suture surface, the less the tissue injury and tissue reaction. Uncoated, wide bore, and braided substances obviously will do more damage than coated, thinner, monofilamented strands.

Elasticity is generally not a desirable quality. Any suture that stretches over time will not hold tissues together in the manner intended at the operating table. True elasticity, i.e., stretching under undue tension rather than cutting through tissues, and then springing back to the original size of tissue inclusion on release of the strain, would be ideal in certain situations. For example, such a material would be perfect for fascial closures of vertical abdominal incisions to compensate for intestinal distention while maintaining integrity of the closure both during the distention and after its disappearance. As will be discussed, today we do have available one such material.

Allergenic properties can be related to almost any substance entering the body through any portal. Essentially the body can react to any agent that is foreign or unnatural to it. This includes suture materials. Natural substances, especially catgut, are known to stimulate allergic responses in certain individuals. On the other hand, sensitivity to synthetic sutures is essentially unknown. Detection of such potential is best learned through the history of events related to any previous operations in a given patient.

Infection can be destructive to both tissues and sutures alike, particularly if allowed to progress to the stage of severe cellulitis. Coated, synthetic, thicker, monofilament sutures do better in the presence of inflammation and infection than do plain, natural, thinner, braided materials. The issue becomes clouded depending on the number of stitches and the number and size of the knots in any given area. When infection reaches the abscess stage, it probably makes no difference what the suture is. Certainly at this point, sutures should be removed, especially if nonabsorbable.

Predictable rates of absorption for individual sutures have been studied and are fairly well known. These will be addressed in the subsequent discussion of particular substances. It must be remembered that, in many cases, rate of absorption is not always related to persistent tensile strength, a common error of presumption.

Breakdown products of sutures are either destroyed or eliminated by the body. If nonallergenic, they probably produce no harm. However, there is currently conjecture that some breakdown products may produce local beneficial antibiotic action,[91,97–99] truly a pleasant surprise.

Improving suture quality by *coating* began many years ago when plain catgut, a very poor suture by all modern standards, was treated with basic chromium salts. The new product, chromic catgut, doubled to quadrupled the tensile strength of the original catgut and correspondingly delayed its absorption. Currently coating is commonly used with the multitude of available synthetic sutures. As already mentioned, additional properties afforded by coating beyond improved tensile strength are easier handling, better knots, and less tissue drag.

Suture Armamentarium

It would be impractical and superfluous for clinically active surgeons in any specialty to be thoroughly knowledgeable about all of the many sutures commercially available for different types of operations in varying circumstances. However, they should feel obliged to understand all of the various properties assigned to sutures in general, as noted in the preceding section of this chapter, so as to be fully geared to select the best sutures for each component of each operation they regularly perform. As implied earlier, however, unfortunately an unacceptably large percentage of operating clinicians have continued to use fairly much the same sutures with which they were taught in their residency training some 10, or 20, or even 30 years ago. Not only do habit and custom prevail, to the detriment of the patient who should be better served with newer and more effective materials, but residents currently in training often become exposed to outmoded sutures as a false standard, so they also get cheated. It is not difficult to understand how busy clinicians, occupied enough with the consuming duties of medical practice, and overwhelmed by the flood of new scientific literature they regularly receive, put a boring subject such as suture evaluation on the back burner and stick with what they "know." Hopefully the information condensed into this book should awaken the reader's awareness and incite appropriate change, particularly in the area of reconstructive and urogynecologic surgery in the elderly, where choice of suture is absolutely crucial to good healing and satisfactory long-term outcome.

Because of commercial competition, duplication of products, tight hospital financial policies, doctors' personal preferences, lack of demand for whatever reason, and the ever-present ubiquitous element of professional politics, rarely if ever does any medical facility offer all varieties of all sutures. Fortunately, many types of sutures manufactured by one company are so similar in properties to those made by other concerns that no gynecologic patient should be deprived of the best materials for her operation providing the doctor is sufficiently knowledgeable. In this regard, tedious as it may be, I will first list commonly used suture materials according to the definitions already described, including proprietary and generic names. Then I will discuss individual sutures as to their similarities and differences and their special properties, including both benefits and deficiencies. Finally, in the exciting practical portion of this section on the critical subject of wound healing, suggestions with supportive reasoning on application of appropriate sutures to specific operations will be presented as exercised by our service at TUH and by authorities at other centers.

Natural substances
    Catgut
    Silk
    Cotton
    Linen
    Stainless steel (metal)
Synthetic materials
    Polyglycolic acid (Dexon)
    Polyglactin (Vicryl)
    Polyglyconate (Maxon)
    Polydioxanone (PDS)
    Polyglecaprone (Monocryl)
    Nylon (Dermalon, Ethilon, Neurolon, Surgilon)
    Polypropylene (Surgilene, Prolene)
    Polyethylene (Dermalene)

Polyester (Dacron, Mersilene, Polydek, Tevdek, Ti-Cron, Ethibond, Ethiflex)
Polybutester (Novafil)
Polytetrafluoroethylene (Gore-Tex)
Absorbable substances
  Catgut
  Polyglycolic acid (Dexon)
  Polyglactin (Vicryl)
  Polyglyconate (Maxon)
  Polydioxanone (PDS)
  Polyglecaprone (Monocryl)
Nonabsorbable sutures
  Cotton
  Silk
  Linen
  Stainless steel
  Nylon (Dermalon, Ethilon, Neurolon, Surgilon)
  Polypropylene (Surgilene, Prolene)
  Polybutester (Novafil)
  Polyethylene (Dermalene)
  Polyester (Dacron, Ti-Cron, Tevdek, Polydek, Mersilene, Ethibond, Ethiflex)
  Polytetrafluoroethylene (Gore-Tex)
Polyfilament or braided substances
  Catgut
  Cotton
  Silk
  Linen
  Stainless steel
  Polyglycolic acid (Dexon)
  Polyglactin (Vicryl)
  Nylon (Neurolon, Surgilon)
  Polyester (Dacron, Mersilene, Ti-Cron, Polydek, Tevdek, Ethibond, Ethiflex)
Monofilament materials
  Stainless steel
  Nylon (Dermalon, Ethilon)
  Polydioxanone (PDS)
  Polyglyconate (Maxon)
  Polyglecaprone (Monocryl)
  Polypropylene (Surgilene, Prolene)
  Polybutester (Novafil)
  Polytetrafluoroethylene (Gore-Tex)

Please note that stainless steel and nylon are the only sutures that come in both monofilament and polyfilament form. All others appear in only one or the other physical configuration.

Chromic catgut elicits a severe inflammatory response. The tensile strength lasts only for 14 to 28 days. Many authorities continue to advocate its use in vaginal, serosal, and visceral closures that heal quickly. A surprising number of reputable gynecologists still use catgut in hysterectomies "because it ties so nicely." Still more amazingly, some outstanding professors persistently claim significant success with catgut in sacrospinous ligament fixation. I feel strongly, as does J. D. Thompson of Emory University,[100] that catgut has had its day of glory when there were no alternatives and that now, in any form and for any use, it should be officially outlawed and removed from the market. Many superior synthetic substitutes work much better.

Thirty to 50 years ago, including my residency days, long before sutures were clinically and scientifically studied to any major extent, and certainly before the advent of all the remarkable synthetic materials at our disposal today, *surgical silk* was extolled and glorified widely as an ideal suture for gynecologic purposes. The love for silk developed because of its low memory, easy handling, and great knot security. It was used extensively in hysterectomies and in skin and fascial closures, and even in repairs. Gradually its capacity to produce intense tissue reaction and severe inflammation, not infrequently followed by infection, often accompanied by later need for removal as cut ends surfaced or sinus tracts developed, became generally recognized. Studies ultimately revealed, despite its classification as a nonabsorbable substance, that silk lost its tensile strength far more rapidly than had been suspected, essentially retaining no effectiveness at 2 years.[82] Along with other highly reactive natural fibers, like cotton and linen, which also enjoyed brief popularity, silk is uncommonly used today and should hold no place in any kind of gynecologic surgery. Astonishingly I have discovered that general surgeons at several major facilities still use fine silk on peritoneal surfaces and some gynecologists do the same.

In days gone by, *stainless steel wire* was used widely for such purposes as rectus abdominis fascial closure associated with obesity and diabetes and for secondary mass closure in abdominal wound dehiscence and evisceration. It was preferred in infected sites.[101] The virtues of stainless steel are its negligible tissue reactivity, its great tensile strength, and its obvious knot security. The polyfilament form replaced the single-wire strand in popularity because it is more flexible and easier to handle, but its cut ends fray and may puncture gloves. The deficiencies of steel suture are its inability to conform and its tendency to kink and to cut through tissue. Synthetic sutures have totally replaced stainless steel in gynecologic use. In today's market, one form of metal suture remains viably superior to others, apparently being used by some general surgeons in special situations and by orthopedists. This material is known as

Flexon (Davis and Geck), a twisted multistrand of a ferrous alloy characterized by exceptional strength, great flexibility, and easy handling. It comes in a coated form if desired, as for cardiac use. It seems to be quite superior to stainless steel.

Dexon (1970) and *Vicryl* (1975) have become entrenched as the most popular so-called rapidly absorbable synthetic sutures. They are similar enough in biologic characteristics to be discussed together. Unlike the absorption of catgut by cellular degradation, the copolymer structures of Dexon and Vicryl are reduced in vivo by slow hydrolysis with concomitant low tissue reactivity. Tensile strength is minimally altered during the first 10 days and apparently is undisturbed even longer in the current coated forms. Then absorption and decrease in tensile strength occur steadily and reliably over the next 15 to 40 days. However, the coated heavier strands, 2-0 to 0, in our experience, can be grossly identified as late as 80 to 90 days, long after loss of effective tensile strength.

Dexon and Vicryl have been modified in various ways since their initial fabrication to reduce memory and make them easier to handle. Once tied, they maintain good knot security, but the tendency to slip if only one turn is taken on the first throw of the knot has caused the manufacturers to advise two turns to start. The latest version of these two sutures, Dexon-II, with a superior coating, requires but one turn on the first throw. If that should slip, the second throw brings both down securely. Overall both have proven to be excellent adjuncts in gynecologic surgery of all kinds.

Maxon and *PDS* were developed in the late 1980s as so-called delayed absorbable sutures to fill the gap between the rapidly absorbable Dexon and Vicryl on the one hand and nonabsorbable synthetics on the other. Both these monofilament sutures are similar enough to be discussed together despite tensiometer tests showing Maxon to be stronger and clinical reports declaring effective tensile strength to last slightly longer in PDS than in Maxon in vivo. Forty to 50% of tensile strength is still present at 28 days and enough remains through 40 to 50 days to allow fascia, the principal site for use of these sutures, time to heal enough to carry the load itself to the point of maximum healing. Dexon and Vicryl are inadequate in this regard. In a large study, polyglyconate (Maxon) was rated superior to polydioxanone (PDS) in lack of drag, tensile strength, and first-throw holding. They were found to be equivalent in knot rundown, knot security, memory, fraying, and curling. Polyglyconate was less supple than polydioxanone.[80]

As monofilaments, Maxon and PDS are slightly stiffer, have more memory, and are more difficult to tie than Dexon and Vicryl, thus requiring strict adherence to very careful manipulation during tying. Knots do not hold well if a double turn is used in the first throw, as in the traditional surgeon's knot because of extra slippage from the coating, which sounds paradoxical but nonetheless is true. Best results, with ultimate good knot security, are obtained when four throws are used, one turn to each throw, to form three squares or reefs. It is essential, especially with the first two throws, that they be placed flat, even in deep places, by opposing index fingers, and that each throw be brought down snugly while each strand is maintained under marked tension.

These two sutures are especially applicable in vaginal surgery[87] because they are inert and strong and act as a poor nidus for bacterial collection. Because the success of pelvic repair depends on complete healing of strong connective tissue components, which must withstand marked pressure and strain in the waking hours and which require a prolonged postoperative period to attain maximum strength, Maxon and PDS are well suited to the task. Their tensile strength, still 50% effective by the 28th day after surgery,[87] allows sufficient time for the healing tissue to take over and continue its progress to full stability some 115 to 120 days postsurgically. Their monofilament structure makes them most applicable for use in areas of high relative contamination, i.e., proximity to the rectum and anus. Monofilaments, like Maxon and PDS, were found to be best for cuff closure in abdominal hysterectomy because, unlike catgut and polyfilaments, they do not induce granulation formation.[102]

At the time of this publication, *Monocryl,* a new monofilament synthetic suture, has come on the market. It seems to lie intermediate to Dexon and Vicryl on the one hand and Maxon and PDS on the other in strength retention in vivo. The manufacturer (Ethicon) claims its benefits are its pliability as a monofilament and its choice applicability to situations requiring a high initial strength and short strength retention profile.

Polypropylene (Prolene and Surgilene) is an established relatively inert nonabsorbable monofilament synthetic material in wide use that has taken the place of silk for many surgeons. Although less pliable and of more memory than silk, it is much stronger. *Polybutester* (Novafil) is newer and somewhat similar to polypropylene but slightly stronger. Most importantly, it is the only substance capable of tolerating stretching under tension, as much as 15%, followed by return to original length after relief of strain. Since dehiscence of abdominal wounds occurs primarily because sutures cut through tissues, not suture breakage or knot slippage, polybutester is a prime choice for vertical abdominal closure when distention or marked coughing or nausea are anticipated. The only drawback is the increased potential for later sinus tracts to the skin.[103] Nonetheless, it is probably not used often enough.

Nylon seems to be more popular with general surgeons than with gynecologic surgeons. Both the braided (Neurolon and Surgilon) and the monofilament (Dermalon and Ethilon) forms consist of polymer fibers that, though easy to handle, are more disposed to knot slippage than polyester. I have observed surgeons make as many as 15 to 17 throws when using nylon for heavy duty. Especially when working in contaminated areas, with such large knots, the monofilament form is more desirable than the polyfilament. A recent study revealed Novafil to undergo significantly less biodegradation over the long term than nylon.[81]

Except for stainless steel, *polyester* sutures are the strongest materials currently available.[84] Dacron is as easy to manage and tie as silk and, as with Mersilene, has the best knot security of this group.[81] However, coated varieties such as Polydek, Ti-Cron, Ethiflex, Tevdek, and Ethibond are slightly easier to handle.[81] Tevdek and Ti-Cron are in wide use because of their flexibility but are slightly less inert and less knot secure than the others. In the presence of infection, both must be removed because they are braided.

Sutures made entirely of *polytetrafluoroethylene* (PTFE), used as a coating for some synthetics, marketed as Gore-Tex, possesses a unique quality that places it in a separate category from all other materials.[103,104] This monofilament nonabsorbable suture has a porous microstructure that proffers the unusual capability of incorporation into the adjacent structures through connective tissue ingrowth during the healing process. All other nonabsorbable sutures become encapsulated. This special microporous structure has helped to make it popular with cardiovascular surgeons who have favored it for almost 20 years, even more so because the diameter of the suture is the same as that of the needle into which it is swedged. Since PTFE material is 52% air, it is compressed at the point of juncture with the needle and then immediately expands to its designated size. All other swedged-on sutures are of narrower caliber than their associated needles. Thus, they cannot fill the hole made by the needle, so tiny blood vessels along the course of the stitch are not blocked, as they are with Gore-Tex. Other qualities are pliability, easy handling, low memory, and minimal tissue reaction. Although Gore-Tex is as easy to tie as silk, strangely its knots tend to slip. So, a minimum of seven throws are required for security, but the total knot size (foreign body mass) is no larger than three or four throws of other synthetics because of the compression afforded by the porous structure. In the presence of infection, PTFE rates similarly to other synthetic, monofilament sutures despite its porosity.[105] The spaces are large enough to allow penetration by macrophages, granulocytes, and leukocytes in pursuit and destruction of bacteria. The bacteria cannot "hide" inside the structure.

Situations

Closure of abdominal surgical wounds is always a matter of major decision.[63,64,84–88] This becomes particularly important when negative factors are present, such as diabetes, obesity, gross contamination, pulmonary disease, or autoimmune deficiency syndromes. Poor healing leading to abdominal wound disruption carries a mortality rate of approximately 20%, ranging from 11% to 35%.[106] Such a serious postoperative complication demands good surgical technique and wise choice of suture for the best efforts in its prevention, even though improvements in technique and suture choice have dropped the overall occurrence of fascial dehiscence to 0.3% to 0.7% for gynecologic procedures.[86] Wound dehiscence occurs less often in gynecology than in general surgery primarily because of the greater use of low transverse and subumbilical vertical incisions. Nonetheless, wound separation down to the fascia and fascial separation itself occur often enough to demand attention.[107–110] The incidence is significantly higher in older than in younger patients, a major reason for including this discussion in this book. Also, despite this volume's concentration on surgery conducted primarily through the vaginal approach, 75% of the greater than four million gynecologic operations performed annually in the United States invoke an abdominal incision.[111] A significant proportion of these cases are in the geriatric population, often with varying degrees of debilitation.

At TUH, the gynecology service generally does not close the abdomen in a layer-by-layer closure. However, the layer-by-layer method has been supplanted anyway generally by mass closure of the Smead-Jones type in vertical midline suprapubic closure. This method uses a much stronger interrupted stitch than does a single loop for mass closure (see Figure 16-2). It is generally accepted today that the strongest wounds are the result of correct placement of stitches that encompass large bites of tissue in mass closure.[29] Smead-Jones suturing uses a far-near–near-far stitch placement involving anterior fascia, rectus muscle, posterior fascia, and peritoneum in the far swings, while fascial edge only is included in the near swings. It is best performed using monofilament nonabsorbable material of relatively heavy caliber. Placement 2.5 cm from the wound edge on each side in the far swing and 2 cm apart, one stitch from the next, has produced an exceedingly low dehiscence rate.[112] As with all tissue closures, overtightening negates good healing by devascularization.[113] Wound strength may be cut 50%.

During the past decade, despite the popularity of the Smead-Jones interrupted stitch closure of the midline vertical incision, there has been a steady swing to use of a continuous en bloc technique. For seemingly countless years, though deemed acceptable for low transverse incision, closing fascia with a running suture in vertical abdominal entries was considered dangerous using absorbable material (catgut). It was erroneously thought that even nonabsorbable threads (silk, cotton) would be more apt to lead to dehiscence if used in continuous fashion. However, the advent of laboratory and clinical studies involving new synthetic materials has steadily brought the use of continuous vertical closure into prominence.[114–120] The dehiscence rate has been reported, in a combined series of 1204 patients closed in this manner, to be only 0.5%, including obese patients and those with cancerous lesions.[28,114–117]

A major problem using nonabsorbable interrupted sutures in abdominal fascial closure, dating back to the days when silk and cotton were widely used for this purpose, has been a significant attendant incidence of sinus tract development to the skin.[28,121,122] Even when using running monofilament syn-

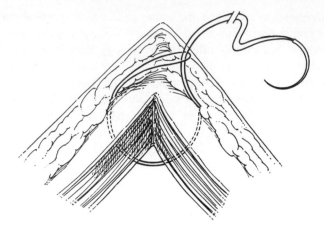

Figure 16-3 Initiating fascial closure with a Maxon looped (double-strand) suture.

thetic nonabsorbable materials, such as polypropylene and polybutester, sinus tracts at the site of knots at the ends of the incisions, and also in the middle if closure was initiated from each end toward the middle, have been irritating consequences. Such problems can be avoided with the use of a newly developed suture configuration that seems to be almost ideal for many reasons, namely, looped 0-Maxon, used in a running almost knot-free technique. Either simple mass continuous closure can be used, as in the average patient, or a running modification of the Smead-Jones method[123] is applicable in patients with compromising factors such as obesity, cancerous lesions, diabetes, and autoimmune problems. As concluded in a major study of this looped running mass closure in which 72% were treated for malignant disease, conducted at three different major institutions,[123] the suture handling was deemed excellent in a majority of cases, the closure time was rapid (only one end knot), and the wound breakdown rate was at least equal to, if not better than, that of the much more tedious interrupted Smead-Jones method. The latter technique, to its disadvantage, involves a much larger amount of foreign body in the wound plus a marked increase in infection potential, considering the number of buried knots. Our experience using the looped 0-Maxon at TUH duplicates the gratifying results of the study above.

The precise system for use of this looped double-strand suture begins with a traditional needle pass at an end of the wound through one edge, outside to inside, then inside to outside at the other edge. The needle is then passed through the loop at the opposite end of the double strand and drawn up securely (Figure 16-3), obviously avoiding a need for a knot. Suturing is continued, taking large bites 1 to 1.5 cm from each edge and a similar distance apart. According to the surgeon's preference, the last two passes can be arranged in such a way that the knot is tied deep or superior to the fascia. Thus after the

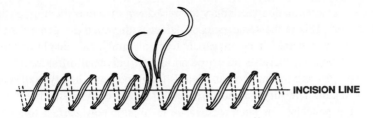

Figure 16-4 Completing the closure started in Figure 16-3, using Maxon looped (double-strand) suture.

next to last pass through the fascia, one thread of the double suture is cut near the needle, the final pass is made with the uncut strand, and it is then tied to its waiting mate on the same side of the incision (Figure 16-4). The latter feature is especially important in vertical incisions because the only tie is made across fascial fibers, not in line with them. At TUH, we actually use two looped double threads, starting at each end of the incision, ending with a single knot, which we bury, for each in the center of the incision, whether it be vertical or transverse. The benefits in using this suture are manifold, including speed, continuous technique, almost certain avoidance of sinus tracts, elimination of a knot at the apex of the incision, markedly reduced infection potential, remarkable suture strength, and cost savings. Perhaps more important than all of these points, the larger cross section of two zero threads measurably reduces the chances of suture cutting through the tissue. Dehiscences occur because of such a mishap, not because knots untie or sutures break.

Closing the "dead space" of subcutaneous fat between fascia and skin, commonly performed in the past using 3-0 chromic catgut, should never be done. It will add nothing to wound strength and merely increases wound infection potential by the addition of increased foreign body.[117,124,125]

Closure of the skin with metal clips is fast, quite efficient, and widely popular. However, it takes time to remove them, often requiring a return trip to the doctor's office for removal, considering how early we send patients home these days after lower abdominal laparotomy. Also, no matter how carefully one withdraws each staple, it hurts the patient substantially. I use a continuous subcuticular synthetic polyfilament, 4-0 skin closure with delightful results. Although requiring slightly more time for placement than do metal staples, the patient loves the immediate look of her incision, the ultimate appearance of the scar is the same, no removal is required, and the patient is not harassed. The positive psychological effects of a buried running absorbable synthetic thread versus staples or interrupted overt skin stitches are of inestimable value in the overall attitude of healing. Additionally, an extra early return visit is avoided, a bonus for older people who often have transportation problems.

As discussed in detail in Chapter 9, any form of prolapse in the pelvis must be regarded as a herniation secondary to breakdown in connective tissue support or suspension. This is the same kind of defect with which the general surgeon deals regularly, whether it be inguinal, femoral, umbilical, diaphragmatic, or incisional. However, there seems to be an almost universal difference between the gynecologist and the surgeon as regards the importance and type of material to use for repair. The surgeon, fully respectful of the weakness in the defective area and the penchant for later recurrence no matter how perfect the surgical technique, generally uses substances of great and enduring tensile strength, most often nonabsorbable. Ironically the attitude of the average gynecologist, commissioned to correct cystoceles, rectoceles, inverted vaginal vaults, hypermotile urethrovesical junctions, and defective perineums, all in areas subject to the worst stress of all connective tissue because of the weight of the erect torso above and inevitable repetitive bursts of intra-abdominal pressure, persists in depending on rapidly absorbable materials like Dexon and Vicryl, and frighteningly yet in some facilities, catgut. An unfortunately persistent naive misconception perceives a rapid creation of strong scar that will more than compensate for the original weakness that allowed the lesion to develop originally. Especially in geriatric patients, nothing could be further from the truth! Fascia, which is really a concentrated sheet of connective tissue, the structural base for all pelvic support in one form or another, regains only 25% of its original strength after 3 weeks of healing. The time has come for gynecologists to emulate surgeons in repair of herniations, particularly since they deal so often with defects secondary to congenital deficiency in connective tissue metabolism and with older and elderly patients whose supportive structures are simply worn out from aging.

In today's gynecologic operating arena, considering the wide range of available materials, anything less than delayed absorbable suture for pelvic reconstruction of any kind is unacceptable. Ideally, if we have learned anything from the general surgeons, we should use only nonabsorbable sutures throughout all reconstructive surgery. However, we work in the pelvis, very close to hollow organs and vital conduits, and thus a combination of common sense and fear force us, despite any developed acceptance of the right stuff to use, to retract and compromise. So we advise the use of delayed absorbable sutures such as Maxon or PDS, at the least, to be the common choice even though nonabsorbable suture is truly the premium.

At TUH, almost 5 years ago, we made the big switch to nonabsorbable suture for anterior pelvic compartment reconstruction. As already discussed, we do three basic types of anterior pelvic repair from below, either alone or in combination, in varying degree, depending on the individual situation. From the start, for the flap sutures of the paraurethral fascial sling urethropexy, the procedure least apt to involve danger of suture intrusion in wrong places, we first chose CV-0 Gore-Tex, for all the reasons already enumerated earlier in this chapter, particularly its capacity for incorporation within the healing scar itself.

About a year later, we expanded from delayed absorbable to Gore-Tex CV-0 suture for all our paravaginal defects repairs also, using it to reattach urethrovesical junction and bladder base to the arcus tendineus fasciae pelvis. Shortly thereafter we followed suit in the standard midline and anterior intracardial vault imbrication. No fistulae or sinus tracts have developed and the surgical outcomes to date have been not only highly satisfactory but apparently better than with absorbable suture.

Since I began doing the Burch procedure in 1980, I have always used nonabsorbable materials. Number one polypropylene (Surgilene or Prolene) and later polybutester (Novafil) were my initial choices. These seemed to present a combination of lasting tensile strength and low likelihood of cutting through tissues. However, I changed to CV-0 Gore-Tex in 1988 and that has been my recommendation for this procedure ever since then.

When repair of paravaginal defects from the suprapubic approach is clearly indicated, again I use CV-0 Gore-Tex for strength, stability, and incorporation into the healed wound. Once again, I think the latter factor makes all the difference in the ultimate long-term results. I have never felt there was any place for absorbable sutures in suprapubic urethral suspensions of any kind, although from fear of potential urethral penetration and poor sequelae if infection developed, I used absorbable sutures in the years when I performed the Marshall-Marchetti-Krantz operation. It is no longer a concern since we (TUH) consider that operation obsolete.

In the posterior compartment, we never use anything less than monofilament delayed absorbable sutures of zero caliber. This is the area of greatest pelvic stress and therefore a dependable colpoperineorrhaphy, the bottleneck for success in cases presenting multiple pelvic support defects, becomes essential. Unfortunately this operation, as mentioned in Chapter 11, is often relegated to the category of "glorified episiotomy" and, usually coming at the end of what may already have been a long procedure, the "tired" operator races through a series of suture placements, usually using rapidly absorbable 2-0 material in a manner totally oblivious to the demands placed on this repair, particularly in the postclimacteric population. This scenario is a prescription for almost certain failure. Precise time-consuming surgical technique, using an orderly and logical sequence of interrupted sutures involving all available connective and elastic tissue remnants, is obligatory with rectocele and perineal body repair. Even thus diligent in the effort to restore the normal vaginal axis, the surgeon still requires strong relatively heavy suture to achieve the best results. We use and recommend either Maxon or PDS, zero caliber, even though we admit this is a compromise choice. The ideal option might be Novafil, the only inert monofilament nonabsorbable substance both resistant to infection and capable of stretching 15% in the presence of edema with guaranteed return to original length. The problems with such a decision are the danger of placing a nonabsorbable suture inadvertently into the rectum and the annoyance of suture ends later protruding through vaginal or, worse, rectal mucosa. However, we compromise again in referral situations to us of cases presenting two or more previous posterior restorative failures. In these instances we do use the nonabsorbable Gore-Tex, the soft cut ends of which will not be troublesome. Unquestionably we do this with trepidation which we try to dissipate by digital rectal examination to check for errant suture placement after every two stitches.

Hysterectomy, whether abdominal or vaginal, as the most common major gynecologic procedure, collectively consumes more suture than all other operations within this field. Because intraoperative and postoperative hemorrhage is the singular most common complication in this surgery, suture selection must be directed at ease of tying and knot security. With the exception of the posterolateral vault stitches involving ongoing support of the upper paracolpium, rapidly absorbable sutures are the only sensible materials for use in hysterectomy where support is not an issue.

In hysterectomies, until relatively recently, catgut has reigned supreme, and still does with some leaders in the field, because unquestionably nothing ties easier or forms a snugger knot than catgut when brought down under tension on a hysterectomy stump. It is perhaps surprising to note how commonly gynecologic surgeons have changed to various synthetic sutures for all their other operations and still have stuck with chromic catgut for hysterectomy because of these qualities of easy handling and knot security. Yet when one considers that all gynecologists with any experience can relate any number of "horror stories" about hemorrhage in hysterectomy, secondary to "knot problems," it becomes easier to understand the reluctance to change from the reliability of catgut. Many operators gave adequate trials to the earliest versions of Dexon and Vicryl and then returned to catgut after repeated episodes of knot slippage limited not just to residents' seeming inabilities to work adequately with these substances but also their own. Thus, despite a series of improvements made in Dexon and Vicryl since their initial manufacture, operators have stubbornly resisted trying again, or trying at all, in making a permanent switch to synthetics. This is a precise description of my own attitude until I finally left catgut behind forever in 1990 with the advent of the absorbable braided Dexon-II, polyglycolic acid material covered with the brand new polycaprolate (1%). This novel coating makes Dexon-II every bit the equal of catgut in both management and snugness, with less drag through tissues, not to mention its inertness compared to the reactivity of catgut. Of great importance is the lack of need for a surgeon's knot, i.e., two turns for the first throw. One turn, under tension, holds, but if it should slip, when the second throw is brought down to form the first of three knots (four throws), it comes down snugly and will not slip back. At TUH, Dexon-II-0 is our suture of choice for any and all hysterectomies.

The next question to ask is, "Why 0? Why not 2-0, or even 3-0?" As related in Chapter 4, at TUH we average only three clamps on each side of the uterus in its removal. This implies wide bites that require more strength to bring down the knots tightly against the tissue than do narrower ones. Also, since hysterectomy stumps consist of soft tissue, a larger bore is less apt to cut through the tissue than a smaller bore. Incidentally, it is timely to mention again that the fewer the bites, the fewer the stitches, which translates into less foreign body, fewer tissue punctures, and fewer knots to act as niduses for infection.

Dexon and Vicryl are excellent sutures for closure of vaginal and perineal operative wounds. When the vaginal mucosa is thick from friction due to eversion, as in the great majority of cases referred to us at TUH, a 2-0 caliber works best. We prefer 3-0 when the mucosa is thin from overstretching or long-term atrophy without estrogen stimulation before preoperative replacement was started within 10 weeks of the scheduled surgery. Except for the area under the urethra, where we use only interrupted stitches to prevent bunching and shortening, vaginal wall closure is accomplished at TUH, both anteriorly and posteriorly, by a continuous locking suture. A little bunching in these surface areas is of no matter considering the looseness and slight excess of tissue anyway. On the perineal skin, the same strand used to unite the posterior wall is carried over the fourchette in nonlocking fashion, completing surface closure of the particular operation. Many surgeons prefer interrupted sutures throughout and others like running submucosal and subcutaneous stitches. Despite a variety of arguments favoring one method over another, we see absolutely no difference in ultimate healing no matter how one closes nor do we see any difference in discomfort from one method to the next. Our locking technique prevents edges from bleeding and never seems to devascularize enough to interfere with prompt mucosal healing. The argument that less pain is produced by subcuticular perineal skin closure than by over-and-over surface running closure does not hold up in our experience. This has been proven in several studies summarized in a major report that also reveals pain levels to be cut in half when traumatized perinei are reunited with synthetic sutures over catgut.[96] Additionally we always cut the perineal surface sutures at the first postoperative follow-up visit (16 to 19 days), thereby giving the patient immense relief. This cannot be done with subcuticular stitching. This is an important consideration because these sutures are not physically absorbed for 75 to 90 days.

During pelvic surgery, particularly via the vaginal approach, and especially if dealing with heavy scar tissue and distortion, the bladder or the rectum may be opened. As long as such instances are recognized, and the surrounding tissue is mobilized freely to avoid tension at the edges, and proper closure is performed, there should be no interference to routine healing. In either case, we recommend a two-layer closure, using Dexon-II or Vicryl, continuous 3-0 for the first layer at the mucosal surface and running or interrupted 2-0 suture for the second layer.

When a vesicovaginal fistula develops after reparative surgery, the Latzko technique of partial colpocleisis is our primary recommendation. This operation is well described in many standard gynecologic textbooks. It is not difficult to perform and good results are noted when the first two layers consist of interrupted 3-0 rapidly absorbable synthetic suture and the third layer of interrupted 2-0 similar material.

Occasionally we receive referred cases of rectovaginal fistulas that have developed after difficult posterior repairs. Initially we invariably convert the fistula into a fourth degree lesion, excise the abnormal tract, and follow with an appropriate extensive meticulous dissection. Then we first close the rectal mucosal edges with a running intestinal submucosal rapidly absorbable synthetic suture, which incidentally also repositions the thin layer of longitudinal fibers comprising the internal anorectal sphincter. Although incidentally providing crucial support for this mucosal reunion, the second layer of stitches primarily is aimed at reestablishing the integrity of all three loops of the external rectoanal sphincter. These consist of a succession of aptly placed (from cephalad to caudad) substantial interrupted stitches of 2-0 monofilament delayed absorbable material. Zero caliber similar suture must then be used in individual stitches designed to restore the perineal body.

Enterocele neck closure involves suturing of peritoneum, which seals and heals rapidly and has no significant inherent strength. Purse-string technique, using 3-0 for the narrow neck and 2-0 for the wide neck enteroceles, always rapidly absorbable polyfilament, is more than adequate. Yet, as already elaborated in Chapter 11, many surgeons close off enterocele necks with nonabsorbable suture. Why this is done is beyond my comprehension because the second layer, supportive of the purse-string suturing, is the one that counts. Such reinforcement should consist of a row of interrupted monofilament zero caliber delayed absorbable or nonabsorbable suture, extending from bladder floor in front to rectum at the "yellow line" in back, bringing together in the midline endopelvic connective tissue from each side while avoiding damage to the ureters.

In our opinion at TUH, sacrospinous ligament fixation absolutely requires nonabsorbable suture. Strangely, many surgeons continue to use absorbable sutures and some still prefer catgut, again a strategy that makes no sense to us, given the major responsibilities for lasting vaginal vault suspension at a deep posterior point in the pelvis. We recommend either number one bore Novafil or CV-0 Gore-Tex as the most reliable materials for this job. Elaboration of this discussion can be found in Chapter 10.

Similarly, because the same predominant requirements are integral to successful abdominal sacrocolpopexy, it is inconceivable to us that anything less than relatively heavy nonabsorbable monofilament suture be used in this operation also.

Knots

Assuming correct choice of material and placement in tissue, the level of efficacy of any stitch becomes dependent on the knot, the weakest point of a suture loop. The type of knot and the particular material used combine to give *knot efficiency*, defined by Zederfeldt and Hunt as the strength of the tied thread as percentage of the strength of the untied strand.[94] Most gynecologic surgeons are not always well versed on which type of knot is required for the material they use, especially since so many new materials are available and manufacturers seldom offer adequate information about knot efficiency for a particular substance. This knowledge is essential in urogynecologic and reconstructive surgery in elderly women more than in any other circumstances because of the already existent compromises in tissue quality and the strength required of suturing in this special kind of surgery. It is in no way comparable to the lesser demands and strains on sutures in such procedures as colon resection, cholecystectomy, or hysterectomy, for example.

As in all branches of surgery, certain principles should govern how one chooses a knot in the special demands of pelvic reconstructive and urogynecologic surgery in older women. Depending on the basic healing properties of the involved tissue, the condition of the wound, the biologic and mechanical properties of the suture material, and the job expected of the stitches, the correct knot should be selected.

To understand and discuss knots, gynecologists should become familiar with some simple relevant terminology which I call "knot language," as follows:

Turn: The ends of the thread are looped once over each other; two turns when they are looped twice, etc.

Throw: This is formed of one or more turns and is really half a knot, generally.

Knot: When at least two throws are laid on top of each other and tightened, a knot is formed.

Formations:
  a. Parallel throws as in a square (reef) knot.
  b. Crosswise throws as in a granny knot. (Figure 16-5, top.)

Knot descriptions:
  a. Arabic numerals indicate the number of turns in each throw.
  b. The method of joining the throws uses the symbols = for parallel and × for crosswise (see Figure 16-5).

Examples:
  a. Square knot: $1 = 1$
  b. Granny knot: 1×1

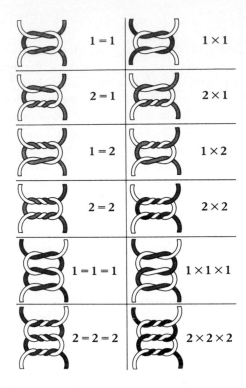

Figure 16-5 Knot table: configurations and symbols. (Reproduced with permission from Davis and Geck.[94])

    c. Surgeon's knot: $2 = 1$
    d. Combined knot: $1 \times 1 = 1$
    e. Inverse surgeon's knot: $1 = 2$

Figure 16-5, as depicted by Zederfeldt and Hunt,[94] illustrates several different types of knots, using this knot language.

In culling the literature on sutures and their knot characteristics[78–95,126–134] over the decade preceding the publication of this book, a series of guiding maxims evolves that should aid the surgeon in choices and actions regarding knots, as follows:

1. The best knot has adequate strength for the assigned task, uses the least amount of suture, and resists slippage.

2. The more throws, the stronger the knot.

3. The more throws, the larger the foreign body.

4. The larger the knot, the greater the possibility of sinus tract.

5. Sutures tied too tightly on tissue or placed too close together inhibit vascularity, nutrition, and oxygenation, thereby interfering with wound healing.

6. Knots very tightly tied in fascia retain only 50% of their usual strength.

7. A stable knot configuration is the number of throws required for the suture loop itself to break rather than the knot to slip loose.

8. The greater the suture memory, the more throws necessary.

9. The stiffer the suture, the more throws required.

10. The softer the suture, the easier to tie.

11. Coated sutures tie easier and their knots hold better.

12. Two-hand ties are better than one-hand ties.

13. Tying under tension helps prevent slippage during the tying.

14. Knots should be tied flat with the strands pulled in diametrically opposite directions.

15. At least one index finger should always be on the knot as it is tied.

16. A granny knot may be better than a square knot and a double granny knot, surprisingly, is safe for all materials.

17. The surgeon's knot, regarded as "old reliable," based on no scientific reasoning, has been dethroned in today's synthetic world:
    a. Unsafe for coated materials
    b. Cannot be tightened
    c. Stands or tolerates only slight strain on the suture loop
    d. If used with Dexon-II, Maxon, or PDS, knot security is severely threatened.

18. In contrast, the inverse surgeon's knot is safe:
    a. Allows tightening by the second throw
    b. Remains stable when strain is placed on the suture loop

19. Half-hitches (tumbled knots; Figure 16-6) offer very poor efficiency:
    a. About 20% of that of a correct knot
    b. Can result unintentionally from careless one-hand ties
    c. May be used intentionally only to tighten the first throw of a knot but then must be complemented, for safety, by two subsequent square throws

20. Coated braided or polyfilament synthetic nonabsorbable materials (Surgilon, Ti-Cron, Dacron) generally have great knot security as well as excellent tensile strength but require four throws ($1 = 1 = 1 = 1$) for safety even though three ($1 = 1 = 1$) will probably hold.

21. Coated monofilament synthetic absorbable threads absolutely demand four throws, one turn only to each throw, for reliable knots because of memory and stiffness.

22. Polypropylene (Surgilene or Prolene), which remain very popular, and polybutester (Novafil), all monofilament nonabsorbable, are best assured of security by a $3 = 2 = 1 = 1$ knot configuration.

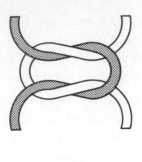

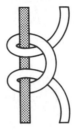

Figure 16-6 Square knot (above) versus tumbled knot (below). (Reproduced with permission from Davis and Geck.[94])

23. When using synthetic absorbable sutures, i.e., Dexon, Vicryl, Maxon, PDS:
    a. A fifth throw is redundant ("hysterical" in knot vernacular) and only increases the size of the knot.
    b. Granny knots probably should be used more commonly in the total configuration, particularly in deeper narrower exposures, ironically to prevent slippage during tying, i.e., 1 x 1 = 1 = 1 or 1 × 1 × 1 = 1.

Finally, in summary, paraphrasing again from the verbal discourses of B. J. Masterson, repairs should be completed and wounds closed with the minimum amount of the most inert suture and its accompanying knots concordant with operative goals and associated hemostasis and anatomic restoration.

REFERENCES

1. Cardozo L. The causes, diagnosis, and treatment of prolapse. *Midwife, health visitor, and community nurse (London).* 1988;24:207–210.

2. Lewis AL. Major gynecological surgery in the elderly. *J Int Fed Gynaecol Obstet.* 1968;6:244–258.

3. Du Nouy PL. Cicatrization of wounds, mathematical expression of the curve representing cicatrization. *J Exp Med.* 1916;24:451–456.

4. Barter RH. *Symposia on Wound Healing.* Sparkman RS, ed. Pearl River, NY:

Davis and Geck, American Cyanamid Co.; 1985:60. Library of Congress Catalog Card No. 85-72109.

5. Eton B. Gynecologic surgery in elderly women. *Geriatrics.* 1973;28:119–123.

6. Jones CM, Eaton TB. Postoperative nutritional edema. *Arch Surg.* 1933;27:159–163.

7. Mecray RM, Barden RP, Ravdin IS. Nutritional edema: its effect on gastric emptying time before and after gastric operations. *Surgery.* 1937;1:53–60.

8. Thompson WD, Ravdin IS, Frank IL. Effect of hypoproteinemia on wound disruption. *Arch Surg.* 1938;36:500–504.

9. Cannon PR, Wissler RW, Woolride RL, et al. Relationship of protein deficiency to surgical infection. *Ann Surg.* 1944;120:514–519.

10. Wohl MD, Reinholdt JJ, Rose SB. Antibody response in patients with hypoproteinemia. *Arch Int Med.* 1949;83:402–408.

11. Brunschwig A, Clark DE, Corbin N. Postoperative nitrogen loss and studies on parenteral nitrogen nutrition by means of casein digestion. In: Symposium on abdominal surgery. *Ann Surg.* 1942;115:1091–1096.

12. Rhoads JE, Alexander CE. Nutritional problems of surgical patients. *Ann NY Acad Sci.* 1955;63:268–273.

13. Rhoads JE. The impact of nutrition on infection. *Surg Clin North Am.* 1980;60:41–47.

14. Sandblom O, Lindstedt E. Wound healing in man: tensile strength of healing wounds in some patient groups. *Ann Surg.* 1975;181:842–846.

15. Dudrick SJ. *Symposia on wound healing.* Sparkman RS, ed. Pearl River, NY: Davis and Geck, American Cyanamid Co.; 1985:80–81. Library of Congress Catalog Card No. 85-72109.

16. Wolfer JA, Farmer CJ, Carroll WW, et al. An experimental study in wound healing in vitamin C depleted human subjects. *Surg Gynecol Obstet.* 1947;84:1–4.

17. Pories WJ, Henzel JH, Rob CG, et al. Acceleration of wound healing with zinc sulfate given by mouth. *Lancet.* 1967;1:121–124.

18. Haley HB, Williamson MB. The healing of human wounds. In vivo studies. *Surg Forum.* 1957;8:62–65.

19. Whipple GH. Protein production and exchange in the body, including hemoglobin, plasma protein, and cell protein. *Am J Med Sci.* 1938;196:609–613.

20. Bump RC, McClish DK. Cigarette smoking and urinary incontinence in women. *Am J Obstet Gynecol.* 1992;167:1213–1218.

21. Last JA, King TE, Nerlich AG, et al. Collagen cross-linking in adult patients with acute and chronic fibrotic lung disease. *Am Rev Respir Dis.* 1990;141:307–313.

22. Polk HC Jr, Simpson CJ, Simmons BP, et al. Guidelines for prevention of surgical wound infection. *Arch Surg.* 1983;118:1213–1217.

23. Polk HC Jr, Fry DE. Surgical aspects of infection. In: Goldsmith HS, ed. *Practice of Surgery.* New York: Harper & Row; 1980:1–33.

24. Polk HC, Lopez-Mayor JF. Postoperative wound infection: a prospective study of determinant factors and prevention. *Surgery.* 1969;66:97–103.

25. Hunt TK. In: Hunt TK, ed. *Wound Healing and Wound Infection: Theory and Surgical Practice.* New York: Appleton-Century-Crofts; 1980: Chaps. 18–21; pp. 214–280.

26. Burke JF. Infection. In: Hunt TK, Dunphy JE, eds. *Fundamentals of Wound Management.* New York: Appleton-Century-Crofts; 1979:170–240.

27. Polk HC Jr. Prevention of surgical wound infection. *Ann Intern Med.* 1978;89:770–773.

28. Cruse PJE, Foord R. The epidemiology of wound infection: a ten year prospective study of 62,939 wounds. *Surg Clin North Am.* 1980;60:27–40.

29. Masterson BJ. Taking steps to promote wound healing. *Contemp OB/GYN,* 1988;March:119–130.

30. Lowbury EJL, Lilly HA, Bull JP. Methods for disinfection of hands and operation sites. *Br Med J.* 1964;2:531–533.

31. Peterson AT, Rosenberg A, Alatary SD. Comparative evaluation of surgical scrub preparations. *Surg Gynecol Obstet.* 1978;146:63–65.

32. Alexander JW, Fischer JE, Boyajian M, et al. The influence of hair removal methods on wound infections. *Arch Surg.* 1983;118:347–350.

33. Branemark PI, Albaktsson B, Lindstrom J, et al. Local tissue effects of wound disinfectants. *Acta Chir Scand.* 1966;357(suppl): 166–168.

34. Glover JL, Bendick PJ, Link WJ. The use of thermal knives in surgery: electrosurgery, lasers, plasma scalpel. *Curr Probl Surg.* 1978;15:1–78.

35. Sowa DE, Masterson BJ, Nealon N. Effects of thermal knives on wound healing. *Obstet Gynecol.* 1985;66:436–439.

36. Hasselgren PO, Hagberg E, Malmer H, et al. One instead of two knives for surgical incision. *Arch Surg.* 1984;119:917–920.

37. Peacock EE Jr. *Wound Repair.* 3rd ed. Philadelphia: WB Saunders; 1984.

38. Hunt TK, Heppenstall RB, Pines E, et al. In: Hunt TK, Hengenstall RB, Pines E, et al, eds. *Soft and Hard Tissue Repair: Biological and Clinical Aspects.* New York: Praeger Publishers; 1984:4–17.

39. Simpson DM, Ross R. Effects of heterologous antineutrophil serum in guinea pigs: hematologic and ultrastructural observations. *Am J Pathol.* 1971;65:79–83.

40. Leibovich SJ, Ross R. The role of the macrophogein wound repair: a study with hydrocortisone and antimacrophage serum. *Am J Pathol.* 1975;78:71–77.

41. Seppa HEJ, Grotendorst GR, Seppa S, et al. Platelet-derived growth factor in chemotactic for fibroblasts. *J Cell Biol.* 1982;92:584–588.

42. Gauss-Miller V, Kleinman H, Martin GR, et al. Role of attachment factors and attractants in fibroblast chemotaxis. *J Lab Clin Med.* 1980;96:1071–1080.

43. Grinnel T, Billingham RE, Burgess L. Distribution of fibronectin during wound healing in vivo. *J Invest Dermatol.* 1981;76:181–186.

44. Grotendorst JR, Change T, Seppa HE, et al. Platelet-derived growth factor is a chemoattractant for vascular smooth muscle cells. *J Cell Physiol.* 1982;113:261–265.

45. Stiles CT, Capone GT, Scher CD. Dual control of cell growth by somatomedins and platelet-derived growth factors. *Proc Natl Acad Sci USA.* 1979;76:1279–1285.

46. Leibovich SJ, Ross R. A macrophage-dependent factor that stimulates the proliferation of fibroblasts in vitro. *Am J Pathol.* 1976;84:501–505.

47. Thakral KK, Goodson WH III, Hunt TK. Stimulation of wound blood vessel growth by wound macrophages. *J Surg Res.* 1979;26:430–436.

48. Knighton DR, Hunt TK, Thakral KK, et al. Role of platelets and fibrin in the healing sequence: an in vivo study of angiogenesis and collagen synthesis. *Ann Surg.* 1982;196:379–388.

49. Van Winkle W Jr. The epithelium in wound healing. *Surg Gynecol Obstet.* 1968;127:1089–1115.

50. Cohen JK, Moore CD, Diegelman RF. Onset and localization of collagen synthesis during wound healing in open rat skin wounds. *Proc Soc Exp Biol Med.* 1979; 160:458–462.

51. Rudolf R, Guber S, Suzuki M, et al. The life cycle of the myofibroblast. *Surg Gynecol Obstet.* 1977;145:389–394.

52. Madden JW, Peacock EE Jr. Studies on the biology of collagen during wound healing: III. Dynamic metabolism of scar collagen and remodeling of dermal wounds. *Ann Surg.* 1971;174:511–520.

53. Forrester JC, Zederfeldt BH, Hayes TL, et al. Wolff's law in relation to the healing skin wound. *J Trauma.* 1970;10:770–779.

54. Edlich RT. *Symposia on Wound Healing.* Sparkman RS, ed. Pearl River, NY: Davis and Geck, American Cyanamid Co.; 1985:8–10. Library of Congress Catalog Card No. 85-72109.

55. Lineaweaver W, Howard R, Soucy D, et al. Topical antimicrobial toxicity. *Arch Surg.* 1985;120:267–270.

56. Elek SD, Conen PE. The virulence of staphylococcus pyogens for man; a study of the problems of wound infection. *Br J Exp Pathol.* 1957;38:573–577.

57. Elek SD. Experimental staphylococcal infections in the skin of man. *Ann NY Acad Sci.* 1956;65:85–89.

58. Edlich RJ, Rodeheaver GT, Thacker JG, et al. *Fundamentals of Wound Management in Surgery: Technical Factors in Wound Management.* South Plainfield, NJ: Chirurgecom, Inc.; 1977:1–76.

59. Phuapradit W, Saropala R. Topical application of honey in treatment of abdominal wound disruption. *Aust N Zeal J Obstet Gynaecol.* 1992;32:381–384.

60. Efem SE, Udoh KT, Iwara CI. The antimicrobial spectrum of honey and its clinical significance. *Infection.* 1992;20:227–229.

61. Meeks GR. Secondary closure. *Contemp OB/GYN.* 1993;February;35–36.

62. Pratt JH. Wound healing-eviscerations. *Clin Obstet Gynecol.* 1973;16:126–139.

63. Alexander HC, Prudden JT. The causes of abdominal wound disruption. *Surg Gynecol Obstet.* 1966;122:1223–1229.

64. Tweedie FJ, Long RC. Abdominal wound disruption. *Surg Gynecol Obstet.* 1954;99:41–45.

65. Gallup DG. Modifications of celiotomy techniques to decrease morbidity in obese gynecologic patients. *Am J Obstet Gynecol.* 1984;150:171–178.

66. Jenkins, TPN. The burst abdominal wound: a mechanical approach. *Br J Surg.* 1976;63:873–876.

67. Fallis LS. Postoperative wound separation: review of cases. *Surgery.* 1937;1:523–528.

68. Douglas DM. *Wound Healing and Management.* Edinburgh: Livingston; 1963:37–38.

69. Hayton HA. Rupture of laparotomy wounds. *Lancet.* 1955;1:919–925.

70. Poole GV Jr. Mechanical factors in abdominal wound closure: the prevention of fascial dehiscence. *Surgery.* 1985;97:631–639.

71. Baggish MS, Lee WK. Abdominal wound disruption. *Surg Gynecol Obstet.* 1975;46:530–534.

72. Joergenson EJ, Smith ET. Postoperative abdominal wound separation and evisceration. *Am J Surg.* 1950;79:282–287.

73. Gilsdorf RB, Shea MM. Repair of massive septic abdominal wall defects with Marlex mesh. *Am J Surg.* 1975;130:634–638.

74. Markgraf W. Abdominal wound dehiscence: a technique for repair with Marlex mesh. *Arch Surg.* 1972;105:728–732.

75. Hiatt JR, Calabria RP, Wilson SE. Septic dehiscence of the abdominal wound. *Infections in Surgery.* 1986;August:429–432.

76. Rodeheaver GT, Nesbit WS, Edlich RT. Novafil: a dynamic suture for wound closure. *Ann Surg.* 1986;204:193–199.

77. Masterson BJ. Personal communication, 1990.

78. Von Fraunhofer JA, Starey, RS, Masterson BJ. Tensile properties of suture materials. *Biomaterials.* 1988;9:324–327.

79. Paterson-Brown S, Cheslyn-Curtis S, Biglin J, et al. Suture materials in contaminated wounds: a detailed comparison of a new suture with those currently in use. *Br J Surg.* 1987;74:734–735.

80. Knoop M, Lundstedt B, Thiede A. Evaluation of physical and biological properties of monofilament absorbable suture materials. *Langenbecks Arch Chir.* 1987;371:13–18.

81. Sanz LE. Wound management-matching materials and methods for best results. *Contemp OB/GYN.* 1987;November:37–46.

82. Swanson BA, Tramovitch TA. Suture materials: 1980's properties, uses, and abuses. *Int J Dermatol.* 1982;21:373–378.

83. Aston SJ. The choice of suture material for skin closure. *J Dermatol Surg.* 1976;2:57–61.

84. Yu GV, Caugliere R. Suture materials—properties and uses. *J Am Podiatr Assoc.* 1981;73:57–62.

85. Backnall TE. Abdominal wound closure: choice of suture. *J R Soc Med.* 1981;74:580–589.

86. Sanz LE, Smith S. Mechanism of wound healing, suture material, and wound closure. In: Bucksbaum HJ, Walton LA, eds. *Strategies in Gynecologic Surgery,* ed 1. New York: Springer-Verlag; 1986:53–76.

87. Sanz LE, Patterson JA, Kamath R, et al. Comparison of Maxon suture with Vicryl, chromic catgut, and PDS sutures in fascial closure in rats. *Obstet Gynecol.* 1988; 71:418–422.

88. Gomel V, McComb P, Boer-Meisel M. Histologic reactions to polyglactin-910, polyethylene, and nylon microsuture. *J Reprod Med.* 1980;25:56–60.

89. Postlethwait R, Willigan D, Ulin A. Human tissue reaction to sutures. *Ann Surg.* 1975;181:144–150.

90. Echeverria E, Jimenez J. Evaluation of an absorbable synthetic suture material. *Surg Gynecol Obstet.* 1970;131:1–14.

91. Edlich RT, Panek PH, Rodeheaver GT, et al. Physical and chemical configuration of sutures in the development of surgical infection. *Ann Surg.* 1973;177:679–688.

92. Chu CC, Kizil Z. Quantitative evaluation of stiffness of commercial suture materials. *Surg Gynecol Obstet.* 1989;168:233–238.

93. Thiede A. Comparison of the physical parameters and handling properties of rapidly and medium fast absorbable suture materials. *Chirurgie.* 1985;56:804–808.

94. Zederfeldt BH, Hunt TK. *Wound Closure: Materials and Techniques.* Wayne, NJ: Davis and Geck; 1990. Library of Congress Catalog Card No. 90-082586.

95. Birdsell DC, Gavelin GT, Kemsley GM, et al. Staying power-absorbable versus non-absorbable. *Plast Reconstr Surg.* 1981;68:742–745.

96. Grant A. The choice of suture materials and techniques for repair of perineal trauma: an overview of the evidence from controlled trials. *Br J Obstet Gynaecol.* 1989;96:1281–1289.

97. Lilly GE, Osborn DB, Hutchinson RA, et al. Clinical and bacteriologic aspects of polyglycolic acid sutures. *J Oral Surg.* 1973;31:103–105.

98. McGeehan D, Hunt D, Chaudhuri A, et al. An experimental study of the relationship between synergistic wound sepsis and suture materials. *Br J Surg.* 1980;67:636–638.

99. Thiede A, Jostarndt L, Lunstedt B, et al. Kontrollierte experimentelle histologische und mikrobiologische untersuchungen zur hemmwirkung von polyglycolsaurefaden bei infektion. *Chirurgie.* 1980;51:35–38.

100. Thompson JD. Personal communication, 1993.

101. Jones TE, Newell ET, Brubaker RE. The use of alloy steel wire in the closure of abdominal wounds. *Surg Gynecol Obstet.* 1941;72:1056–1059.

102. DiSaia PJ, Rettenmaier MD. Reduction of granulation tissue with a monofilament absorbable suture made from polyglyconate (Maxon). *J Gynecol Surg.* 1989;5:279–284.

103. Seeto R, Ng S, McClellan KA, Billson TA. Nonabsorbable suture material in cataract surgery: a comparison of Novafil and nylon. *Ophthalmic Surg.* 1992;23:538–544.

104. DiMarzo MD, Hunter WJ, Schultz RD, et al. In vivo study of expanded polytetra-fluoroethylene vascular suture. *Vasc Surg.* 1989;23:77–82.

105. Patterson-Brown S, Cheslyn-Curtis S, Biglin J, et al. Suture materials in contaminated wounds: a detailed comparison of a new suture with those currently in use. *Br J Surg.* 1987;74:734–735.

106. Stillman RM, Bella FJ, Seligman SJ. Skin wound closure—the effect of various wound closure methods on susceptibility to infection. *Arch Surg.* 1980;115:674–675.

107. Wallace D, Hernandez W, Schlaerth J, et al. Prevention of abdominal wound disruption utilizing the Smead-Jones closure technique. *Obstet Gynecol.* 1980;56:226–230.

108. Greenburg AG, Saik RP, Peskin GW. Wound dehiscence: pathophysiology and prevention. *Arch Surg.* 1979;114:143–146.

109. Sanz LE. Choosing the right wound closure technique. *Contemp OB/GYN.* 1983;21(Surg):142–151.

110. Sanders RJ, DiClementi D, Ireland K. Principles of abdominal wound closure II. Prevention of wound dehiscence. *Arch Surg.* 1977;112:1188–1191.

111. Rutkow JM. Rates of surgery in the United States. *Surg Clin North Am.* 1982;62:559–578.

112. Corman ML, Veidenheimer MC. Controlled clinical trial of three suture materials for abdominal wall closure after bowel operations. *Am J Surg.* 1981;141:510–513.

113. Stone IK, von Fraunhofer JA, Masterson BJ. The biomechanical effects of tight suture closure upon fascia. *Surg Gynecol Obstet.* 1986;163:448–452.

114. Archie JP Jr, Feldman RW. Primary wound closure with permanent continuous running monofilament sutures. *Surg Gynecol Obstet.* 1981;153:721–722.

115. Knight CD, Griffin FD. Abdominal wound closure with a continuous monofilament polypropylene suture. *Arch Surg.* 1983;118:1305–1308.

116. Shepherd JH, Cavanaugh D, Riggs D, et al. Abdominal wound closure using a nonabsorbable single-layer technique. *Obstet Gynecol.* 1983;61:248–252.

117. Gallup DG. Opening and closing the abdomen. In: Phelan JP, Clark SL, eds. *Cesarean Delivery.* New York: Elsevier; 1988:171–181.

118. Orr JW Jr, Orr PF, Barrett JM, et al. Continuous or interrupted fascial closure: a prospective evaluation of No. 1 Maxon suture in 402 gynecologic procedures. *Am J Obstet Gynecol.* 1990;163:1485–1489.

119. Gallup DG, Talledo OE, King LA. Primary mass closure of midline incisions with a continuous running monofilament suture in gynecologic patients. *Obstet Gynecol.* 1989;73:675–677.

120. Gallup DG, Nolan TE, Smith RP. Primary mass closure of midline incisions with a continuous polyglyconate monofilament absorbable suture. *Obstet Gynecol.* 1990;76:872–875.

121. Irvin TT, Koffman CG, Puthie HL. Layer closure of laparotomy wounds with absorbable and nonabsorbable suture materials. *Br J Surg.* 1976;63:793–796.

122. LoCicero J, Robbins JA, Webb WR. Complications following abdominal fascial closure using various unabsorbable sutures. *Surg Gynecol Obstet.* 1983;157:25–27.

123. Montz TJ, Creasman WT, DiSaia PJ, et al. Running mass closure of abdominal wounds using absorbable looped suture. *J Gynecol Surg.* 1991;7:107–110.

124. Ferguson DJ. Clinical application of experimental relations between technique and wound infection. *Surgery.* 1968;63:377–383.

125. DeHoll D, Rodeheaver GT, Edgerton MT, et al. Potentiation of infection by suture closure of dead space. *Am J Surg.* 1974;127:716–720.

126. Trimbos JB. Security of various knots commonly used in surgical practice. *Obstet Gynecol.* 1984;64:274–278.

127. Trimbos JB, Booster M, Peters AA. Mechanical knot performance of a new generation polydioxanon suture (PDS-2). *Acta Obstet Gynecol Scand.* 1991;70:157–159.

128. Van Rijssel EJC, Brand R, Admiraal C, et al. Tissue reaction and surgical knots: the effect of suture size, knot configuration, and knot volume. *Obstet Gynecol.* 1989;74:64–68.

129. Van Rijssel EJC, Trimbos JB, da Costa A, Fleuren GJ, Brand R. Assessment of tissue reaction at suture knots; an adaptation of Sewell's scoring system. *Eur J Obstet Gynecol Reprod Biol.* 1988;27:165–172.

130. Tera H, Aberg C. Tensile strength of twelve types of knots employed in surgery, using different suture materials. *Acta Chir Scand.* 1976;142:1–7.

131. Holmlund DEW. Knot properties of surgical suture materials. *Acta Chir Scand.* 1974;140:355–362.

132. Trimbos JB, van Rijssel EJC, Klopper PJ. Performance of sliding knots in monofilament and multifilament suture material. *Obstet Gynecol.* 1986;68:425–430.

133. Tera H, Aberg C. Strength of knots in surgery in relation to type of knot, type of suture material and dimension of suture thread. *Acta Chir Scand.* 1977;143:75–83.

134. Thacker JG, Rodeheaver G, Moore JW, et al. Mechanical performance of surgical sutures. *Am J Surg.* 1975;130:374–380.

Surgical

Complications

J. Michael Breen
James L. Breen

> Have you not a moist eye? A dry hand? A yellow cheek? A decreasing leg? An increasing belly? Is not your voice broken? Your wind short? Your chin double? Your wit single? And every part about you blasted with antiquity and will you yet call yourself young?
>
> **William Shakespeare**

More and more of those born into the world survive the vicissitudes of infancy, adolescence, and maturity.

The percentage of the population that reaches age 85 and beyond is growing at a faster rate than the population aged 65 to 84. As this phenomenon accelerates, the advantage in female survivorship will become more pronounced. This has led Dr. Robert Butler, former Director of the National Institute of Aging, to call the next century "the Century of the Older Woman." Today there are 2.8 million persons over age 85—2 million women and 800,000 men—a 5:2 advantage. By the year 2000 this population group will grow by 82% to 5.1 million, made up of 3.7 million women, an increase of 85%. By midpoint of the next century the number of people age 85 or over will reach more than 16 million, an increase of more than 57%. In the year 2050 we can expect to see 11.4 million women and 4.6 million men who have reached their 85th birthday.[1]

One dramatic indication of this trend is the number who reach their 100th birthday. In the past decade we could see this shift develop clearly and suddenly. In 1970, according to the Social Security Administration, 4574 persons reached this landmark; by 1985 more than 25,000 Americans had become centenarians, and more than two thirds of these were women.

As gynecologists, we must increase our skills in those areas that apply to the aged. Our purpose in this chapter is to address primarily those complications that we encounter in the older gynecologic patient.

There exists little literature on gynecologic surgery in elderly women. Smith and Pratt in 1959 reported on elective vaginal surgery in older women which represented less than 6% of their population.[2] In 1947, Lash found that patients older than 75 comprised 7% of his study[3] and McKeithen, in 1977, found that 33% of his patients were greater than 75 years of age, thus showing a trend in the amount of surgery being performed on elderly women.[4] Breen and Osofsky reported that the overall mortality rate for major gynecologic surgical procedures was 1.4% with major morbidity being 10%.[5] It has been reported that there are fewer complications among the elderly with symptomatic pelvic relaxation as compared to younger women. The elderly, however, do not tolerate surgical complications as well.[6] Extensive preoperative testing and evaluation becomes mandatory in the aged patient scheduled for surgery.

PREOPERATIVE MANAGEMENT

Surgical procedures may be carried out very well in older people, but it is imperative that extensive preoperative evaluation be applied to the medical conditions prevalent in the aging population. Preoperative preparation should include an extensive history and physical examination carried out both by the surgeon of record as well as by the responsible internist. Although we as gynecologists are considered primary care providers, the internist usually has a more intimate knowledge of the patient's current medical problems as well as any medications that she may be taking. Laboratory screening should include the following: complete blood count, prothrombin time, partial thromboplastin time (PTT), electrolytes, blood urea nitrogen (BUN), creatinine, and liver studies. These will provide a baseline and reveal any preexisting conditions. Electrocardiograms (ECG) as well as chest x-rays will rule out chronic or new conditions associated with cardiac and pulmonary function.

Perioperative cardiac and pulmonary complications related to elective surgery are major causes of morbidity and mortality in the United States and these problems are particularly common in the aged population.[7] There is approximately a 0.2% risk of myocardial infarction or cardiac death associated with surgery and anesthesia. Increased risk is associated with recent myocardial infarction (within the last 6 months), arrhythmias, congestive heart failure and aortic stenosis.[8]

When evaluating a cardiac patient, an extensive history and a thorough physical examination, as well as a chest x-ray and an ECG, are mandatory. Evidence of any cardiac anomaly should be further evaluated by a cardiologist. If the patient has had a recent myocardial infarction, elective surgery should be postponed for at least 6 months. Hemodynamic monitoring is indicated in patients who have had recent myocardial infarctions, congestive heart failure, significant arrhythmias, and aortic stenosis, and are well advanced in age.

Any medications that the patient may be taking, such as antihypertensives or digitalis, should be continued up until the morning of surgery. Diastolic blood pressures should be maintained at less than 100 mm Hg. In a patient with complete heart block or sick sinus syndrome, temporary pacemakers may be used. Endocarditis prophylaxis must be given to patients who have valvular replacements. Current recommendations are ampicillin, 2 g, and gentamycin, 1.5 mg/kg, administered intravenously 30 minutes before surgery and 8 hours after the initial doses.[9]

If the patient is currently on anticoagulant therapy, i.e., coumadin, it should be stopped at least 3 days before the procedure and, instead, full heparinization should be instituted up to approximately 3 hours prior to surgery. This can be resumed 12 hours postoperatively.

Pulmonary risk factors consist of obesity, restrictive lung diseases, cigarette smoking, and any acute respiratory infection. Chronic obstructive pulmonary diseases such as protracted bronchitis or emphysema are probably the most important factors that increase the risk of postoperative pulmonary complications.[10]

Preoperative evaluation of pulmonary systems consists of the history, physical examination, and chest x-ray. Those patients in an extremely high-risk group should have arterial blood gases (ABGs) and full pulmonary function studies prior to surgery.

Preoperative management of any pulmonary condition should involve discontinuing smoking for 2 to 3 weeks before surgery. Additionally, the patient should be sworn to a nonsmoking commitment for life at the same time. The problem of smoking has been discussed more extensively in Chapter 3. Bronchodilators may be given to aid in the management of asthma or emphysema. If required, traditionally theophylline, terbutaline, and acrosolized bronchodilators have been used. Corticosteroids may also be given and are recommended in those patients who are on steroid management.

Diabetes mellitus is a common medical condition found in the aged population and insulin-dependent patients should receive one third to one half of their daily dose of long-acting insulin subcutaneously prior to surgery with an intravenous line containing dextrose solution.[11] The best approach for the older diabetic patient, of course, is strict control and surveillance by an expert in diabetes management.

Another channel by which to reduce the risk of potential intraoperative or postoperative complications is prophylactic management. Since most benign gynecologic disease does not involve major risks of injury to the bowel, antibiotic bowel preparation is not indicated. A mechanical preparation, however, should be instituted before surgery. An empty bowel also certainly makes surgery in the pelvis easier to accomplish than does a full one.

Prophylactic antibiotics reduce the incidence of operative site infections, but they will not prevent infections such as cystitis or pneumonia. Because all pelvic procedures are considered potentially contaminated procedures, at least a single dose of a first-generation cephalosporin should be given intravenously about 30 minutes before surgery.[12]

Skin preparation should include abdominal/perineal hair removal performed in the operating room with hair clippers, not by a razor. Shaving or hair removal the night before surgery increases the rate of infection significantly.[13] Scrub preparations should be performed with povidone-iodine solutions or chlorhexidine gluconate. Both will effectively sterilize the skin, as will 70% alcohol.

This population is also at risk for increased deep vein thrombosis and pulmonary embolism; therefore, antiembolic prophylaxis is indicated. Several large multicenter studies have shown a reduced postoperative complication by giving a low-dose prophylactic heparin. A standard prophylactic regimen is 5000 U heparin subcutaneously 2 hours perioperatively and every 12 hours until the patient is totally ambulatory.[14] Approximately 15% of patients appear to be hypersensitive to low-dose heparin and may develop prolonged PTT or decreased platelet counts. This is not felt to be clinically significant, however. Another preventive measure is external pneumatic calf compression, which is used both intraoperatively and postoperatively until the patient is completely ambulatory.[15]

POSTOPERATIVE MANAGEMENT

The aged patient tolerates invasive procedures as well, for the most part, as younger individuals but does not manage so well if postoperative complications occur. In any operative procedure, on young or old, meticulous tissue handling and hemostasis must be observed with an eye toward preventing or minimizing postoperative complications. In the immediate postoperative period, acute respiratory failure, shock, and oliguria are major problems to anticipate or to contend with in the elderly.

Respiratory Failure

Respiratory dilemmas of failure potential require acute clinical assessment and may necessitate emergency mechanical ventilation. Acute respiratory failure has been defined as a PaO_2 of less than 50 mm Hg, a PCO_2 of more than 50 mm Hg, and a pH less than 7.3 on room air. In a top-flight facility, the decision to maintain a patient on ventilatory support postoperatively is usually made by the anesthesiologist in charge and the consulting critical care manager.

It is crucial to point out, in aged patients with marked fluid shifts during surgery, in an aura of potentially diminished cardiac and pulmonary function, that weaning or immediate extubation are not often in the patient's best interest.[16] If there is any question, the patient should be transferred to the recovery room, intubated, and placed on ventilatory support. Patience and caution are imperative.

Shock

The second complication often seen immediately in the postoperative period is shock, defined best as generalized inadequate tissue perfusion. The several types of shock fall into three main categories: hypovolemic or hemorrhagic shock, septic shock, and cardiogenic shock. The warning signs of hypoperfusion or shock are systolic blood pressure less than 90 mm Hg, urine output less than 30 mL/h, metabolic acidosis, and cold, clammy integument. When assessing any patients who might be in shock, ABGs, serum electrolytes, creatinine, and a complete blood count should be drawn immediately. An ECG and chest x-ray should be performed on an emergency basis as well. If the hypotension does not respond quickly to volume expansion, invasive monitoring techniques should be performed. A relatively simple one available to most physicians is the central venous presure (CVP) monitor, performed by inserting a catheter into the internal jugular or subclavian vein. Pressures of less than 5 cm H_2O indicate hypovolemia on a CVP monitor. Pressures greater than 15 cm H_2O reflect congestive heart failure or fluid overload.

In an unstable patient, Swan-Ganz catheterization should be used. This allows electronic monitoring of pulmonary artery wedge pressure, which gives an accurate assessment of the intraluminal status. Pulmonary wedge pressures of less than 6 mm Hg indicate hypovolemia, whereas pressures greater than 18 mm Hg indicate heart failure or fluid overload.

When approaching any patient in a hypotensive situation, the immediate concern should be restoration of the circulatory volume. Initially this can be established through crystalloids in normal saline or lactated Ringer's solution administered at a rapid rate of infusion. Care must be taken not to overload the patient. The hypotensive state and the urine output must be closely monitored. Colloids may also be used, i.e., 25% albumin in a 200-mg dose, which equals approximately 1 L crystalloids.[17] Colloid may also be used as a plasma expander. There has been some mention of adult respiratory distress syndrome occurring when colloids are used as volume expanders, but this is controversial.

When dealing with a hemorrhagic state, blood transfusions of packed red blood cells should be administered. The old criterion of 10 g/dL or a hematocrit of less than 30% does not necessarily hold up in today's increasingly widespread environment of hepatitis and acquired immunodeficiency syndrome. If in a 24-hour period there is a loss of 3 g hemoglobin or a drop in hematocrit of 6 points, transfusion should be considered. Transfusions can be withheld in patients with hemoglobins as low as 8 g or with a 24% hematocrit if active bleeding has essentially stopped.

When transfusing more than 5 U packed red blood cells, monitoring of platelet function and PTT is important. Due to changes in hematologic profile, it has been recommended in the past that 1 U fresh frozen plasma be used for every 5 U packed red blood cells transfused, but this is somewhat controversial.

After circulatory volume is restored, if the patient's hypotensive status persists, then vasoactive drugs are indicated. Those most commonly used are dopamine and dobutamine. Dopamine has α- and β-adrenergic activity and increases cardiac output, heart rate, and blood pressure. One advantage of dopamine is that low doses increase renal perfusion. At high doses it causes systemic vascular resistance. Dobutamine is a β-adrenergic agent that also increases cardiac output, heart rate, and blood pressure. Dobutamine at lower doses decreases cardiac filling pressure by decreasing systemic vascular resistance. Combining the two drugs is controversial as to benefit.

Military antishock trauma (MAST) suits may be used if the problem is secondary to acute intra-abdominal hemorrhage. This works by diverting blood from the lower body to augment venous return via increased peripheral resistance.

Quite different from hemorrhagic or hypovolemic shock is cardiogenic shock, a condition of decreased cardiac output. In these cases, administration of intravenous fluid should be restricted. Diuretics such as the popular furosamide should be used, thereby drawing fluids from the general body tissues to produce venous dilation. Inotropic agents should also be given in this situation, the drugs of choice again being dobutamine and dopamine. Digitalis may be used, but inotropic agents have a greater potency and a more rapid onset of action.

The last area in the shock category is septic shock. This is managed similarly to hypovolemic shock, but broad-spectrum antibiotics should be added to the regimen of fluid expansion. It should be noted that there is little evidence that corticosteroids enhance or alter the outcome in this situation.

Oliguria

The third area of anxiety in the immediate postoperative period is oliguria, defined as significant diminution in excreted urine and is quantified as less than 30 mL urine per hour. When evaluating oliguria, we deal essentially with three potential problems. Postrenal oliguria is rarely the cause of postoperative oliguria. Nonetheless one must first ensure that there is no obstruction to urinary outflow. Total anuria may be related to bilateral ureteral injury.

The most common cause of postoperative prerenal oliguria is hypovolemia secondary to inadequate hydration. Insufficient hydration may be related to hemorrhage or third spacing of fluids at the operative site. If prerenal oliguria is suspected, the initial response should be an intravenous fluid challenge of approximately 500 to 1000 mL normal saline or lactated Ringer's solution over 30 to 60 minutes depending on the patient's age and physical condition. If an increase in urine output is noted, this indicates a prerenal component.

The main cause of renal oliguria is acute tubular necrosis (ATN). In the immediate postoperative period, ATN is usually due to hypotension and hypoxia.[18] Laboratory findings are consistent with a BUN/serum creatinine ratio of less than 15, urinary plasma/creatinine ratio of less than 20, a specific gravity of less than 1.16, or a urine sodium level of more than 40 mEq/L. If this condition is suspected, both immediate discontinuation of any nephrotoxic medications and rapid correction of hypotension are indicated. It is essential that fluid and electrolytes be monitored continuously. Accurate input and output measurements as well as daily weights should be taken. When all these measures fail, and BUN levels rise over 100 mg/dL, dialysis is indicated. Hypokalemia of more than 7 mOsm/L, pseudoacidosis, electrolyte disturbances, fluid overload, and uremia constitute additional criteria for decision-making.

Other Problems

The converse of the hypotensive state, hypertension, often appears in the aged postoperatively, manifesting approximately 24 to 48 hours after surgery. The mechanism of this action is related to the mobilization of intraoperative fluids. Aged patients are also apt to be taking antihypertensive medications, so propranolol rebound may also occur in approximately this time frame. If hypertension is noted, antihypertensives should be administered to bring the elevation down to a stable but not excessively low level.

Pulmonary embolism is probably one of the most life-threatening late postoperative causes of morbidity or mortality.[19] This commonly presents as chest pain, dyspnea, and tachycardia. The affected patient may or may not have clinical evidence of deep vein thrombosis, but the sudden onset of these symptoms is strongly suggestive. Once these signs and symptoms present, aggressive assessment must be instituted. The most common first line laboratory evaluations are ABGs and ECGs. Common ECG abnormalities are ST-T wave changes and possible right bundle branch block or right axis deviation.

The ABGs will often show a PaO_2 less than 80 mm Hg. Chest x-rays are also indicated in this situation but are often normal or may show nothing more than atelectasis. If any question still remains, ventilation and perfusion pulmonary scanning is indicated. If there are perfusion defects in the area of normal ventilation, then pulmonary embolism should be suspected. When high suspicion for deep vein thrombosis arises, venograms or Doppler flow studies may be performed on the lower extremities.

Treatment is most commonly directed toward anticoagulation therapy initially with continuous low-dose heparin and monitoring of the PTT followed by subsequent institution of oral coumadin therapy. If anticoagulation fails or if the patient develops recurrent pulmonary emboli or septic emboli, interruption of inferior vena caval flow can be accomplished by intracaval umbrella, caval ligation, or clipping. Thrombolytic therapy is usually contraindicated in the postoperative period and pulmonary embolectomy is only indicated in patients with large pulmonary emboli compromising the hemodynamic status of the patient.[20]

The final postoperative complication of note is postoperative febrile morbidity. An initial febrile response in the first 24 to 48 hours in the postsurgical patient is usually secondary to the hypermetabolic state of surgery. If the patient continues to demonstrate temperatures greater than 38° C (100.4° F) after the initial postoperative period, thorough evaluation should be performed including pelvic examination, blood cultures, urine cultures, and sputum cultures if the patient has a productive cough. In the first 2 to 5 days postoperatively, the common infections seen are in the urinary tract or in the lungs (pneumonia). Wound infections and intra-abdominal abscesses as well as thrombophlebitis tend to present as a later complication.[21] However, surgery through the vaginal approach carries a significant incidence of cellulitis. This should be recognized and treated at the earliest possible time so as not to jeopardize the effectiveness of a reconstructive procedure and to prevent abscess formation.

CONCLUSION

The concept of the "whole patient" applies to the aged more than to any other group. Evaluation of the assets and liabilities of all systems, including the emotional status of the patient, must precede any proposed gynecologic surgery. The individualization of therapy, with occasional deviations from accepted modalities, is required when treating the aged patient with multiple disease processes and impairments. Normal babies perhaps can be cared for by the wholesale; not so old men and women. They need individual attention; no two cases are alike. Moreover, the treatment suitable for younger patients becomes progressively unsuitable for the aged. Their comfort and not their impossible rejuvenation should be the physician's aim.

One may conclude, since it has become obvious that surgical intervention in our elderly population is becoming more and more common, that a clear understanding of the patient's medical condition before surgery, coupled with awareness of the aged patient's inability to tolerate and combat postoperative complications, make it imperative that meticulous individual attention be paid to the preoperative, intraoperative, and postoperative care of these patients.

REFERENCES

1. Breen JL. *The Gynecologist and the Older Patient.* New York: Aspen, 1990; preface;xv–xvii.

2. Smith LR, Pratt JH. Vaginal hysterectomy in the geriatric patient. *Obstet Gynecol.* 1959;13:84–89.

3. Lash AF. Surgical geriatric gynecology. *Am J Obstet Gynecol.* 1947;53:766–775.

4. McKeithen WS Jr. Major gynecologic surgery in elderly females 65 years of age or older. *Am J Obstet Gynecol.* 1975;123:59–65.

5. Breen JL, Osofsky HJ. *Current Concepts in Gynecologic Surgery.* Baltimore: Williams & Wilkins; 1987: 33–39.

6. Cruse PJ, Foord R. A five year prospective study of 23,649 surgical wounds. *Arch Surg.* 1973;107:206–212.

7. *Vital and Health Statistics.* U.S. Department of Health and Human Services, series 13, no. 88. Washington, DC: U.S. Government Printing Office; 1983;17–19.

8. Goldman L. Cardiac risks and complications of non-cardiac surgery. *Ann Intern Med.* 1983;98:504–519.

9. Mills P, et al. Long term prognosis of mitral valve prolapse. *N Engl J Med.* 1977;297:13–18.

10. Grersen MC, et al. Prediction of cardiac and pulmonary complications related to elective abdominal and noncardiac thoracic surgery in geriatric patients. *Am J Med.* 1990;88:101–104.

11. Meyers EJ, et al. Diabetic management by insulin infusion during major surgery. *Am J Surg.* 1979;137:323–336.

12. Sevin BU, et al. Antibiotic prevention of infections complicating radical abdominal hysterectomy. *Obstet Gynecol.* 1984;64:539–545.

13. Seropian R, Reynolds BM. Wound infections after preoperative depilatory versus razor preparation. *Am J Surg.* 1971;121:251–253.

14. Kakkar VV, Corrigan TP, Fossard DP. Prevention of fatal postoperative pulmonary embolism by low doses of heparin. *Lancet.* 1975;2:45–51.

15. Clarke Pearson DL, et al. Prevention of postoperative venous thromboembolism by external pneumatic calf compression in patients with gynecologic malignancy. *Obstet Gynecol.* 1984;63:92–98.

16. Jung R, et al. Comparison of three methods of respiratory care after abdominal surgery. *Chest.* 1980;78:31–36.

17. Moss GS, et al. Colloid or crystalloid in the resuscitation of hemmorrhagic shock: A controlled clinical trial. *Surgery.* 1981;89:434–438.

18. Grillon G, Stanton SL. Long term follow-up of surgery for urinary incontinence in elderly women. *Br J Urol.* 1989;56:478–483.

19. Hertzer NR. Vascular problems in urologic patients. *Urol Clin North Am.* 1985;12:493–498.

20. Barzilui B, et al. Avoidance of embolic complications by ultrasonic characterization of the ascending aorta. *Circulation.* 1989;80:275–279.

21. Harbrecht PJ, et al. Role of infection in increased mortality associated with age in laparotomy. *Am Surg.* 1983;49:173–178.

Postoperative Management

Marvin H. Terry Grody

The postoperative course for any surgical patient begins while the last suture is being tied. The surgeon in charge and the assistant staff should already have discussed the continuing care of the patient. I feel strongly that this is not a time for the "relaxed" (semi-detached?) attitude so pervasive in operating rooms (often occurring throughout the procedure, not just at the end) wherein piped-in or radio music takes over, jokes are told, or irrelevant conversation ensues. Mistakes are made because attention is diverted from the business at hand and errors of omission and commission are attributed later to lack of communication. Although such loss of focus is inexcusable in any case, the margin for error is slimmest in the older patient. In fact, many operating rooms allow the playing of music throughout the entire operating day and I think this is a travesty. The very idea that music promotes tranquility and relieves tension is utterly ridiculous since the young resident staff almost always demands the rock variety anyhow and, regardless of the type of music, it invariably distracts the operating team from concentration on the surgery. It is my considered opinion that any divergent element, including extraneous conversation, should be eliminated from the operating room from the moment the patient enters until she leaves. Not only is it not fair to the patient, but it interferes with the fixed attention mandatory for good resident education.

As the procedure reaches completion, discussion and determination of the precise orders, both in general and in particular, for that operation and that patient, should be occurring. Where applicable, explanations by the surgeon in charge should be given for certain orders so that understanding for the reasoning behind them promotes their proper expedition, obviously simultaneously educating students and residents—for example, how and why a catheter should be taped in a certain way and when it should be removed, or the purpose of packing and when it can be extracted, or why and when certain blood tests should be monitored. Experience dictates that adherence to a prescribed regimen is much more likely to happen with than without explanation and repetition. Especially poor form occurs when the surgeon, racing off to office hours, or to the delivery room, or to a social engagement, blurts out as he or she disappears, "Just give her my usual routine!" Tomes could be written on errors in management resulting from such irresponsible behavior, especially in elderly patients who always require more individual and elaborate and precise care than do younger people.

Primary objectives for all patients immediately after surgery, all things considered, really narrow down to maximum patient comfort and shortest reasonable hospital stay. Expressed differently, the goals are rapid surgical recovery and quick return to usual systemic stability. The two most commonly occurring major concerns center on possible postoperative hemorrhage, usually very early, within hours after leaving the operating room, or fever, later in the hospital course. Especially in the older patient, the additional potential for deep vein thrombosis can never be forgotten. Thus, it follows, a rational sequential approach, leaving nothing to chance, should be developed. As with preoperative preparation, since such a large proportion of surgical procedures on the older patient are performed, or should be performed, through the vaginal approach, the postoperative recommendations will be weighted in that direction.

VAGINAL PACKING

Except for isolated vaginal hysterectomy involving no repair, and surgery confined to the abdominal route, I adamantly feel that packing is essential to both an immediate and long-term good outcome. Inevitably when I make my usual declaration in this vein in educational conferences, a significant faction rises in opposition, proclaiming, always vehemently, that good surgery with meticulous hemostasis obviates the need for packing. Such an attitude is disconcerting because I usually find that these outcries arise from operators (I hesitate to call them surgeons) who invariably do grossly inadequate dissection, both anteriorly and especially posteriorly, and also often overuse cauterization (in the process of which an inordinate amount of dead tissue and detritus is created, thereby increasing infection potential). Unless repair is confined only to simple perineorrhaphy, reconstructive vaginal surgery, properly conducted, creates large areas of raw dissected surface which can lead to significant postoperative collections of serosanguinous fluid. Although these raw surfaces are thereby individually forced apart by this seeping fluid, a problem in itself, the greater dilemma lies with an increased probability of infection, the major nemesis in all reparative operations.

A 2-inch gauze strip, soaked in antibiotic (i.e., bacitracin) solution, packed snugly between two ribbon retractors through the full vaginal length will accomplish two major objectives. By compression it will minimize fluid accumulation, but just as importantly it will protect the integrity of the crucial stitches of the reconstruction by resisting sudden jolting increases in downward pressure arising from nausea or coughing in the immediate postoperative phase. Most surgeons remove the pack in 1 day, but I retain its protective effects for 2 days. The longer presence of packing does not alter the patient's course adversely and discomfort over the second day is minimal compared to the first. I feel it distinctly discourages infection and enhances healing, significantly more so in 2 days than 1.

POSTOPERATIVE CATHETER MANAGEMENT AND VOIDING ASSESSMENT

Urinary drainage becomes a concern almost from the moment incisions are initiated in most major gynecologic procedures. Such anxiety becomes exaggerated the closer our work draws us into the sphere of ureters, bladder, and urethra. Once the surgeon feels comfortable that no direct damage has been inflicted on these organs, and the operation is completed, focus shifts to facilitation of postoperative bladder drainage. Because voluntary micturition is improbable, at best, in the immediate postsurgical phase, and bladder overdistention is most undesirable, the catheter suddenly becomes the patient's and the doctor's best friend. Catheter care will vary based on the type of operation, on its placement transurethrally or suprapubically, and on the level of available nursing attention. The best of circumstances occurs with simple straightforward uncomplicated hysterectomy, either abdominal or vaginal, accompanied by one-on-one nursing care, in which case retention catheter use is virtually precluded. Abdominal explorations of a benign nature fall into the same category, requiring usually, at the most, constant drainage through the first night, when nursing care is minimal, followed by catheter removal from the fully alert patient in the morning.

Extensive reconstructive and urogynecologic cases require more attention. In the presence of full vaginal packing, spontaneous voiding cannot be expected before the packing is withdrawn. If the surgery has not involved the anterior pelvis, transurethral catheters are usually adequate and may be removed at the same time as pack extraction. However, in a small percentage of these cases, either because of a high sensitivity range or because the surgical inflammatory reaction of wide dissections has extended circumferentially, spontaneous voiding is postponed one or more days. When this occurs, the patient should be reassured at once that such a delay is common (much more settling than "is not uncommon") and that it will in no way interfere with the healing process or the integrity of the surgery. Thus explained, she will accept the retention catheter with more patience and less disappointment.

In any anterior repair, whether performed vaginally or suprapubically, even if limited only to a simple cystourethral angle elevation, I feel strongly that temporal assisted continuous bladder drainage should be used, even if only for a matter of hours, in all cases. Assuredly a small number of patients, having undergone a minimal repair involving the lower urinary tract, will void after recovery from anesthesia. However, based on more than 40 years of both wide personal experience and observations of the work of many other physicians, I have always been firmly convinced that bladders and urethras, traumatized either directly or indirectly by restorative work in the anterior pelvis, require significant time for recovery from the expected resultant inflammatory reaction to the surgery itself. Such a judgment is particularly applicable to the postreproductive woman. One hopes that the positive anatomic readjustment from the surgery acts to help speed up the localized recovery.

Young practitioners should not allow themselves to be intimidated, as I have seen happen so often, by the tales of some of their elders proclaiming, "All my patients void at once," or "I never need a catheter more than 2 days, no matter how old she is." Surgeons of any experience know this to be an outright lie. If the patient has been properly counseled preoperatively, then bladder drainage by catheter for several days, even extending through immediate recovery at home, as is occasionally necessary, to use the vernacular, is no "big deal." Lumping all patients into the same category becomes unrealistic and harmful; no two operations are precisely alike and certainly each patient is significantly different from the next, especially in the older age group, in all kinds of ways.

Methods of catheter management in gynecologic surgical patients, with accent on the older and the elderly, seem almost as myriad as the number of doctors performing the surgery. In open discussion, any proposal always invokes controversy and none is universally applicable anyhow. Because our major concern lies with reestablishment of normal bladder function and urinary control in major operative reconstructions in the sixth decade and beyond, a most challenging situation, I will confine my remarks to that segment of our management program.

Experience has taught me always to use, in these cases, a suprapubic catheter. At the outset of the procedure, I very simply, carefully but rapidly, thrust a long narrow uterine dressing forceps transurethrally, with vaginally placed finger guidance, through the anterior bladder wall, forcing the tips to emerge in the midline just under the skin 1 to 2 cm above the symphysis pubis. A scalpel nick allows for protrusion far enough so that towel clips, with tips inverted, can open the arms of the forceps enough for a number 16 Foley catheter to be grasped and pulled entirely through the bladder and out the urethral meatus. The catheter is then retracted back into the bladder as noted by a palpating index finger under the urethra. To ensure against inadvertent withdrawal of the Foley balloon through the bladder wall during the operation, the catheter should immediately be taped to the side of the abdomen and then connected appropriately to provide constant drainage from that point on. The entire maneuver consumes about 90 seconds as opposed to the much longer time spent using alternative methods involving initial bladder installation of 500 to 600 mL saline followed by suprapubic puncture through the abdominal wall into the bladder for the insertion of a Silastic catheter with associated adhesive apparatus to fix the catheter in place. For one reason or another, I have always encountered trouble with the Silastic retention catheters but none with the Foley. Occasionally, using the transurethral uterine forceps, the external urethral meatus will tear slightly as the arms are spread. This is no problem and healing is prompt.

When restitutional surgery is limited to a simple essentially suprapubic elevation of the cystourethral angle, even with accompanying paravaginal defects repair from above, or to hysterectomy by either route, or to an isolated posterior pelvic repair of any magnitude, postoperative urinary catheter management rarely presents difficult problems. When surgery includes significant restorative work on the anterior pelvis from below, an approach I feel we must encourage, the conduct of catheter control until normal physiologic voiding is attained becomes more exacting. The extensive dissection that I feel is so often necessary to precede efficacious anterior pelvic reclamation usually generates considerable inflammatory reaction and capillary extravasation. These unavoidable surgical companions can be expected to exert a muting effect of greater or lesser degree on detrusor muscle activity, as alluded to earlier. So, a practical regimen, leading ultimately to catheter withdrawal and continued temporal bladder accommodation, as recovery progresses, must be instituted.

Before I expand on such a routine, the advantages of suprapubic over transurethral bladder drainage demand discussion. Cystitis hardly ever occurs with suprapubic retention catheters, but it is not uncommon in transurethral usage. Patient discomfort is minimal with the former as compared to the latter, when the Foley balloon also is much more apt to irritate vesical mucosa. Spontaneous voiding occurs earlier when the transabdominal pathway is used and residual urine volumes are very easily and quickly measured by simply unclamping the catheter for release of the urinary balance as soon as the patient has finished voiding. The patient does this herself. In the case of the urethral catheter, once it is removed, a nurse must be summoned after each voiding to recatheterize the patient to check for the residual urine. Repeated catheter insertion is most annoying to the patient, is time-consuming for the nurse, is often inaccurate because of time delay before the nurse arrives, can potentiate infection, and certainly is not cost effective.

When the patient, for whatever reason, must go home with a catheter in place, unquestionably the upper outlet wins the vote over the lower. Not only is it more comfortable, but it averts guesswork in determining the correct time for removal because it affords the patient herself a method, through self-measurement at home after unclamping, of checking residuals. Unless the patient is adept at self-catheterization, such is not the case when the urethral catheter has been used. After having drained the balloon and removed the catheter, spontaneous voiding is attempted. She must return to the doctor's office about 2 hours later to learn how she's doing. Then, if the residual urine is too high, back in goes the catheter for another few days, only to run through the same routine later. In summation, using the suprapubic catheter is the only way to go.

Depending on the extent of the anterior pelvic surgery, ranging from the simplest Pereyra type of suprapubic correction to the combination of urethropexy, paravaginal defects repair, and central imbrication done from below, clamping of the suprapubic catheter can be started on the second, third, or fourth postoperative day. Certainly the extent of the original preoperative distortion plays an equivalent determining role in timing the testing for resumption of spontaneous voiding. Above all, in the postreproductive age group, especially the very elderly, there is no need to rush the program. Extensive reparative work in this category of women, regardless of third-party pressures and diagnosis-related group standards, requires a 5-day hospital stay in most cases, especially if there is no help at home. So it is much better to wait an extra day to initiate attempts to void rather than disappoint the patient.

At Temple University Hospital, on the particular morning that is selected for trial at spontaneous voiding, the patient is given a printout written in laymen's terms instructing her precisely on the regimen to be followed, beginning with clamping of the catheter and detaching it completely from the drainage apparatus. The nurses work with the same instructions on a regular basis, so their response once the catheter is clamped is routine. An ordinary medium-sized paper clasp (Figure 18-1) is used because this is easy for the patient to manage as opposed to the regular catheter clamps that require fine strong hand manipulation of a screw mechanism. This method of catheter closure is leak-proof when the catheter end is bent on itself, as pictured. Using a plastic plug is easy for the patient to manage, but it promotes infection.

Fluid intake is regulated to 6 to 8 glasses during the waking hours and deliberate voiding attempts are made every 30 to 40 minutes or earlier if urge occurs. Immediately after successful freely flowing spontaneous urination, which need not be measured, the patient must climb back into bed, roll well over onto her side, and open the clasp to allow the residual urine to flow into a cup for measurement. The patient must be made to understand the need for positioning on the side in such a way that the bladder is at the highest elevation possible for accurate collection because water only runs downhill. When voluntary freely flowing micturition appears to be satisfactory and the immediate residual urine measures 50 mL or less for at least four consecutive times, then the catheter may be removed. The need for the amount to be at least as low as

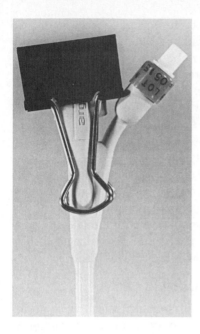

Figure 18-1 Medium-sized paper clasp clamps the bent drainage end of Foley catheter.

50 mL is because in this position, on the side, at least an additional 50 mL will still remain in the bladder since mechanical drainage is incomplete. Transurethral emptying of residual urine is straight down and thereby more thorough, so catherization may be discontinued when the transurethral channel is used at sustained residual levels of 100 mL or less.

While following such a bladder drill when in the hospital, the catheter should be connected to direct continued bag drainage during the night to allow the patient uninterrupted sleep. Direct bag drainage should be reinstituted otherwise, however, if the patient is not able to void at all spontaneously within 3 hours of trial. Assuming she is ingesting adequate fluid, inability to void by 3 hours simply means the detrusor muscle is not yet ready to respond and needs more time for recovery to normal contraction status. After another day or two the patient will try again. To let the patient go longer than 3 hours while still trying to void spontaneously risks bladder overdistention which, though not at all serious, may set the patient back a few more days. As it is, sometimes it may take 3 weeks for spontaneous micturition to happen. Inability to void spontaneously adequately or not at all is no reason to delay discharge to home if she is otherwise ready. The bladder drill is easily continued by the properly instructed patient in the psychologically more inducive atmosphere of her own home. Restraint from fluid intake after supper, unless truly thirsty, is ordered so as to avoid overfilling during the night. This dilemma is also prevented by directing the patient to empty the bladder two to three times during the night when she wakes for any reason, i.e., to turn over. At Temple University Hospital, we feel bag drainage at home is generally unnecessary. The regimen is continued until the required low level of residual urine is reached. Then the patient calls to schedule catheter removal.

When this time arrives, the bladder should be thoroughly emptied first to reduce postremoval leakage through the abdominal wall aperture to a minimum. If this occurs, it will cease completely within 2 to 4 hours if the patient keeps the bladder empty and does not allow overfilling. To avoid postremoval overdistention, the patient is instructed to void deliberately about every 60 to 75 minutes during the waking hours for the first 2 days. Again, fluid intake should be avoided after dinner and one to two emptyings during each of the 2 nights act as prophylaxis against the occasional race to the emergency room in the wee hours to transurethrally empty a distressing overdistended bladder, which now requires constant drainage once more, this time transurethrally.

The drainage orifice heals quickly and usually cannot be found in a few months because it lies below the hairline and the ultimate scar is negligible.

Occasionally one encounters cases of long standing which preoperatively reveal astounding postvoiding residual urine volumes of as much as 400 to 750 mL. A suprapubic retention catheter is ideal for these women, who require several weeks of postoperative bladder training, assuming no underlying neurologic basis. Postvoiding bladder emptying is necessary after every micturition to allow the detrusor to recover from its long-term overdistention. Parasympathomimetic drugs may speed up the process to normal. The physician must be alert to medications the patient may be taking in treatment of other body systems that might also cause detrusor laxity or urethral muscle hyperactivity.

Certainly the reverse situation can occur as a result of the surgery, or may have preexisted the operation, namely, the hyperactive bladder symbolized by urge incontinence. A different kind of bladder training is necessary here to decrease spasticity and often to enlarge bladder capacity. When such a postoperative patient, particularly one who has demonstrated via preoperative urodynamics a maximum bladder capacity of 250 mL or less, feels the urge to void, she must go to the bathroom at once. Knowing then in mental comfort that she will now not spill urine on the floor uncontrollably, as she sits or stands over the commode, the patient must deliberately try to restrain from voiding for at least 5 minutes more. Usually in conjunction with anticholinergic medication, 3 to 6 weeks of this exercise can prove to be an amazingly effective regimen in simultaneous recovery from frequency, urge incontinence, and small bladder capacity. Surgical eradication of funneling of the proximal urethra (see Chapter 7) may be crucial to success in these cases. Assuming normal anatomy has been restored surgically, an unstable bladder hopefully should be more apt to respond to control anyhow, often with the aid of appropriate drugs.

A few additional remarks regarding catheter management might be helpful. In instances of unintended intrasurgical cystotomy, recognized at the time, healing after surgical closure is known to be best when the urinary drainage tube emerges through a separate bladder puncture. In retropubic operations it should be brought through the abdominal wall separately from the surgical incision. Occasionally in instances of extensive retropubic dissection, an active drain, i.e., Hemovac or Jackson-Pratt, is appropriate. When associated with both a suprapubic catheter and a snugly packed vagina, as in cases with accompanying posterior repair done vaginally, the resident staff often is astonished to view copious urine being pulled through the suction drain. This occurs because the pressure of the vaginal pack induces urine to seek the path of least resistance, i.e., around the catheter and through the space of Retzius into the drainage tract, the suction effect of which has caused this startling but benign phenomenon. This is not a problem. Ultimately removal of the vaginal pack establishes the expected urine flow through the catheter.

If urine flow through a suprapubic catheter stops, an investigation is in order. Most commonly the catheter is bent or kinked acutely, secondary to positional change by the patient, an easily correctable condition with instant resumption of urine flow. More uncommonly a small blood clot may obstruct the tubal lumen. A saline lavage through the tube readily clears the barrier in this instance and urine will flow again. However, if the saline cannot be withdrawn from the bladder, then inadvertent traction of the catheter balloon through the bladder wall, placing the tip between the bladder and the rectus fascia, must be strongly suspected. If this proves true, then the catheter should be removed and replaced by transurethral drainage. Although disappointing, this is not a serious event. Prevention can be effected by properly securing the catheter to the abdomen to avoid any traction on the bulb and informing the patient to check on this attachment, as well as to look for inadvertent kinking that could block flow and cause backup.

Most unusually, assuming the absence of neuropathies, infections, and so on, some patients are unable to void spontaneously or at all adequately after anterior pelvic reconstruction at 3 weeks postsurgically for no obvious reason except the effects of the surgery itself. Certainly a complete review of the steps used during the operation is in order. A careful examination is equally important to rule out a disruptive subvesical fluid collection or a neglected foreign body. If this effort proves negative and the patient is otherwise recovering nicely, the best formula is one of patience, encouragement, and continued training techniques to coax the bladder back to normal action. Many active operators disagree with this nontampering approach of mine and advocate more active measures in situations of apparent nonresponsive bladders. These investigations include intravenous pyelogram, pelvic sonogram, urology consultation, and cystoscopy. In 40 years of experience, in the absence of distinct suspicion, I have yet to uncover fruitful findings from any of these proceedings, unless it be the satisfaction of the patient and her family "everything is being done to help her." The physician should double the efforts to inspire an attitude of hope and optimism in the patient, and in time, aided by appropriate pharmacologic resources, as necessary, the bladder will work again. A recent study lends credence to the belief that prostaglandins, administered either intravesically or intravaginally, may speed up the return of normal bladder function.[1] In the end, perhaps the strongest corollary to good postoperative management coupled with comprehension and understanding by both patient and family is the preoperative installation of faith and confidence by the surgeon.

Regardless of age, but particularly in the elderly, once spontaneous voiding has been established within reasonably normal limits after anterior pelvic correction, a form of simple lifetime bladder drill is imperative for comfort and prophylaxis. Even though some patients may exult in their rediscovered capacity to extend voiding intervals to 4 or 5 hours in association with average fluid intake without any incontinence, such conduct is best discouraged. All patients should be directed to void deliberately, with or without urge, every 2 to 2.5 hours. If urge develops earlier, generally it should be satisfied at once. If urge and shortened interval become repetitive, the patient must understand the need to consult the doctor.

In my mind, the practicing gynecologic surgeon who becomes too scientific by running postoperative urodynamic and cystometric tests on the patient who is satisfied and happy with her results as is does her a gross disservice for a variety of reasons. Under these circumstances, the doctor should be delighted with the achievement and should leave well enough alone. Many doctors test postoperatively as a routine. I think this is too much science at the patient's expense, both literally and figuratively. Only when the patient continues to complain, with or without objective evidence of surgical failure, after an adequate interval of observation, are further testing measures in order.

RELIEF OF POSTOPERATIVE PAIN

Pain relief is primary in postsurgical care. Over the past 4 years, we have developed a routine, aimed particularly at the postmenopausal patient, that seems to be ideal in the relief of suffering from the moment the patient leaves the operating room until she goes home.

Anecdotally speaking, from the start of my residency in 1949, I have felt that patients rarely ever receive adequate medication for pain relief, at least in the first 48 hours postoperatively. Through pointed questions of countless colleagues over many years, I have yet to find any one to disagree with me. Marks and Sachar, in a directed study,[2] bear out this contention but I still feel their results are far too conservative. During close observation and contact with patients by both my residents and myself in the first 4 to 6 hours after leaving the operating room, we ask repeatedly, "How are you doing?" almost invariably the answer comes back, "in terrible pain." Certainly this is nothing new to any of us, nor is the endless battle with anesthesiologists who universally seem to abide in such a well of deadly fear of respiratory depression that they allow nothing but placebo-like doses of narcotics while they remain in charge in the recovery room. Because we cannot beat the anesthesiologists in their domain, we have found the only answer: insist on moving the patient at the earliest possible time to the regular nursing floor. There immediately the patient is placed in command as the patient-controlled analgesia (PCA) pump is attached and activated. The combined psychological as well as pharmacologic benefits are enormous, the former also to the doctor.

Actually we begin pain control in the preoperative preparation for the surgery that lies ahead. We explain in some detail, especially when the approach is entirely vaginal, that there will be abundant stitching in the internal areas for hysterectomy and for repair but that these will give minimal to negligible discomfort. Then we describe the external suturing required in the perineum in completion of the posterior repair as being most akin to that of the episiotomy of the first vaginal delivery. We tell them frankly that this will give them pain, augmented somewhat in the beginning by the presence of packing, but that we will concentrate on alleviating pain from the very outset with all the correct medications. That we bring up the subject and stress our intent to pay attention to their comfort in itself proves to be a wonderful psychological ploy. As described in a major treatise by Bonica on management of pain, uncertainty, fright, and a feeling of helplessness, augmented in the older patient by a fear of death, drop the pain threshold markedly postoperatively.[3] In contrast to this, the fully informed patient, again especially in the postmenopausal group, made totally aware of all aspects of the surgery, the expected early ambulation and the very short recovery phase, plus anticipated good results, develops a positive attitude that carries through the entire course. Fear and anxiety are allayed and, correspondingly, perception of pain is remarkably diminished. The pain threshold indeed becomes significantly elevated and the end result objectively becomes a markedly reduced need for ancillary medication.

What can the surgeon do intraoperatively to help reduce postoperative pain? Foremost is the concerted effort to handle tissue as gently as possible. The primary admonition is to avoid crushing of tissue by keeping clamping and grasping with heavy and sharp instruments to a minimum. As discussed thoroughly in Chapter 16, any use of natural substances for suture, all markedly tissue reactive, principally catgut, in today's surgical milieu is not only archaic, it is almost barbaric. Many experts believe the change to synthetic sutures, which have been proven to be minimally tissue reactive (see Chapter 16), in itself cuts postsurgical pain in half. Whenever an indwelling catheter is indicated for more than 24 hours, so often necessary, in benign surgery in older patients, suprapubic placement should always be chosen over transurethral insertion. Not only is the latter very uncomfortable and annoying as compared to the former, the patient almost invariably has heard "stories about traditional catheter management from below and is often more in dread of this aspect of the surgery than all others. When informed in advance of her operation that she will absolutely not have to endure such "the change in attitude is perceptibly remarkable.

When considering choices and dosages of narcotics and analgesics, supplemented by antidepressants and so-called mood elevators, in postreproductive and elderly patients, extreme care and caution with particular attention to each individual case must be exerted.[4] The older the patient, the more delicate the situation, and the primary fear of the anesthesiologist, respiratory depression, despite their reluctance to give adequate medication for pain relief, must be respected. Pulmonary and cardiac reserves are apt to be decreased in a significant number of patients, as discussed in Chapter 3, and all medications for pain relief and anxiety reduction must be adjusted accordingly. Similarly, recognition of probable increased sensitivity to analgesics and sedatives indicates in many instances lower dosage schedules than in younger people. Add to these issues the likelihood that older patients are much more apt to be sustained on drugs, frequently mimetic of the autonomic nervous system, in compensation for medical deficiencies, and there rises the dilemma of synergistic or conflicting action with medications used routinely for comfort and recovery in the immediate postsurgical phase. However, with common sense and deep concern, and armed with our current remarkably adaptable armamentarium of drugs, no patient should receive less than the maximum of pain relief and solace at this crucial time of recovery.

Certain factors operate in postmenopausal women that reduce requirements for pain relief and in many ways make them easier patients to take care of postoperatively than premenopausal patients. Firstly, all have denervation of varying extents that makes them progressively less sensitive to pain. More specifically, the greater the parity, the older the age, and the larger the number of previous pelvic operations, the more the denervation. Secondly, since the overwhelming number of procedures in this age group are performed for prolapse of organs or urinary incontinence or both, the prospects of clearing themselves once and for all of these problems that they regard as disgusting are so positively motivating that they are willing to tolerate a considerable amount of discomfort with a philosophically positive attitude. Since many have already stated preoperatively, "I'd rather be dead than go on living like this," or less dramatically, "I'd go through anything just to get rid of this awful condition,"it is easy to understand how such an affirmative posture can deter the cry for pain relief. Finally, in general, older people have a different philosophy about life than even they themselves have had in earlier years. They have witnessed friends and relatives die at ages younger than their own. They are satisfied that they have been fortunate enough to reach their present stage of life and many are content that they have survived long enough to witness happy events they had hoped to live to view. Although they still have the fear of death, it is not so compelling as in younger people, and when they wake up after the surgery to find themselves still alive, they are so grateful that nothing else seems to matter.

Then, when their doctor tells them that "All went well with the operation,"an-algesic requirements drop significantly. I can write and speak about this with absolute affirmation after countless participations in major surgery in this age group, including my own hip replacement.

The PCA pump is a wonderful adjunct to patient care. Geared to deliver a predetermined amount of drug intravenously for rapid action over a given unit of time, it provides an automatic safety factor as well as immediate relief without demanding the nursing attention implicit in PRN (given on patient's request, when needed) orders, usually by intramuscular injection.[5–11] At Temple University, on the gynecology service, we feel that PRN orders for pain relief are archaic and should be abandoned as a general routine during the usually short (5 days or less) current postoperative hospital course. Because the PRN dose of narcotic ordered is usually insufficient for relief of established pain, augmented almost always by a considerable time delay between request and administration, the patient suffers unnecessarily. Making matters worse are the wide variability from patient to patient in the dose-response curve based on the divergent blood levels achieved by intramuscular injection.[12,13] The situation is further magnified by the broad differential of blood level required by patients for relief as well as the time needed to attain top blood levels in different patients. The PCA pump, which titrates analgesic medication on an individual basis, seems to conquer most of these problems at the same time that it overcomes fear of respiratory depression by the use of well-calculated drug release. As noted by Keenan, when the patient is in control, titrating what she needs, she prevents the wide swings from intense pain to sedation and back again, as observed with PRN intramuscular narcotic administration.[14] Additionally, she does not have to watch the clock as she waits with anxiety and anguish for her next dose. However, although the PCA pump unques-tionably makes things easier, caution via close monitoring to be certain the correct dosage allowance is offered, especially in the more fragile older patient, is still necessary to prevent respiratory depression. Obviously this is most important in the first 12 to 24 hours after anesthesia is terminated in the operating room.

Our favorite narcotic is morphine. We use it routinely unless some specific contraindication is present. We do not seem to get the same levels of pain relief with meperidine (Demerol), even with standard recommended dosages, and if it must be given intramuscularly, it hurts.

Somewhere between 8 AM and noon of the first day after surgery we stop analgesia via narcotics and change abruptly to oral medication in most cases. Our experience of the past 5 years reveals that our system of management has an incidence of nausea and vomiting of less than 5% by noon of the day after surgery, and this enables us to make a rapid switch from parenteral to oral therapy.

We readily recognize that nausea and vomiting are apt to be more pro-nounced both in intensity and duration in abdominal than in vaginal cases. The same is true regarding pain simply because of the trauma inflicted on pain receptors in the abdominal wall, especially in the skin, and because of the effects on intraoperative manipulation of bowel and inadvertent peritoneal irritation. However, it is not difficult to equate the pain of an extensive posterior compartment repair with that of the pain from an abdominal laparotomy, both of which call for adequate dosages of narcotics, such as morphine, for relief. Yet morphine, despite the low level of postoperative nausea induced by modern anesthetics and the mitigating effects of parenteral antiemetics, still provokes significant nausea in a minority of patients. Since we discontinue narcotics of all kinds anyhow now by 24 hours postsurgery, the emetic influence of morphine will generally disappear within 12 to 16 hours. In the meantime, the patient will require continued effective pain relief. Today we bridge this gap most efficiently by using ketorolac (Toradol), a parenteral medication that can be used either intramuscularly or intravenously. It is not a narcotic drug and is classified in the medication group assigned the acronym NSAID (nonsteroidal anti-inflammatory drug) that exhibits analgesic and antipyretic as well as anti-inflammatory action. These analgesic medications do not sedate, thus do not depress respirations, nor do they effect rectal or bladder elimination. Ketorolac is the only drug of this nature approved by the U.S. Food and Drug Administration at the time of the writing of this book. Ketorolac has been shown to be more effective than meperidine,[14] and some clinicians have found that opioid derivatives give the most complete pain relief when supplemented by ketorolac. Combined with ketorolac, the dose of morphine can be cut in many cases.

Once we have moved from parenteral analgesic administration to oral capabilities of medication ingestion, beyond the type of drug and the dosage, the key to successful pain relief is an absolutely "by the clock" regular intake. Depending on the individual characteristics of the chosen drug or drugs and dosage, orders are written for it to be given without fail every 3 or 4 or 6 hours. For example, Motrin (ibuprofen) 600 or 800 mg, or Anaprox (naproxen sodium) 550 mg is ordered for every 6 hours automatically ("by the clock"). Extra-strength Tylenol (acetaminophen) can be ordered every 3 or every 4 hours "by the clock." As already discussed, we never use PRN orders any longer for analgesic therapy and we regard such choices as poor treatment.

We have not used restricted drugs such as codeine or perocodan or any of their derivatives for more than 4 years. Our concentration has been centered on the ever-growing list of acceptable NSAIDs, which have been proven to be at least as effective, if not more so, than opioid drugs. Ketorolac is available in oral and parenteral forms and is remarkably effective, as are ibuprofen and naproxen, our favorites. However, equally effective available agents are etodolac (Lodine) and ketoprofen (Orudis). The patient and the nursing staff must be reminded that none of these medications should be taken on an empty stomach, that each time food of some sort must be taken simultaneously to buffer against gastritis. None of the NSAIDs has any potential for addiction.

Although covered later in this chapter, it must be mentioned here that our obsession in stopping opioids as soon as possible is part of our prophylaxis against the development of constipation, a major problem in recovery from reconstructive surgery.

A considerable number of surgeons use continuous epidural or spinal analgesia as their favorite method for pain relief. We do not use these routes simply because we feel the methods already presented are much less complicated.

FLUID INTAKE

The need for adequate fluid intake and electrolyte balance is basic to all surgery. The subject is well covered in several surgical texts and will not be discussed in depth in this book, especially since, with rare exception, the patients in our attention take fluids by mouth so soon. In the older person, however, two precautions are worthy of note. In many of this age group, having come to the operating room without oral intake for several hours, leading to minor dehydration, and functioning physiologically considerably more slowly than their younger counterparts, often urinary output during the procedure and shortly thereafter seems alarmingly low to the anesthesiology team. Usually without notifying the surgeon, intravenous fluids are then flushed in much too rapidly, and the older patient, with a decreased margin for safety, stands in jeopardy of pulmonary edema. So long as ureteral obstruction can be ruled out, patience will be rewarded by adequate urinary output.

Catheters out of position or obstructed can also lead to false impressions of inadequate fluid output while in truth the bladder becomes markedly overdistended. Either through incompetence or carelessness, an intended transurethral catheter can be placed in the vagina rather than the bladder. When suprapubically placed, the catheter balloon and tip can be inadvertently pulled through the bladder wall to lie under the fascia. A defective nonpatent catheter may have been inserted without preliminary testing, or a small blood clot from the bladder may plug the catheter lumen. Most commonly, a catheter may become twisted on itself and urine flow ceases. Incredibly often neither nursing or house staff check adequately, and the patient is subjected to an intravenous "fluid challenge" test, potentially disastrous to the patient if the challenge goes well over 500 mL. All of the events noted above are well within my experience and fortunately the problem has been discovered "in the nick of time." I know of less fortuitous situations. Although not desirable, dehydration is far less dangerous than fluid overload, considering the oft-compromised preexisting cardiovascular, pulmonary, and renal systems in older patients.

Finally, with rare exception, such as instances of severe nausea, my patients generally have begun taking fluids by mouth on the same day as surgery or, at the latest, by the next morning. Again, unless unusual circumstances dictate otherwise, in cases of benign pelvic surgery, I do not wait to hear adequate full normal bowel sounds before starting oral fluid intake. Patients almost always handle the situation well and the beneficial psychological effects are enormous, especially if simultaneously the patients have risen from their beds.

CAFFEINE WITHDRAWAL SYNDROME

When making rounds on the first postsurgical day, it is particularly discouraging and disturbing to the operative team to hear complaints of headache, fatigue, and muscle pain and stiffness, or to witness unexpected lethargy or noncharacteristic mood changes in an ordinarily upbeat patient in whom the surgery went well. These are all symptoms of caffeine withdrawal,[15] which not infrequently also includes nausea and vomiting or a feeling similar to that of affliction with "the flu." Studies have revealed these problems to occur after discontinuing the customary daily intake of 1 cup of coffee, or 2 cups of tea, or 3 cans of caffeinated soft drinks, each the equivalent of only 100 mg caffeine. A report on caffeine consumption in the United States, principally mediated through coffee drinking, has revealed that 82% of adults ingest an average of 227 mg caffeine per day (roughly equivalent to 2 cups of coffee) and 99% consume less than 563 mg/d.[16] These figures are in line with the habits of our surgical patients.

Our attention to the problem of caffeine withdrawal came abruptly through the publication of a report by Silverman and colleagues in 1992 who pointed out the need to be aware of the syndrome described above when patients are deprived of their regular coffee or tea intake before operations.[17] Obviously this situation of deprivation is carried over to the first postoperative morning by which time the patient will have had no coffee, tea, or cola drinks for a maximum of 36 hours. As a result, we are now quick to recognize the syndrome and have become thoroughly amazed at the remarkable change in patients in less than an hour after that first postsurgical cup of coffee. Currently, when we can all remember, we try to make certain that coffee is offered to all patients at the first moment of resumption of ability to take fluids by mouth.

RESPIRATORY EXERCISE AND AMBULATION

In older patients, prevention of atelectasis and promotion of active vascular flow are lifesaving ingredients of the postoperative menu. Within a mere 2 to 3 hours at the most after surgery, not by the next morning, an active program of deep inhalation and full exhalation is instituted, with or without the aid of ancillary respiratory mechanics, such as incentive spirometry, and the patient is policed by the house staff and nursing personnel to enforce such pulmonary exertion. Over the first 24 hours postoperatively, relevant instructions on this activity are repeated three to five times to the patient, along with dire predictions of what can happen to her if she ignores our insistent instructions.

Simultaneously and similarly, orders are given directly to the patient regarding the necessity of periodic (every 20 to 30 minutes) pumping of the lower extremities alternately by flexing and extending about ten times. Encouragement to change position in bed frequently must be standard. Sitting at the side of the bed with legs dangling and moving should begin in the same evening of the day of operation; those with hysterectomy only, whether abdominal or vaginal, but particularly the latter, generally have no excuse not to be walking short distances to a chair that first evening. This activity must be graduated within 18 to 20 hours of the operation, regardless of its extent and the presence or absence of packing, catheters, and intravenous tubing, to full ambulation about the room and sitting in a chair. I militantly pursue the monitoring of this forced exertion through the assistance of nursing personnel, house staff, and relatives. Again the possible grave consequences of indolence in this regard are made crystal clear to both patient and relatives. Besides the obvious prophylactic effects of such activity, the associated attention pays additional dividends. Invariably the patient feels better, becomes more motivated, and gets well faster, and both she and her relatives are inspired to adoring confidence by the intense interest of the surgeon.

After the first 36 hours or so, we never allow our patients to sit in bed. Elevation of the upper half of the hospital bed, without exception, slides the patient downward so that sitting angulation and stress center at the lumbosacral area rather than at the level of the hips. Of course, I would rather see my patient sitting up than lying flat in bed all the time, but the sitting must be done in a chair. Beds should be kept flat for sleeping and resting, not manipulated into skeletally distressing positions that send the patient home with a backache she does not deserve and that the doctor breezily but wrongly ascribes to aftereffects of surgery.

LABORATORY TESTS

Unless unusual circumstances develop, and except for concomitant medical diseases, as diabetes, following benign pelvic surgery in well-prepared patients, young or old, only two laboratory tests are really necessary. The first is either a hematocrit or hemoglobin, obviously to reflect the amount of blood loss related directly to surgery. When the charge physician deems it necessary, the patient can always be given back her autologous blood if it has not already been given during the operation. However, since it has been established that postoperative anemia has no influence on infection one way or another, even if fever develops, I have become loathe even to return the patient's own blood if there is no active bleeding, her vital signs are normal, and nutrition becomes positive within 48 hours. Correct diet and oral iron bring the patient back to normal rapidly.

The second test I make mandatory is a creatinine level. No matter how careful and meticulous our surgery may be, unless we are working only in the posterior pelvis below the level of the ischial spines, we may unintentionally cut or capture a ureter. Urine flow by itself is not a good indicator if the patient had two functioning ureters before surgery. If urine output is zero, a thorough investigation is required at once.

If one ureter has been tied off or blocked because of surgery, even if the other is working well, it will be reflected within hours by a creatinine blood level significantly elevated over the preoperative result. Such a laboratory signal should initiate exploration and correction.

White blood cell counts are not helpful. They will be elevated in many cases initially in reaction to the traumatic effects of the surgery and are basically meaningless at that time. If fever develops, as will be discussed, the level of temperature elevation and the patient's clinically reversed response tell us enough by themselves. White blood cell alterations may not change until later and therapy cannot be withheld that long. However, to satisfy most third-party payers, both a white blood cell reading and vaginal culture, although neither is truly helpful at the outset of significant fever, pragmatically speaking, may have to be done.

THROMBOSIS AND EMBOLIZATION PROPHYLAXIS

Carelessness in measures directed at the prevention of the development of thrombosis and subsequent pulmonary embolus in association with pelvic surgery, particularly in the postreproductive woman, is absolutely unacceptable by today's standards. Although use of surgical stockings starting preoperatively is almost automatic at most facilities, it is far from adequate. The stockings plus early ambulation unquestionably go a long way prophylactically, but the older the patient, with known or unknown progressive propensity to atherosclerosis or vascular stasis, as a group, in general, deserve better protection and should receive it routinely. Stockings and activity are not enough.

Prophylactic regimens vary widely from one doctor to another and from one institution to another despite the rigid standards established by the Consensus Conference sponsored by the National Institutes of Health in 1986.[18] Clearly the level of risk of deep vein thrombosis and pulmonary embolus in the age group identified in this text is high, rising ominously with each decade of life. The doctor has no right to gamble, even in the presence of overt good health in the patient who walks almost immediately after surgery and enjoys a short hospital stay. I must interject at this point that, although there is growing sentiment to send women, after isolated vaginal hysterectomy, home within 24 hours of surgery, and I do not disagree, such rapid dismissal can very well jeopardize the life of the patient in the postreproductive category. Close observation and continued care for at least a few days, in my opinion, are mandatory in the older group after major pelvic surgery, regardless of extent, especially if they live alone or some distance from the hospital.

Deep venous thrombosis is relatively common, perhaps far more than most physicians are aware. Serious pulmonary embolus appears much less often and therefore generally is ignored until the catastrophe strikes. To bring this subject to the level of concern it demands, conclusions of the 1986 Consensus Conference stated that (1) deep venous thrombosis and pulmonary embolism constitute major health problems in the United States and (2) in high-risk patients, like the elderly undergoing major pelvic surgery, these disastrous events can be significantly reduced through prophylactic regimens. Further recommendations included more extensive use of prophylactic regimens with emphasis on low-dose heparin and gradient elastic stockings (TEDs). The addition of external pneumatic compression (sequential compression devices or SCDs) was urged in cases of the highest degree of suspicion. It was noted that there is no evidence of benefit from aspirin.

Chapter 3 throughly reviews the subject of postsurgical thrombosis and embolism. As noted, because of our strong feeling at Temple University, as at many other major institutions, that significantly increased bleeding occurs during surgery in association with heparin, generally we combine high TEDs, SCDs, early ambulation, and deep respiratory exercises as our prophylactic regimen. We also feel, as described in a recent publication,[19] that significant postoperative oozing of blood from the large raw surfaces created in reconstructive surgery occurs in association with heparin. We no longer use prophylactic heparin as a routine. Generally speaking, regardless of whether or not SCDs or heparin or both are used, it is strongly recommended, especially in the postreproductive woman, particularly those with any history of cardiovascular disease, that they be continued on a specific prophylactic regimen for a minimum of 4 days. When hospitalization is less than 4 days, discharge orders must emphasize adequate progressive ambulation at home.

MITIGATION OF VALSALVA EFFECTS

In all cases of pelvic reconstruction, any postoperative increase in intra-abdominal pressure jeopardizes the integrity of the repair. This particularly applies to those with older and more attenuated tissue, especially if estrogen replacement has been neglected for considerable time, and to those with a record of one or more failed previous procedures. Constipation, most notably occurring in conjunction with extensive posterior repairs, is the principal cause of voluntary expulsive efforts that can inaugurate destruction of even the best surgical endeavors. Additionally, constipation relatively commonly has been a habitual problem in older people for a variety of reasons beyond that of anatomic aberration. It must be remembered always that, although posterior pelvic relaxation can help to cause bowel movement difficulties, the reverse is just as apt to be true. Thus, logically, a preoperative investigation into bowel habits followed by attempts then to initiate positive corrective measures where necessary before surgery can significantly reverse a trend to failure if such habits continue post-surgically.

Obviously prudence dictates anticipation and prophylaxis. An abundance of innocuous stool softeners are available, any one of which should be started two or three times a day on the first or second full postoperative day. Narcotic analgesics, as already discussed, should be discontinued at the earliest possible moment to avert interference with return to normal peristalsis. Oral fluid intake, followed soon thereafter by solid food, especially in vaginal cases, essentially devoid of bowel manipulation, seems to promote peristalsis, especially in association with the anabolic effects of early ambulation. I also routinely give a simple Fleet enema immediately after the pack is removed about 48 hours after surgery. Although some critics might feel such a routine asks too much of the bowel too soon, I have seen no ill effects result from it and constipation has been a rare occurrence. The stakes are too high to afford waiting too long and then to have to wrestle with the problem of initiating bowel movements without increasing intra-abdominal pressure. This may become especially aggravating if, while waiting and hoping for something to happen, the rectum and distal colon fill up with solid feces.

Occasionally loose stools develop, but this problem is easily and quickly remedied by limiting the measures used to promote bowel movements. Although not desirable, loose movements present no strain on the operation and are therefore preferable to the antithesis, constipation. Despite all my standard methods, in some cases, especially those with considerable bloody extravasation from wide areas of raw surfaces and in those that develop associated cellulitis, bowel stimulus is slowed down or postponed and solid food should be curtailed until an extra day or two passes. This approach usually will lengthen the hospital stay, ordinarily short enough anyway, about a day, but undesirable expulsive efforts by the patient can thereby be avoided. In recalcitrant cases of absent excretory results despite apparently adequate bowel activity, as heard through the stethoscope, and an accompanying good appetite, the judicious use of suppositories or oil enemas can bring a turnabout. When impaction is suspected, examination must not be delayed. If found, clearly it must be broken up, but this must be accomplished ever so gently so as not to disturb the integrity of the repair. In short, close continuous scrutiny of bowel function is imperative in all cases involving any reconstruction.

Inadequate fluid intake, often a problem with older patients, especially in the summer when water loss through the skin is at its peak, can lead to inspissated stools and impaction. When the total body fluid balance becomes negative because of inadequate supply of water, after intravenous lines have been removed and dependence is placed on the oral route, compensatory withdrawal of water from the intestines to equalize the imbalance will leave both bowel and stool dry. Thus, adequate fluid intake by the patient must be absolutely demanded to avoid this preventable threat to good recovery.

Severe postsurgical nausea, especially if associated with convulsive vomiting, can make a good reconstructive pelvic surgeon cry. Such a situation is capable of creating extreme increases in intra-abdominal pressure with possible explosive consequences on the best of restorative efforts. A disaster of this nature can and should be avoided at all costs, especially when one considers that no effective healing actually begins till after the first 4 days and reaches a maximum so begrudgingly slowly only at 115 to 120 days in both the abdominal and pelvic fascial tissues. The incidence of dehiscence of abdominal surgical wounds, although more likely in the presence of cancer, still is higher in older patients than in the young even when only benign problems are involved. Potentiation of this undesirable event by severe vomiting, especially if prolonged, must be a matter for concern. Therefore, it behooves the gynecologic surgical staff to write for appropriate antiemetic orders and to maintain themselves and the nursing personnel in a constant state of alert for the appearance of nausea. If the patient has ever had any surgery previously, she must always be questioned as to any reaction to anesthesia. How often, when this is not done, have we all heard the patient tell us later, "I vomited like this after my last operation, too." Guilt really sets in if she adds, "I tried to tell everyone this had happened, but no one was listening." The greatest assistance can come from the anesthesia department but do not hope that they will pick up the pertinent information. Call attention to everyone involved to the postanesthetic nausea of previous experience and address the subject before surgery begins. An attentive anesthesiologist can be a formidable ally in these situations.

Coughing falls into the same category as nausea and vomiting as a factor in producing increased wound strain. If it occurs, it must be ameliorated at once. Experience reveals that the hazard of postsurgical respiratory problems, with or without tracheitis or bronchitis, is much less apt to appear when a seasonal "flu shot" has been given several weeks before surgery. Some of the recently occurring strains of influenza have been disastrous, often fatal, in the elderly, and so it follows that protection must not escape the scope of surgical care. Certainly in these cases of elective surgery there is adequate time preoperatively for administration of influenza vaccine so as to afford prophylaxis from this threat to operative wound healing.

HEMORRHAGE

Even in the best hands, for a variety of reasons, postoperative bleeding of serious magnitude can occur. Whether abdominal or vaginal in approach, or young or old patient, danger is ever present. Vigilance for the possibility must be relentless for the first 48 hours, especially if overt external manifestations are absent. Detection may be earlier in the elderly because vital sign changes happen faster than in younger patients. Most common causes are suture slippage or release of constriction or pressure after surgery is completed. Progressive changes in pulse and blood pressure must never be ignored. Judicious serial hematocrits may play a strong role. False low results, however, when the blood is drawn from the same site used for intravenous fluid replacement, can be misleading.

Bleeding from the vault cuff after abdominal or vaginal hysterectomy or from vaginal mucosal edges after repair is easily detectable because of manifest external bleeding. Placement of a single stitch, without need for either anesthesia or the operating room, usually is all that is necessary. When blood is noted to be coming through the pack while the patient is still in the recovery room, after a vaginal reconstructive procedure, often all that is necessary is constant strong digital pressure against the pack for 20 minutes while the patient's natural clotting mechanisms take over in conjunction with the compression of developing edema of surgically traumatized tissue. When this does not work, then, and only then, should the pack be removed in the operating room after conditions are preset for active intervention.

If hemorrhage is occurring intraperitoneally after an abdominal case, exploration after taking down the abdominal wall sutures may readily reveal the free vessel stump. Obviously, a well-fixed ligature can solve that problem quickly. However, if the bleeding activity is low down and retroperitoneal, hematoma formation, bloody infiltration into tissues, and edema may produce enough obscurity to mask the precise bleeding point or points. A stubborn search in such cases is foolhardy because of possible ureteral damage. Bilateral hypogastric artery ligation or ligation of its anterior branch should be resorted to without hesitation in these cases.

When serious bleeding occurs after vaginal cases, all vaginal edges should be swiftly inspected, turning them outward if necessary for better viewing. If this possible source is ruled out, usually a quick determination, the operative site should not be taken apart for further inspection, especially in wide repairs, but not even if only a vaginal hysterectomy has been performed. I have never heard of any one finding the bleeder in these cases. Almost always, by the time the decision is made to take operative intervention, the combined edema and hematoma have produced enough obliteration to render the search for the bleeder fruitless. Additionally, there is always the possibility of damaging the ureters, new bleeders can be opened up, and the integrity of a fine repair may be destroyed. I cannot emphasize strongly enough that, having discovered no active source in a vaginal edge, in the face of obvious copious bleeding pouring out from somewhere inside, the abdomen should be opened at once for bilateral internal iliac artery ligation, foregoing any exploration beneath the vaginal surface. Going after the internal iliac arteries takes only minutes for the experienced and anatomically knowledgeable gynecologist to perform without inflicting further damage. It can thwart tremendous blood loss very quickly and concommitantly a good repair is not torn apart.

FEVER

Excluding the expected low raised levels in the first 36 to 48 hours after surgery, postsurgical temperature elevation over 37.7°C (100°F) may prove to be a vexing problem. I strongly feel that traditional criteria for a diagnosis of true postoperative pyrexia are in no way applicable to postmenopausal women who have undergone reconstructive surgery of any extent, with or without hysterectomy, because of the threat of destruction of the repair by even small degrees of infection. Whether or not the patient has already experienced a previous pelvic operation, with or without a repair, but especially in those with some sort of sequela, i.e., failure of vaginal surgery or development of subsequent massive eversion, should make no difference in the management plan. Considering that we are dealing in these cases almost always with aging well-compromised tissues, the situation is tenuous at best. Even the slightest threat to the integrity of the restored anatomy could imperil the ultimate result and pelvic cellulitis manifested principally by fever constitutes the most common and most worrisome such jeopardy to good healing. Again, the stakes are high and there is no margin for delay. Incipient cellulitis must be recognized at once and attacked vigorously before it has gained the slightest foothold. Every moment of active infection significantly decreases the overall healing obligatory to the ultimate best outcome.

In my experience, if potentially serious pyrexia will become a factor to thwart a smooth recovery, all the signals seem to materialize during the third full day after surgery in 95% of cases and, at the latest, in the next day in the remainder. Even before the temperature has risen over 37.2°C to 37.3°C (99.0 to 99.2°F), still within normal range, the patient often reflects some early toxic effects when, on rounds on the third morning not quite 48 hours after the operation, she states that the appetite that joyfully returned the evening before has disappeared today at breakfast. If true cellulitis is developing, this early warning will shortly thereafter be amplified as the day goes on by lassitude in getting out of bed, sharply contrasting to activity easily and progressively accomplished in the previous afternoon and evening. At this point you can count on it; by evening two or more consecutive temperatures over 37.7°C (100°F), the second higher than the first, will almost certainly be recorded.

My resident staff remains in constant alert for these signals. We do not wait for white blood cell elevation or "shift to the left," to occur, nor do we wait another day just to be sure. The importance of immediate action under this ominous potential cannot be emphasized enough. Without delay we rule out other common causes of postsurgical fever, such as atelectasis, upper respiratory infection, urinary tract involvement, and phlebitis. Simultaneously, the patient is started on a full gamut of parenteral antimicrobial therapy, covering a full aerobic and anaerobic bacterial slate. I have been criticized roundly for this dashing approach, one considered most unscientific by many experts, but I stand firm in my belief that, after weighing all the pros and cons, physicians must now and then deviate from pure science to render the best possible care to their fellow human beings. Logic dictates such a pragmatic attitude, especially since the patients, even as their temperatures continue to rise to levels as high as 39°C (102.5°F) on the second pyretic day, already are feeling better with a return of appetite and activity. Not only is the surgical effort protected but additionally such a jump into the breach has uniformly guaranteed the patient a hospital discharge date in line with the preoperative projection and she can then finish her antibiotic course via oral administration at home.Lest we forget, the primary goal is preservation of the reconstructive surgery, not the early hospital dismissal. Also, it must be repeated that the dramatic, though subtle in the first few hours, change in the clinical picture is the real key to the institution of a strong antibiotic regimen, certainly therapeutic, not prophylactic, at this point. Critics offer that we probably are giving unnecessary medication, to which there is a small but significant potential for reaction, to some patients. We contend that this is not so, in full recognition of the analysis of normal temperature ranges as discussed by Mackowiak and colleagues in 1992.[20] Clinical responsibility could never be more important.

What about cultures? It has long been demonstrated that routine vaginal vault cultures are essentially of no value, but we all are forced to do them because of the demands of third-party payers. In one hospital laboratory after another in case after case, predictably five to ten aerobic and anaerobic organisms, thriving in symbiosis, are uncovered. This ridiculous waste of money and time, when treatment is delayed while waiting for results, is underscored by the fact that cultures of patients without fever and cellulitis reveal the same combinations of organisms. They are the fortunate ones, unlike the 10% to 15% of patients where circumstances, for reasons mostly unknown to us, give rise to bacterial invasion into the operative site. Yet, with alertly administered therapy, without delay, they all go home at the same time and achieve the same level of outcome, whether fever has developed or not.

There is an exception, fortunately generally uncommon. If in any of these cases of cellulitis a positive clinical response of some sort is not observed by 48 hours, whether or not a culture has been planted before, one must be taken at that time in dead earnest. Almost certainly one particular microbe, or more, will be revealed as resistant to the antibiotics being given, demanding change in accordance at once.

A special word or two about lower urinary tract infection (UTI) upsetting an otherwise serene course is necessary. Susceptibility to UTI, especially in the elderly, where resistance is more apt to be lower, is easily understandable in association with pelvic surgery. In almost every case, this affliction, usually not serious, but annoying and demanding of attention, is promoted through the use of indwelling bladder catheters and by the traumatic manipulation during surgery of tissues directly adjacent to or part of the bladder and urethra. Often, despite a low-grade temperature elevation, these patients can easily be differentiated clinically from those with true early cellulitis because they rarely appear toxic. Generally neither appetite nor activity is curbed and, coupled with immediate positive evidence from a urinalysis, not waiting for the results of urine culture to be reported, routine oral treatment, preferably nitrofurantoin (Macrobid), can be instituted with good response to be expected rather quickly with twice daily dosage for a week.

In summary, infection remains, throughout all surgery, the greatest single hazard to good healing. In the cases concerned in this text, it can ruin the entire procedure despite a meticulous performance. There is no margin for error or delay.

FURTHER DETAILS

Sitting in a chair and walking must take place by the first morning after surgery at the latest. There is no excuse for any other course. Return to normal mobility and ambulation as rapidly as is reasonably possible promotes anabolic metabolism throughout the body and leads to expeditious recovery. A false notion persists in many centers that reparative procedures, especially when extensive, or deep into the pelvis, demand a very slow and gradually progressive schedule to full normal ambulatory motion. When one considers the disturbing catabolic effects of inactivity plus the decidedly increased threat of deep vein thrombosis, plus awareness of the absence of any true healing for the first 4 days followed by 4 months for maximum restitution anyhow, restriction of activity seems positively silly. The ultimate success of restorative surgery has nothing to do with any perceived strains due to the erect posture but rather depends entirely on the quality of the tissues in the particular case, full surgical reestablishment of normal vaginal axis and dimensions, elevation of the levator plate to its naturally horizontal position in the erect body, and correct choice and deployment of sutures.

After the first 24 to 36 hours, having already been activated out of bed, my patients may sit up only in a chair and not again sit in bed. When the head of the typical hospital bed is elevated and the patient tries to sit, she inevitably slides downward, creating an abnormal convexity of the lumbodorsal region, as mentioned earlier. If this posture is maintained, even intermittently, over a long enough period of time, the patient often will go home with a backache. In postreproductive women, the resultant discomfort can be exaggerated often secondary to preexisting lumbodorsal arthritis. Within 24 hours, I have my patients sitting in a chair where the normal flexion at the hip will occur in a right angle formation. From that point on, the bed is kept flat and all sitting is restricted to chairs. Backache is avoided and patients are mobilized more rapidly in the process.

The number of medications taken by patients over age 50 seems, on average, to grow as a direct arithmetic progression as age increases. These usually relate to cardiovascular, respiratory, metabolic, and digestive tract disorders, but drugs covering diabetes, neuropathies, arthritis, nephropathies, dermatitic problems, thyroid deficiency, and many other chronic diseases have also been taken regularly before surgery. They all should be reinstituted at the earliest most propitious time.

The most important drug of direct concern gynecologically in the older woman, and particularly so in those undergoing reconstructive surgery of any kind, as so adequately covered elsewhere in this book, is estrogen. Without question, adequate replacement therapy must be restarted before the patient leaves the hospital. She must be reminded of her preoperative agreement to lifetime estrogen commitment as the prime essential for prophylaxis against breakdown of her surgery. How it is administered is of little matter, i.e., orally, vaginally, or dermally. My preference over all my years of practice is daily oral equine natural conjugated estrogens (Premarin). However, effective pelvic tissue response can be sustained with as little as one half an applicator full of Premarin cream intravaginally twice a week. Never forget that a major etiologic factor bringing the patient to the operating room is hypoestrogenism, and postoperative deprivation can bring her back in short order, but most likely under the care of another physician. I have been that next physician in more cases than I choose to remember. Finally, a small but significant percentage of women, very sensitive to the fluid retention effects of daily oral estrogen, even in the accompaniment of salt restriction, can be relieved by small doses of diuretics, usually three times per week.

Initiate oral vitamin C therapy in doses of 500 mg daily as soon as is feasible in all patients after surgery, with particular emphasis on the older elderly patients. The beneficial effects of ascorbic acid in the healing process have long been known, as well as its positive effect in promoting red blood cell repopulation. It is nontoxic and will cover dietary deficiencies, which we must presume will be likely. My feelings are similar regarding the need for supplemental calcium, which has usually become an intrinsic accompaniment to estrogen replacement preoperatively anyhow. I make certain that the patient goes home on the daily dose of 1000 to 1200 mg elemental calcium added to her regular diet.

If the postoperative hemoglobin is less than 11 g or the hematocrit is lower than 36%, I also discharge the patient on a dose of 325 mg ferrous sulfate three times daily for a month. This may need coverage with stool softeners to avert constipation.

Simple local analgesic therapy after surgery involving the introitus and perineum, although not objectively essential to good healing, offers a varying degree of comfort and considerable amount of psychic enhancement. Where applicable, I routinely order ice packs, sitz baths, or lidocaine or nupercaine ointment, and occasionally analgesic sprays when requested by the patient. Many of us categorize such measures as just good "doctoring," like removing a dressing yourself, or reaffixing a catheter while talking to the patient, or personally taking the pack out, instead of giving the order to a resident or nurse for such action. A caring display by the surgeon does much to build a good doctor–patient relationship, and, perhaps more than anything else, builds a positive attitude in the patient.

Kegel's exercises (isometric pubococcygeal contraction), designed to strengthen the skeletal muscles of the pelvis to overcome disuse atrophy, thereby augmenting pelvic tone in conjunction with estrogen-promoted new vitality in pelvic tissues in general, may be helpful in producing the best long-term results in a significant number of patients.[21–23] They are easily taught but care must be taken to teach patients to squeeze up and in rather than to bear down, a not uncommon mistake in patients in the eighth and ninth decades where difficulty in muscle group isolation is not uncommon. Make no assumptions that they know what you are talking about; have them demonstrate during the examination at the first postoperative outpatient visit. Kegel's exercises are best understood when the patient is told to do the same thing she does when stopping urination in midstream. A routine that she can easily follow should become a daily habit to be effected while doing other things, such as watching television, or reading the newspaper, or sitting in an automobile waiting for a red light to change. I feel Kegel's exercises are helpful adjuvants to good healing.

I am a strong advocate of return to normal activity as fast as possible. My patients are all geared to this positive approach long before the operation itself. Ordinary house cleaning, cooking, taking short walks, and driving a car are encouraged at once. Except for those whose jobs require extensive stretches in the erect posture or a moderate degree of physical activity, patients who regularly work are back at their positions within a week after leaving the hospital, albeit with a soft cushion if desired. However, strict instructions include a lifetime ban on such activities as heavy lifting, wearing a girdle, smoking, pushing heavy objects, and aerobic jumping.

A brief mention of "donut ring" cushions is pertinent. I used them routinely until recently on the presumption that the hole in the middle of this type of cushion would eliminate pressure on the sore perineum in cases of perineal repair. Actually the donut configuration may void the pressure amelioration by creating even more discomfort from its indirect stretching effect on the stitches in the perineum. So I advise only a plain soft cushion in the recovery phase.

Showers or baths are permissible from the outset, whether or not any catheter is in place. Daily walks are imperative on both a physical and mental basis. Long deprivations from the patients' previous usual athletic participation makes no sense. Depending on her own inclinations, she may slowly and steadily, within a few weeks, return to such activities as swimming, golfing, and bicycle riding. Aerobics minus jumping can be integrated into her schedule as desired, as can tennis, fairly limited at first with slowly progressively increasing involvement over 3 months, but with permanent restriction of jumping for overhead balls. Sexual activity need not be deliberately delayed, even in the most extensively repaired cases, beyond 4 weeks. Adjunctive lubricants should be encouraged for the first several ventures. Even when the best efforts have been made at the operating table to ensure a functional vagina, occasionally overscarring in healing will occur sufficient enough to impair comfortable sexual function. A simple series of gentle dilating maneuvers can quickly overcome this problem, using Premarin cream as the lubricant.

Maintaining a good relationship with the patient's close relatives is considered good form for the caring physician in all cases but particularly so with older patients. Doing so and simultaneously keeping them informed can reap a myriad of benefits for the practicing physician and will reflect well on the medical profession in general.

Finally, I offer some very special admonitions and advice to the gynecologist who has performed the surgery on a postmenopausal woman in elective benign situations. Schedule the case always such that you will not leave on vacation until at least 10 days postoperatively. Make daily rounds on this patient yourself; do not relegate this obligation to a partner or a resident, unless the colleague has been directly involved and known to the patient and her family from the outset. When discharging the patient, give her your home telephone number. You will become an angel in her eyes. I have done this for over 40 years and not once has the patient or her relatives abused the privilege of knowing this number. They have always gone through the office or answering service channels first. In the very few times I have been called directly, the patient has been unable to make connections through these lines in situations in which she felt desperate and she thought she deserved rapid or emergency attention. Under these conditions, believe me, you will be glad they could reach you. Lastly, when the patient telephones and seems particularly concerned, even though you may feel she is unduly alarmed, always offer her the opportunity to see you at that time. Thus reassured, usually she will renege on the offer and wait for her regular appointment. Nonetheless it behooves you to write a brief note in her chart of your solicitous response; if you do not do this, you may have later regrets. It takes but a few moments, as do so many little things that makes the doctor bigger and better in the patients' eyes.[24]

REFERENCES

1. Bergman A, Mushket Y, Gordon D, David MP. Prostaglandin prophylaxis and bladder function after vaginal hysterectomy: A prospective randomized study. *Br J Obstet Gynaecol.* 1993;100:69–72.

2. Marks RM, Sachar EJ. Undertreatment of medical inpatients with narcotic analgesics. *Ann Intern Med.* 1973;78:173–181.

3. Bonica JJ. Postoperative pain. In: Bonica JJ, ed. *The Management of Pain.* Philadelphia: Lea & Febiger; 1990:461–463.

4. Bellville JW, Forrest WII, Miller E, et al. Influence of age on pain relief from analgesics. *JAMA.* 1971;217:1835–1841.

5. White PF. Use of patient controlled analgesia for management of acute pain. *JAMA.* 1988;259:243–247.

6. Keeri-Szanto M. Apparatus for demand analgesia. *Can Anaesth Soc J.* 1971;18:581–582.

7. Forrest WH, Smethurst PWR, Kienitz ME. Self-administration of intravenous analgesics. *Anesthesiology.* 1970;33:363–365.

8. Sechzer PH. Studies in pain with the analgesic demand system. *Anesth Analg.* 1971;50:1–10.

9. Graves DA, Foster TS, Batenhorst RL, et al. Patient controlled analgesia. *Ann Intern Med.* 1983;99:360–366.

10. Bennett RL. Patient controlled analgesia. *Ann Surg.* 1982;195:700–705.

11. Parker RK, Holtmann B, White PT. Patient controlled analgesia. *JAMA.* 1991;266:1947–1952.

12. Austin KL, Stapleton JV, Mather LE. Relationship between blood meperidine concentrations and analgesic response. *Anesthesiology.* 1980;53:460–466.

13. Austin KL, Stapleton JV, Mather LE. Multiple intramuscular injections: a major source of variability in analgesic response to meperidine. *Pain.* 1980;8:47–62.

14. Keenan DL. The active management of postoperative pain. In: Thompson JD, Rock JA, eds. *TeLinde's Operative Gynecology Updates.* Philadelphia: Wyeth-Ayerst; 1992;1:1–11.

15. Griffiths RR, Woodson PP. Caffeine physical dependence: a review of human and laboratory animal studies. *Psychopharmacology (Berl).* 1988;94:437–451.

16. Graham DM. Caffeine—its identity, diet sources, intake and biologic effects. *Nutr Rev.* 1978;36:97–102.

17. Silverman K, Evan SM, Strain EC, Griffiths RR. Withdrawal syndrome after the double-blind cessation of caffeine consumption. *N Engl J Med.* 1992;327:1109–1114.

18. NIH Consensus Development. Prevention of venous thrombosis and pulmonary embolism. *JAMA.* 1986;256:744–749.

19. Clarke-Pearson DL, Synan IS, Dodge R, et al. A randomized trial of low-dose heparin and intermittent pneumatic calf compression for the prevention of deep thrombosis after gynecologic oncology surgery. *Am J Obstet Gynecol.* 1993; 168:1146–1154.

20. Mackowiak PA, Wasserman SS, Levine MM. A critical appraisal of 98.6 degrees F, the upper limit of the normal body temperature. *JAMA*. 1992;268:1578–1580.

21. Kegel A. Physiologic therapy for urinary stress incontinence. *JAMA*. 1951;146:915–917.

22. Klarskov P, Nielsen KK, Kromann-Andersen B, Malgard E. Long term results of pelvic floor training and surgery for female genuine stress incontinence. *Int Urogynecol J*. 1991;2:132–135.

23. Koelbl H, Strassegger H, Riss PA, Graber H. Morphologic and functional aspects of pelvic floor muscles in patients with relaxation and genuine stress incontinence. *Obstet Gynecol*. 1989;74:789–795.

24. All too often, the doctor isn't listening, studies show. *New York Times*. 1991; November 13:C-1.

Anatomical-Surgical Synopsis

Marvin H. Terry Grody

PELVIC CONNECTIVE TISSUE

1. Delicate interlacing interdependent network extending from pelvic brim to pelvic floor.
2. At varying locations forms "fascial" sheets, septa, and "ligaments" varying in dimension, strength, and elasticity.
3. Principal constituent is collagen, but elastin predominates in some areas; reticulin is the third major component.
4. Smooth muscle and striated muscle fibers are frequently interspersed, depending on location.
5. Surrounds and anchors pelvic organs at strategic levels of support and suspension.
6. An attenuated or weakened segment in any one area, over time, may lead to imbalance and deficits elsewhere ("weak link" analogy).
7. Surgical correction of one impairment may unmask others in a different pelvic compartment. A good surgeon will detect all defects preoperatively, whether symptomatic or not, and rectify all of them at the same time.

VAGINAL AXIS

1. Forms a central core of the pelvis.
2. In the erect position:

    a. Lower one-third of vagina almost vertical

    b. Upper two-thirds of vagina almost horizontal

3. The four major components of vaginal axis stability:
   a. Cardinal-uterosacral ligament complex
   b. Rectovaginal septum (fascia of Denonvillier)
   c. Perineal body
   d. Levator plate

4. The natural position of the posterior vaginal vault is well posterior to the anterior edge of the levator plate.

5. A surgical correction inadequate in reestablishing the above relationship is likely to fail.

MAJOR LEVELS OF PELVIC SUPPORT

1. *Upper:* Cardinal-uterosacral ligamentous complex.
   Suspends:
   a. Cervix and isthmus of the uterus
   b. Upper paracolpium (upper vagina)

   Extensions:
   a. Anterior bladder base extensions (bladder "pillars")
   b. Posteroinferior extensions into the cul-de-sac and rectovaginal septum

2. *Lower:* Levator ani muscular complex, including the puborectalis muscle, and associated enveloping connective tissue—"pelvic floor"

ANCILLARY IMPORTANT PELVIC STRUCTURES OF SUPPORT BETWEEN OR CONNECTED TO THE MAJOR LEVELS OF SUPPORT

1. Posterior pubourethral ligaments

2. Pubovesicocervical (pubocervical; paraurethrovesical) "fascia"

3. Urogenital diaphragm

4. The fibers of Luschka (middle paracolpium)

5. Rectovaginal septum

6. Levator plate

PRESSURE, POSITION, AND PROTECTIONS OF PELVIC ORGANS; ERECT POSTURE

1. A line down from the sacral promontory to the junction of the middle and anterior thirds of the symphysis pubis is almost 100% vertical! Most texts

still show the symphysis to lie in a plane well forward of that of the promontory in the erect posture.

2. The pelvic organs lie behind this imaginary line except for the anterior bladder.

3. The symphysis pubis lies *flat, not* semivertically, as shown in most texts.

4. The levator plate lies essentially *flat.*

5. Intra-abdominal pressure bombards principally the lower abdominis recti muscles and the more lateral muscles of the abdominal wall.

6. Intra-abdominal pressure dissipates significantly before it affects the pelvic organs and their supportive and suspensory mechanisms.

7. The pelvic connective tissue apparatus could never tolerate *direct* abdominal pressure, whether in female or male, in the erect human being, even under absolutely optimal conditions.

THE BLADDER

1. This hollow organ lies supported by a hammocklike sheet of thin but very strong connective tissue in the anterior pelvic compartment.

2. This supportive layer is ill-defined by anatomists but can be demonstrated surgically with relative ease and is called various names by surgeons (i.e., pubovesicocervical, pubocervical, vesicocervical, or paravaginal fascia).

3. The bladder is attached by this connective tissue bilaterally to the arcus tendineus fasciae pelvis, which runs from the mid-symphysis to the ischial spines on the medial surface of the obturator internus muscle, which is essentially divided by it into anterior and posterior halves.

4. Additional bladder support arises from extensions of the pelvic floor foundation, principally fascia off the levator ani musculature and the urogenital diaphragm.

5. The levator ani muscles, which especially support the bladder almost directly laterally, originate in a line from the pubic area to the ischial spine off the arcus tendineus levator ani, which blends almost contiguously with the arcus tendineus fasciae pelvis, except in the pubic area where it angles slightly anteriorly.

6. Cystoceles are herniations of the bladder formed from breakdown of its fascial supports.

7. A distention cystocele occurs more or less centrally because of a linear split in the pubocervical fascia anterior to the vagina, under the bladder.

8. A displacement cystocele occurs paravaginally from either unilateral or bilateral paravaginal defects in pubocervical fascia attachments at the arcus

tendineus ("white line"; arcuate line). When discovered, such lesions must be corrected by appropriately placed sutures to reestablish as much as possible the normal hammock-sling lateral suspension apparatus of the bladder. This should be effected, at the least, in the regions of the urethrovesical junction and the bladder neck (WREBS procedure). When possible, further bolstering sutures adjacent to the proximal urethra and above the bladder neck give the best guarantee for good lasting results.

9. In severe cases of denervation and atrophy of the levator ani musculature, for example, as a sequel to traumatic birth events many years earlier followed by aging over a period of years, even levator attachments may be disrupted from obturator fascia. In such cases, during dissection from the vaginal approach, the surgeon's fingers can easily wander directly to the superior ramus of the pubis.

10. Anterior descending extensions of cardinal-uterosacral fibers and paracervical fascia attach to the pubocervicovesical tissue at the uppermost bladder base. At the sides these connections are called the "bladder pillars." An unrecognized and uncorrected defect at this level can later lead to an anterior enterocele. Surgical repair at this level could be termed an anterior "intracardial imbrication."

11. Cystoceles have long been thought by surgeons to be central or distention in type and, consequently, reparative efforts have been concentrated on midline plications of connective tissue under the bladder. Recognition of paravaginal defects in recent years has helped to explain the high level of short-term failures of traditional (midline) anterior compartment repairs. Today both types of cystoceles can be recognized and assessed preoperatively, often found to coexist, and can be repaired appropriately either from above and/or below by capable surgeons at the same setting.

12. When bladder defects occur in posthysterectomy cases, especially when the vaginal length anterior to the hysterectomy scar seems short, the innermost bladder base should be dissected free from the scar and reanchored 2 to 3 cm behind it. This works out anatomically through appropriate posterior wall dissection and readjustment, designating a new vault in line with the reestablished vaginal axis and functional vaginal dimensions.

13. The ureters enter the bladder musculature relatively medially and run fairly deep to the fascial layers. Since the targeted connective tissue is thin, yet strong, at no time are deep bites into it required and, as a result, the ureters should not be jeopardized.

14. Branches of the inferior vesical arteries and veins occasionally present problems on extensive dissection from below. Cautery must be used judiciously when offending vessels are visualized. Bleeding from these vessels, though infrequent, may unfortunately not be directly accessible. In such cases one must rely on pressure, patience, and placement of coagulating substances, that is, oxidized regenerated cellulose [avitene (best used in

sheet form)]. The operation can be continued with further dependence on ultimate efficient post-operative packing, extraperitoneal confinement, and the patient's natural coagulating mechanisms.

THE URETHRA

1. This tubular, 3.5- to 4.0-cm-long organ angulates slightly backward from its origin at the bladder neck where its proximal portion is held within the same sphere of equalizing intra-abdominal pressure as the bladder, above the level of the urogenital diaphragm.

2. When urethral support fails, this angle becomes more obtuse and the proximal urethra falls outside the direct influence of intra-abdominal pressure, thereby presenting a pressure differential with the bladder and setting the stage for stress incontinence.

3. The external suspensory-supportive mechanism of the urethra, with which we are concerned surgically, consists of two parts:
   a. Posterior superior pubourethral ligaments, which are extensions from the levator fascia and the urogenital diaphragm, but which can be demonstrated as well-defined entities when undamaged
   b. Pubourethral fascia, which is merely the distal extension of the same pubourethrovesicocervical connective tissue layer already described in conjunction with the bladder

4. The term *urethrocele* is a distinct misnomer that unfortunately continues to be used. It erroneously suggests that the urethra balloons through a defect in its fascial supports in the same manner as does the bladder when a cystocele is formed. What really happens in genuine stress incontinence is the relaxation or destruction of support at the urethrovesical junction (cystourethral angle). This leads to the much more accurately descriptive designation of *rotational descent of the urethrovesical junction or cystourethral angle,* currently also termed *hypermotile urethra.*

5. Although a true vesicovaginal space exists between the vagina and the bladder, allowing each to dilate or contract independently of the other, the urethra is directly attached to the vaginal wall. This close association requires significant sharp dissection, much more so than that usually required in freeing up the bladder when surgery is performed in these areas.

6. In many cases where true obvious rotational descent exists concomitant with a hypermotile urethra, the expected associated stress incontinence does not occur. This usually happens when an associated cystocele is sufficiently large enough that it dominates the defective urethrovesical angle and produces a "kinking" effect, cutting off involuntary urine loss. However, if

the surgeon ignores the hypermotile angle area and repairs only the cysto-cele, stress incontinence may well be initiated. Although it is not the ultimate reliable test for stress incontinence and urethral rotational descent, the simple Q-tip test can contribute to establishing an anatomic diagnosis of urethral hypermotility even in the absence of stress incontinence. When the urethra becomes very short, as in marked funneling, the Q-tip test is not valid. Incidental information: kinking can also be caused commonly by a markedly prolapsed uterus or a severe post-hysterectomy enterocele.

7. Funneling is a relatively common anatomic defect of the proximal urethra in which the internal os of the urethra opens up and disappears, literally extending the bladder neck into urethral territory. An acceptable analogy to this problem could be the incompetent internal os of the cervix. When funneling occurs and the proximal urethra literally becomes funnel shaped, urine comes in contact with unnatural constancy with urethral mucous membrane, leading reflexly to urgency and frequency. These two symptoms are generally thought to be functional, but in funneling, an anatomic cause is indicated. This is proved by the disappearance of urgency and frequency when the funneling is corrected surgically in cases where functional com-ponents are not present.

8. The above phenomenon can shorten the urethra by anywhere from 1 to 3 cm, which can easily be measured as part of the Q-tip test and sometimes, when shortening is marked, it may render the Q-tip test invalid. Some authorities mockingly state that urethral lengths should be of no concern and that any anxiety about it is simply an expression of machismo. This is misdirection of thinking. When the shortened urethra is a direct conse-quence of funneling, as explained above, it will automatically be lengthened on correction of the funneling. Therefore, measuring an increased urethral length can be a good indicator of successful correction of funneling.

9. Paraurethral fascial sling urethropexy is a reparative technique, significantly effective performed entirely vaginally, using only attached adjacent connec-tive tissue. This method uses bilateral flaps of delicately dissected pubour-ethral fascia, which is extremely strong, in overlapping fashion to elevate the proximal urethra as much as 2.5 cm without impingement on urethral lumen, especially if no funneling is present. Metaphorically speaking, arranging flaps in this way can be likened to changing a single-breasted jacket to a double-breasted one. Traditional Kelly sutures, in contrast, invariably produce an artificial kinking with accompanying abnormal narrowing of urethral lumen.

10. Funneling of the urethra is a common lesion and yet it probably has never been emphasized enough. Traditional vaginal methods, that is, Kelly sutur-ing, have been aimed at angle reformation and elevation and, without direct intention, by obstruction may have helped, if only temporarily, to relieve

this distortion. All methods of suprapubic urethral suspension, which attempt to reestablish an intra-abdominal position of the proximal urethra, do nothing to decrease the ballooned lumen of the proximal, and often also the middle, urethra. The paraurethral sling, made of bilateral connective tissue overlapping flaps, seems to be the only type of correction for the funneled dilation that allows for a steady postoperative natural retraction of the bulging lumen. The elimination of this defect, of course, automatically lengthens the urethra.

11. A final word on the triple combined anterior pelvic compartment restitution, described herein, which includes: (1) paraurethral fascial sling urethropexy (Grody urethropexy), (2) paravaginal defects repair (WREBS procedure) of displacement cystocele, and (3) extended intracardial imbrication correcting both deep vault defects and distention cystocele:

    a. All done through single vaginal entry without need for suprapubic incision

    b. Obstructive techniques, involved in all other methods of control of urethral rotational descent and stress incontinence except for suprapubic paravaginal defects repair, are avoided

    c. Most orthodox adherence to a return to normal anatomy as compared to all other surgical method

    d. Only method that allows for correction of both types of cystocele through one approach

    e. Only method specifically designed to allow "natural" recovery from funneling

THE VAGINA

1. The term *paracolpium* is today commonly accepted as a reference to vaginal supportive tissue. It is divided into three parts.

2. *Upper paracolpium:* Cardinal-uterosacral complex fibers that fix the upper third of the vagina to the posterior and posterolateral pelvic walls.

3. *Middle paracolpium:* Connective tissue (collagen and elastin) strands (Luschka) that attach the vagina bilaterally to levator fascia.

4. *Lower paracolpium:* Interlacing fibrous extensions from the urogenital diaphragm, the perineal body, and the levator fascia that fix the lower vagina in relation to the pelvic floor and allow for functional relationship with the urinary system anteriorly and the lowermost digestive tract posteriorly.

5. The vagina itself, a hollow tubelike organ closed at one end by either the

cervix or a posthysterectomy scar, consists of a mucosa of varying thickness depending on the level of estrogenic stimulation or friction, if everted. It has a fibroelastic-muscular encompassing base the quality of which also depends on the amount of estrogen stimulation present and, additionally, on aging plus antecedent trauma, for instance, childbirth.

6. An associated neurovascular supply, subjected to all the same influences, ultimately determines the vitality of all the organ's components.

7. No reconstructive surgery should be performed on the vagina without a thorough assessment of these factors in advance, plus supportive corrective measures preoperatively where possible, for example, estrogen replacement therapy, good nutrition, weight loss, and cessation of smoking.

8. The thickening of a vagina by the friction of slowly progressive eversion, although certainly more substantial than one much thinner after relatively rapid protrusion and overstretching, in the absence of adequate estrogen priming, appears stronger than it really is.

9. A universal concept has persisted, even among "experts," that there are two different methods of vaginal reconstruction for the same condition depending on a predetermination of whether or not the woman will participate in future coital activity. With rare exceptions, no notion, for many reasons, could be more irrational. Yet day after day, in operating rooms everywhere, pontifical blueprints of misdirection are laid out on such basis without thought to the total pelvic anatomic havoc that lies ahead.

10. The psychosocial poignancy of this subject, although germane, and apt to fill countless pages, will not be included in this concentrated discussion on surgical anatomy. Specifically, indicated surgical restoration is directed at the alleviation of disabling symptoms of one or more of the three pelvic systems, that is, lower urinary, genital, and lowermost alimentary, each of which is interdependent on the others, both anatomically and physiologically. Therefore, considering the long life expectancy of women today, and assuming a goal of the very best long-term symptomatic relief, it is inconceivable that pelvic surgeons today would pursue any path short of the most natural anatomic restoration possible. Short cuts, substantiated by coverup excuses, particularly if hiding technical inadequacy, are not acceptable. *Conclusion:* Whether or not future coital performance is anticipated is irrelevant. All things considered, as normal a vagina as possible, in conjunction with as normal a vaginal axis as possible, will give the best and most enduring symptomatic relief for the entire pelvis. As with all things in life, there are exceptions. In some cases, fortunately uncommon, the only wise choice may be colpocleisis. *Final word:* Because of interdependence, the best function in any one pelvic compartment is best reestablished when the best restitution to normal anatomy in all three compartments has been achieved.

11. A common mistake still widely taught in surgery involving prolapse of all kinds through the urogenitorectal hiatus is the need "to trim (generous) portions of excess vaginal mucosa" prior to closure. Clearly, because it sticks out (everts), particularly when the introitus is markedly widened with a fourchette rotated down and back, to assume that vaginal wall is automatically in excess and literally needs to be chopped off is fallacious, even stupid. Almost automatically the surgeon then commits him or herself to the result that the vagina is only 4 to 6 cm long and that it might also be too narrow. Of course, this also obviates any possible restoration of normal vaginal axis and is a good prescription for later surgical breakdown. So many of the "old masters" used to say, "Worry not, repeated strong coital activity will provide adequate length." What false reassurance! Even if such suggested activity were available, and often it is not, considering the age group, the lengthened vaginal vault will have no support and merely will telescope back on itself, starting the eversion again. Although simplistic, this is what actually happens due to an absence of understanding of sound surgical and anatomic principles. Think about it—an airport windsock blown west is the same size when it is blown east in the opposite direction. Would you be more apt to shorten it in one direction than the other?

12. Another problem which, if not managed correctly, can lead to a foreshortened inadequate vagina is that of the wide-open vaginal introitus emitting a semicylindrical semiconical eversion, with or without a uterus. Once again there rises the tendency to remove too much vaginal mucosa because of an apparent excess of tissue, but, in truth, the total square surface is almost always just about the correct amount required to allow for a refashioned, functionally and anatomically normal vagina. What is vital in these cases is wide free dissection accompanied by extensive shifting of vaginal wall for proper accommodation. For the most part only a small amount of mucosa need be removed in the anterior area and, except for the extremely large protrusions, none should be removed posteriorly so as to provide for deep posterior fixation of a newly positioned vaginal vault without tension. Undoubtedly all these ideas about vaginal conservation will shake up a lot of people and will cause a lot of negative head wagging, but direct observation of corrective surgery which follows these concepts has converted innumerable observers.

THE CARDINAL-UTEROSACRAL COMPLEX

1. These are thickened bands of connective tissue on which the isthmus uteri, cervix uteri, and upper vagina (upper paracolpium) depend for suspensory elevation and attachments to the posterolateral pelvic sidewalls.

2. Play an important role in the maintenance of the normal vaginal axis.

3. When these fibers are attenuated or devitalized, the uterus will prolapse, the vaginal vault will invert, and the vaginal axis will become disrupted.

4. In hysterectomy, whether vaginal or abdominal, cardinal-uterosacral complex stumps must be firmly united with their respective posterolateral corners to include peritoneum, rectovaginal septal edge, and vaginal cuff, employing delayed-absorbable sutures.

5. In vaginal hysterectomy, the cardinal ligaments, when being clamped and tied, can be and should be shortened as much as 3 to 4 cm.

6. In vaginal hysterectomy, the cardinal-uterosacral fibers can be shortened an additional 1 cm by inversion of the stumps posterolaterally at the termination of the procedure in a maneuver that also affords further hemostasis and further ensures support of the vault toward the hollow of the sacrum, especially if delayed-absorbable suture is used for anchorage.

7. The cardinal-uterosacral stumps should never be crossed over to their opposite corners. This not only is anatomically incorrect but will accentuate the attenuation and create weaknesses, especially at the sides, which might provoke future enterocele.

THE RECTOVAGINAL SEPTUM (AND RECTOCELE)

1. A very thin but very strong sheet of fibroelastic tissue first described by Denonvilliers that lies just behind the posterior vaginal wall.

2. Begins in the area of the cul-de-sac, with direct connections to posterior extensions of the cardinal-uterosacral complex, and ends below by inserting directly into the perineal body.

3. Bilaterally attaches to the medial aspects of the levator ani fascial coverings.

4. As might be expected, in line with the requisite distensibility of the third stage of labor, it is heavily endowed with elastin, perhaps exceeded elsewhere in the body only by the ligament of Treitz.

5. Lacerations of this septum are the direct cause of rectoceles. The locale and extent of the tear, it follows, determine the site and magnitude (width and length) of the rectocele. The amount of protrusion of the rectocele, its third dimension, is determined both by time and the intensity of increased intra-abdominal pressure.

6. Lacerations are most usually thought to be linear, not necessarily in the midline, and repairs are generally concentrated in repair of this longitudinal disruption.

7. Transverse separations, however, particularly at the junction of the rectovaginal septum with the perineal body, are just as common, if not more so,

and obviously must exist in the presence of any appreciable perineal body defects.

8. Although it is possible for low rectoceles to develop as a consequence of either or both low linear or transverse rectovaginal tears in the absence of perineal body defects, it is unusual. Regardless, the operator must always consider, for an "airtight" repair, after reuniting rectovaginal lacerations and reconstituting the perineal body, using a few interrupted up-and-down stitches to ensure reassociation of the rectovaginal septum with the perineal body.

9. In the case of upper level rectocele, or full-length rectocele, midline reunion of the innermost and uppermost endopelvic fascial fibers from each side is mandatory to correction. This surgical exercise guarantees continuity of the top of the rectovaginal septum with the posterior cardinal-uterosacral fibers and helps complement and sustain an associated sacrospinous ligament fixation whenever it is included in the total operative plan.

THE PERINEAL BODY

1. This is a dense pyramid-shaped structure lying between distal posterior vaginal wall in front and lowermost rectum and anus behind. The base of the pyramid lies directly on the perineum. Length is usually about 3.5 to 4.0 cm. It varies in size naturally from one woman to another.

2. This structure consists principally of collagen but contains substantial elastin, smooth muscle, and striated muscle in the healthy nulliparous state in which it also includes considerable nerve tissue.

3. It acts as a core in the pelvic floor into which fibers from the levator, deep and superficial transverse perineal, and bulbocavernosus muscles are incorporated. It is connected anteriorly to the distal vaginal supportive fascia and to posterior extensions paravaginally of the urogenital diaphragm. The rectovaginal septum mediates its association with the upper pelvis. The anchorage to it of the levator plate through pararectal extensions, in the normal status, affords it a stabilized relationship to the sacrum and coccyx.

4. It is probably the most traumatized structure during childbirth, particularly when torn as opposed to being incised at the appropriate time before being damaged by the delivering vertex.

5. Despite arguments to the contrary by perinatologists favoring the absolute minimum of interference at delivery, all anatomic and clinical perceptions point to a progression of destruction of substance and innervation after each delivery. The best recovery occurs after the first delivery, on average, but subsequent deliveries reveal significantly lower healing potential.

6. Permanent damage to this bottleneck entity, the perineal body, is multiplied by inadequate repairs of episiotomy or lacerations at delivery, compounded by poor choice of suture or inadvertent infection.

7. Perineal body defects constitute a distinct lesion separate from a rectocele. Each can exist independently or they can occur together.

8. An intact perineal body is necessary to a normal vaginal axis.

9. A seriously defective perineal body is often accompanied by a fallen levator plate. In such situations, a complete perineorrhaphy accompanied by a low colporrhaphy, at the least, should elevate the levator plate to normal horizontal position.

10. It is now well recognized that an isolated restoration in the anterior pelvic compartment will widen the vaginal aperture and this, in the presence of asymptomatic perineal defects, sets the stage for future posterior enterocele development. It would be prudent to perform a perineorrhaphy, when significant defects are present, simultaneously with any suprapubic urethral suspension (retropubic urethropexy), for example. The prophylactic effects for the future are well worth the effort. Unfortunately, this additional surgery is uncommon.

11. Severe perineal defects with associated widened introitus and significant loss of vaginal axis, all asymptomatic, often coexist in situations demanding indicated hysterectomy, as in disabling adenomyosis or uterine descensus, for example. Every effort should be exerted preoperatively to convince the patient to agree to an accompanying full perineorrhaphy when associated perineal body defects, even though asymptomatic, have been detected preoperatively. Considering the tremendous potential for the future development of posthysterectomy enterocele, with or without rectocele, under these circumstances, particularly in view of current long life expectancy, such a plan represents solid common sense. The additional operating time is but 20 to 25 min and the current hospital stay of only one to 2 days is not likely to be lengthened. Avoiding future aggravation and hospitalization for extensive reconstruction by this simple prophylaxis seems most prudent. Unfortunately, such a course is not often pursued.

12. Not infrequently one can be fooled, if perineal examination is limited to observation only and not touch, in the presence of a broad expanse of perineal skin between fourchette and anus. An examination with index finger in the vagina and thumb on the skin may reveal no intervening perineal body tissue at all. In such cases, the perineal body has split completely and widely, and the only solid tissue that may remain between lower rectum behind and distal vagina in front may be the sphincter ani. The initial appearance suggests falsely that a good perineal body lies internal to the perineal skin.

THE LEVATOR ANI MUSCLES

1. The pubococcygeus, iliococcygeus, and coccygeus (ischiococcygeus) muscular complex constitutes the levator ani musculature. Far back in the phylogenetic scale, the only job these muscles had to do was wag the tail.

2. The immediately subjacent puborectalis muscle is generally included with the levator group.

3. This striated muscle quartet, more or less in a tonic ("slow twitch") state of activity and ever ready reflexly to resist ("fast twitch") sudden increases in intra-abdominal pressure, together with its fascial components, comprises the major structure of the pelvic floor.

4. Artists always depict these muscles to be thicker and heavier than they truly are. Nonetheless, they are essential to the support of the pelvic organs and, all things considered, they do a surprisingly good job in resisting pressure from above. Obviously the stronger they are, mostly a congenital endowment, and the more posteriorly recessed into the sacral curve are the pelvic structures, the more effective is this muscle group.

5. The levators of the multiparous woman have quite often taken a terrible beating. If, in addition, they were on the weak side to start, and then were subjected to other negative influences, such as smoking, pulmonary disease, obesity, poor nutrition, hypoestrogenism, and aging, the pelvic floor may collapse. Associated denervation can lead to disastrous atrophy and even the best reconstructive surgeon is hard put to find any decent tissue to place back together again. This becomes startlingly evident in posterior repairs when one expects dissection to reveal levator muscle and fascia and instead only ischiorectal fossa fat pops into view. In such discouraging situations, one must compensate by sacrospinous ligament fixation and plication of deep endopelvic fascia behind the fixation. Hopefully some of the bilateral remnants of old posterior cul-de-sac extensions of cardinal uterosacral fibers can be united medially also. Since the disintegrated levators have probably taken with them any retrievable rectovaginal septum remnants, although one must search for them anyhow and use them if found, the balance of salvage rests on a meticulous high, strong perineal body repair. Fortunately, if coupled with stringently followed good habits by the patient postoperatively, satisfactory anatomic results can be had. If later breakdown occurs, synthetic mesh must be considered if further correction is attempted.

6. Levator disruption can be noted frequently in thorough anterior dissection when the examining fingers, wandering forward over the obturation internus medial surface, from the vaginal approach, find no levator attachment at its line of origin, the arcus tendineus. In such cases palpation extends without resistance to the superior ramus of the pubic bone and the obturator neurovascular canal is easily identified. Such a situation of total arcuate line

disruption, which may be unilateral or bilateral, represents the worst kind of paravaginal defects, demanding reestablishment of the arcus onto the obturator internus fascia in a line between the mid-symphysis and the ischial spine. The latter can be rather easily palpated through a thoroughly dissected anterior pelvic compartment. Thus, when necessary, whether paravaginal defects are corrected from below or above, levator attachments of origin must be restored as well as those of the disengaged pubovesicocervical hammock supporting the bladder laterally (WREBS Procedure).

THE LEVATOR PLATE

1. This structure is a thick fibrous horizontal midline strap of tough connective tissue, the interlacing union of the levator muscles from each side between the coccyx and the anus, extending forward around the anus into the perineal body.

2. When the pelvic anatomy is intact, this anteroposterior sling lies horizontally in the female adult. On it rests the rectum, the upper two thirds of the vagina, and the cervix and isthmus of the uterus.

3. When the levator muscles become attenuated, especially in association with significant perineal body defects, the pelvic floor descends and the levator plate rotates downward and backward while still attached to the coccyx. The urogenitorectal hiatus then widens, the normal vaginal axis disappears, and the middle and posterior pelvic organs literally slide downward on the tilted plate.

4. During the surgically correct performance of colpoperineorrhaphy, when only the deepest sutures have been placed, evidence of progressive restoration of the levator plate to a normal flat position can be visually demonstrated as each successively more distal suture is pulled upward, thereby also illustrating the interdependence of the pelvic connective tissue network.

5. Uncommonly the levator plate may detach from its coccygeal mooring points. In these cases it must be surgically refastened as a retrorectal levatorplasty. This condition is most uncommonly recognized and the procedure is rarely done.

PELVIC INTERORGAN SPACES

1. These are spaces, which can be likened to bursae, between the bladder and vagina anteriorly and the rectum and vagina posteriorly.

2. These spaces allow the hollow pelvic organs to function independently by sliding one over the other. Coupled with the distensibility and pliancy of the

bladder, the vagina, and the rectum, when one of these three organs is in a state of activity, this lack of direct attachment allows the other two organs to lie at rest. The most graphic example is the absence of urination and defecation during coitus in the presence of normal anatomy.

3. Obviously, then, it is surgically incorrect, when reuniting transected vaginal wall at the termination of a reconstructive procedure, to attempt to close off the "dead space" external to the vagina both in front and in back.

4. *Exception:* The vagina is directly adherent to the urethra anteriorly and to the perineal body behind the fourchette posteriorly.

THE SACROSPINOUS LIGAMENT

1. This is a condensation of dense connective tissue fibers within the coccygeus muscle at its posterior border.

2. It varies in thickness, density, and strength from one woman to the next.

3. Paradoxically it usually becomes progressively more of an identifiable visible ligament, assuming appropriate surgical exposure, as aging transforms muscle into white connective tissue so that there is less muscle and more ligament.

4. Not uncommonly in the postmenopausal patient, this "ligament" becomes as thick as the small finger of the hand and, as a result, cannot be grasped by the ordinary Babcock clamp.

5. Tugging on it will move the whole patient.

6. It runs posteromedially and upward from behind the ischial spine to the sacrum.

7. It represents a vital fixture point in surgical correction of structural lesions involving pelvic prolapse, the most glaring example of which is massive vaginal eversion.

8. In the operation called sacrospinous ligament fixation, only one, either right or left, ligament needs to be used. One side is more than adequate and no significant deviation off the midline results. Using both sides in the same case may cause a midline weakness. The surgical risk is also doubled.

9. The right side is preferable to the left because of proximity of descending distal large bowel on the left.

10. Attachment usually is made to the raw vaginal undersurface of the posterior vaginal vault, one suture on either side of the midline of the vagina, in such a way as to ensure direct contact of vagina with the ligament.

11. Proper vaginal fixation points are determined before suture placement to avoid either tension or laxity on the anterior wall. This precaution is often neglected. Urinary symptoms not present preoperatively may result.

12. Direct visual placement of sutures into the ligament is mandatory because of the serious danger potential when sacrospinous ligament fixation is improperly performed, for instance, blindly.

13. Use of correctly chosen instruments decreases the danger, particularly to retract for adequate exposure, to elevate peritoneal cavity containing small bowel superiorly, and to displace upper rectum from the field medially.

14. Piercing suture-carrying instruments should go through the ligament substantially (two thirds) but never around it to avoid injury to the inferior gluteal vessels which descend immediately behind the coccygeus muscle.

15. Laterally, improper placement of sharp instruments can produce serious consequences because the pudendal vessels and nerve run under the ischial spine and the sciatic nerve lies slightly further out, lateral to the ischial spine, but close enough for constant worry.

16. Sacrospinous ligament fixation is considered by many as the technically best method, in appropriate cases, for restoration of normal vaginal support and normal vaginal axis plus restoration of functional vaginal dimensions when caution has been applied to disposition of vaginal mucosa, as already discussed.

17. The fixation should always be complemented by associated deep posterior sutures uniting endopelvic fascia in the midline in juxtaposition to the fixation just distal and behind the fixation in front of the coccygeus muscle.

18. Often much of the success accompanying sacrospinous fixation depends on the bony configuration of the pelvis. This should not be surprising. When the pelvis is shallow, from top to bottom, the ligament, disappointingly, is not so internally sited as in the deep pelvis and hence vaginal length is shorter. Also, the further back the sacrum tilts, or the more hollow the sacral curve, the further posteriorly will lie the ligament. Attachment in these cases brings the vaginal vault more posteriorly behind the anterior edge of the levator plate than when the sacrum tilts more forward or when the curve is flatter.

THE "YELLOW LINE"

1. Retroperitoneal fat descends posteriorly but stops abruptly at the junction of abdominal peritoneum with cul-de-sac peritoneum. Such a delineating border is colloquially called the "yellow line."

2. This boundary is a landmark to designate the uppermost level for posterior closure when obliterating the cul-de-sac or closing the neck of an enterocele sac.

3. Suturing in this area should bite slightly more deep than the peritoneum itself medially. There is a safe enough margin between peritoneal surface and large bowel lumen (4.5–5.0 cm).

4. Closure at this line posteriorly should be complemented by anterior obliteration to the uppermost posterior bladder verge to avoid vulnerability toward later anterior enterocele. This line can easily be determined by the placement of a metal catheter in the bladder which can point out the precise level for suturing.

5. A prudent addendum must be interjected at this point. In closure of an enterocele sac, posterolateral bites into the peritoneum must be superficial to avoid the ureters.

THE CUL-DE-SAC

1. This is the most dependent and weakest area of the peritoneal cavity, hence it is highly vulnerable to herniation, particularly if congenitally deep.

2. It should be routinely obliterated by any of several methods at all hysterectomies, whether vaginal or abdominal, as an integral part of the operation.

3. Cul-de-sacs become classified as enteroceles when they deepen and contain small intestine. Current theories suggest that a deep cul-de-sac, sometimes almost to the perineal body, occurs congenitally and is of no consequence if it remains empty. Nonetheless, if discovered by chance at hysterectomy or other pelvic surgery, even though asymptomatic, prudence dictates excision.

4. Anatomists tell us that small intestine will not enter a cul-de-sac, no matter how deep, because its mesentery is, at the most, normally only 15 cm in its longest dimension. So, logically, questions arise as to how enteroceles develop. Does the patient have a congenitally abnormally long intestinal mesentery, which allows the small bowel to slowly eke its way down over time as it forces the normal or congenitally weak cul-de-sac to descend? Alternatively, can the cul-de-sac be congenitally abnormally deep and, over time, does a mesentery of normal length slowly stretch as its small intestine, through gravity, drops downward into the chasm? Can it be that both abnormalities must coexist for enteroceles to happen? At this time we can only conjecture. No one really knows, but who cares? The trick is to detect it, especially if symptomatic, and fix it.

THE ANAL SPHINCTER COMPLEX

1. Fecal incontinence occurs secondary to anatomic or innervating incompetence of the sphincter mechanism located at the very end of the digestive tract.

2. In the presence of fecal incontinence, anatomic defects should be searched for and, if uncovered, repaired.

3. The anal canal begins at the dentate line (anorectal junction), about the level of the puborectalis muscle, and extends downward to the perineum.

4. The involuntary internal and voluntary external sphincter systems are the controlling muscle groups. The complex sophisticated balance between the two groups is quite remarkable, including the capacity to distinguish between gas and stool of varying consistency.

5. The internal muscle fibers are smooth and circular, lying within the wall of the anal canal. The innervation is autonomic, maintaining tone in a constant state of contracture. It remains relatively collapsed until the canal fills. The distention acts as the sensory stimulus to initiate evacuation of stool.

6. The external sphincter of the anal canal consists of three muscular groups classified as loops surrounding this terminal fecal channel. The upper loop is the puborectalis muscle, encircling the canal posteriorly and beginning and ending at the pubis. The forward angulation of this configuration is considered a major factor for fecal continence. The middle loop of the external sphincter consists of fleshy skeletal muscle fibers that encircle the medial portion of the canal in front and are attached by a strong tendon to the coccyx, in balancing contrast to the puborectalis. The base loop is the totally encircling subcutaneous sphincter muscle which almost all of us have always considered the external sphincter, disregarding the roles played by the two loops above in the sphincter system.

7. For anatomic completeness, the hiatal ligament, fibers off the pubococcygeus, must be mentioned. They encircle the rectum just above the dentate line anteriorly and come together in back as the anococcygeal raphe, which attaches to the coccyx.

8. Finally, between the external and internal sphincters, longitudinal muscle bundles descend to the perineum from the levator plate on either side, acting as an intermediary connecting force between the two groups.

9. Only when this complicated integrated muscle network is intact and fully innervated can fecal evacuation be controlled. When the patient complains of anal incontinence, this system must be carefully evaluated both preoperatively and intraoperatively, including examinations always with a finger in the rectum. Repair of defects can only be most effective when a gloved finger is placed rectally. When the posterior compartment is opened above the perineum and the defects extend through the internal sphincter, the gloved finger can almost be seen through the anal mucosa.

10. Sphincterpexy is as small or as big a job as the extent of the lesion demands. Obviously careful scrutiny must be exercised to identify the defects. Despite the increased number of knots, interrupted sutures are advised to prevent bunching and distortion. Delayed absorbable materials ranging in bore from 4-0 to 2-0, depending on the particular layer, offer the best potential for good outcome.

DENERVATION AND TISSUE QUALITY

1. Denervation of pelvic tissues, particularly muscle, both smooth and striated, plays a powerful role in deterioration of general pelvic function and in decreased capacity for anatomic recovery in pelvic reconstructive surgery.

2. Denervation is primarily the combined product of trauma and aging.

3. Trauma refers principally to childbirth via the vaginal route. All studies reveal significantly less permanent pelvic nerve damage in patients delivered only by cesarean section than in those delivered vaginally.

4. Trauma to the pelvis causing nerve damage also includes prior pelvic surgery, accidents involving the pelvis directly, and chronic pelvic insult from long-term conditions of increased intra-abdominal pressure.

5. Deterioration with aging occurs in all tissues, including nerve tissue, and the pelvis is no exception. Multiple factors may speed up the process, differing from one individual to the next.

6. Hypoestrogenism is a major factor in deficient physiology and anatomy in pelvic supportive structures and pelvic organs, affecting connective tissue, muscle, vasculature, nerves, and mucous membranes alike. Although significant neurologic regeneration is unlikely, exogenous estrogen over time can do a surprisingly good job of rejuvenation of the other tissues. Without question, all states of hypoestrogenism must be remedied preoperatively in pelvic reconstructive and urogynecologic surgery to attain the highest level of return toward normal function and structural integrity. By the same token, continued estrogen replacement must remain a lifetime commitment in order to maintain maximum tissue health, else a slide backward is inevitable.

7. Recent studies have proven beyond all doubt that the quality of tissue and the capacity for healing are significantly reduced in chronic smokers. Intelligence dictates that permanent cessation of the smoking habit is mandatory, for multiple reasons, before corrective pelvic surgery of any kind is undertaken.

8. Kegel's (isotonic pelvic muscle) exercises can substantively, in many cases, enhance the results of restorative surgery. They are not always so helpful when the anatomy has gone awry. Once pelvic supportive structures, including muscles, especially the levators, which are striated, have been operatively restored toward normal positioning, these exercises can help improve results markedly in many cases if nerve pathways remain at all intact. Logically, striated muscle anywhere in the body will respond and strengthen if the correct stimulus can be directed to it, so why not in the pelvis?

9. Current studies are revealing that loss of innervation in one part of the pelvis is usually reflected in other areas. Specifically, urinary incontinence probably is accompanied in many cases by some degree of fecal incontinence, no matter how slight, and vice versa. Both deficiencies are probably due to combined neurologic and anatomic breakdown. Since we cannot create new nerves, our best efforts must be directed at anatomically restructuring sphincter mechanisms, both in front and in back. Then, with the aid of estrogen, good habits, good nutrition, and good luck, we must pray for the best possible result.

10. *Final note:* The very best surgery, which may seem objectively to provide the very best anatomic restitution, may not ultimately provide the best long-term function and anatomic results. Because of factors over which doctors have no control, promises to patients must always be governed by information, explanation, and caution. The trap is set; do not let ego, pride, imprudence, and foolishness push you into it. Hyperbole and false optimism have no place in pelvic reconstructive and urogynecologic surgery. Promise only the very best efforts to attain the maximum long-term results with the tissues at hand, emphasizing the rigid ancillary role of incessant good habits to be followed by the patient herself.

INDEX

Page numbers followed by a *t* indicate tables;
page numbers followed by an *f* indicate figures.